AF876719

# NEURAL TUBE DEFECTS

# PEDIATRIC HABILITATION

*Series Editor*

**ALFRED L. SCHERZER**
*Cornell University Medical Center*
*New York, New York*

1. Prevention of Mental Retardation and Other Developmental Disabilities, *edited by Michael K. McCormack*
2. Developmental Disabilities: Management Through Nutrition and Medication, *Eric Denhoff and Steven Feldman*
3. Early Diagnosis and Therapy in Cerebral Palsy, *Alfred L. Scherzer and Ingrid Tscharnuter*
4. Parenting Children with Disabilities: A Professional Source for Physicians and Guide for Parents, *Peggy Muller Miezio*
5. Visual Disorders in the Handicapped Child, *John L. Goble*
6. Early Diagnosis and Therapy in Cerebral Palsy: A Primer on Infant Developmental Problems, Second Edition, Revised and Expanded, *Alfred L. Scherzer and Ingrid Tscharnuter*
7. Attention Deficit Disorders and Hyperactivity in Children: Early Diagnosis and Intervention, *edited by Pasquale J. Accardo, Thomas A. Blondis, and Barbara Y. Whitman*
8. Medical Care in Down Syndrome: A Preventive Medicine Approach, *Paul T. Rogers and Mary Coleman*
9. Manual of Developmental and Behavioral Problems in Children, *Vidya Bhushan Gupta*
10. Attention Deficits and Hyperactivity in Children and Adults: Diagnosis • Treatment • Management, Second Edition, Revised and Expanded, *edited by Pasquale J. Accardo, Thomas A. Blondis, Barbara Y. Whitman, and Mark A. Stein*
11. Early Diagnosis and Interventional Therapy in Cerebral Palsy: An Interdisciplinary Approach, Third Edition, *edited by Alfred L. Scherzer*
12. Autistic Spectrum Disorders in Children, *edited by Vidya Bhushan Gupta*
13. Genetics of Developmental Disabilites, *edited by Merlin Butler and F. John Meaney*
14. Neural Tube Defects, *edited by Sonya G. Oppenheimer*

# NEURAL TUBE DEFECTS

EDITED BY

SONYA G. OPPENHEIMER
*Cincinnati Children's Hospital Medical Center*
*Cincinnati, Ohio, U.S.A.*

**informa**
healthcare

New York London

Informa Healthcare USA, Inc.
270 Madison Avenue
New York, NY 10016

© 2007 by Informa Healthcare USA, Inc.
Informa Healthcare is an Informa business

No claim to original U.S. Government works
Printed in the United States of America on acid-free paper
10 9 8 7 6 5 4 3 2 1

International Standard Book Number-10: 1-57444-859-5 (Hardcover)
International Standard Book Number-13: 978-1-57444-859-7 (Hardcover)

This book contains information obtained from authentic and highly regarded sources. Reprinted material is quoted with permission, and sources are indicated. A wide variety of references are listed. Reasonable efforts have been made to publish reliable data and information, but the author and the publisher cannot assume responsibility for the validity of all materials or for the consequences of their use.

No part of this book may be reprinted, reproduced, transmitted, or utilized in any form by any electronic, mechanical, or other means, now known or hereafter invented, including photocopying, microfilming, and recording, or in any information storage or retrieval system, without written permission from the publishers.

For permission to photocopy or use material electronically from this work, please access www.copyright.com (http://www.copyright.com/) or contact the Copyright Clearance Center, Inc. (CCC) 222 Rosewood Drive, Danvers, MA 01923, 978-750-8400. CCC is a not-for-profit organization that provides licenses and registration for a variety of users. For organizations that have been granted a photocopy license by the CCC, a separate system of payment has been arranged.

**Trademark Notice:** Product or corporate names may be trademarks or registered trademarks, and are used only for identification and explanation without intent to infringe.

**Visit the Informa Web site at**
**www.informa.com**

**and the Informa Healthcare Web site at**
**www.informahealthcare.com**

# Preface

Neural tube defects are one of the most complex birth defects and require an understanding of the interactions of multiple systems: the central nervous system, the urological system, and the musculoskeletal system. Because of this, a truly multidisciplinary team of specialists, including neurosurgeons, orthopedists, urologists, nephrologists, physiatrists, orthotists, pediatricians, physical therapists, occupational therapists, nurse coordinators, advanced practice nurses, geneticists, genetic counselors, and now perinatologists, fetal surgeons, and ethicists, are required to provide comprehensive treatment.

Before the 1960s, a complicated team was not needed because the majority of infants born with this defect died from infection and/or hydrocephalus. Once surgical techniques were improved and survival increased, there was a realization that helping these children required many different disciplines communicating with each other and the family. Interdisciplinary teams were established in many medical centers. All team members soon recognized that each member had to have knowledge about all areas.

My intent in editing this book is to provide information that will allow all the different disciplines to gain understanding of how the problems of each system relate to the other systems. The therapists need to know what the reason is for a child to develop progressive orthopedic deformities and to question whether it is due to possible tethering of the spinal cord, not a failure of therapy. Development of poor handwriting and progressive hypotonia may be caused by a syrinx of the cord. Development of decubitus may be due to a change in orthopedic status, including progressive scoliosis. Deterioration of schoolwork may be due to a subtle shunt malfunction.

Though there are separate chapters written by authors in different disciplines, the subjects interdigitate with each other. Not only is the knowledge within individual disciplines important, but it is necessary to recognize that communication with all team and family members is essential so the child and young adult can reach their potential.

This book represents my commitment of 35 years of experience with people with spina bifida but, most important, shares what I have learned from the families, children, and young adults with this most complex birth disorder.

I want to thank my own family: my husband, Frank, and sons, Michael and Peter, who over the years not only allowed me to spend time with families of children with spina bifida, but also developed an understanding of people with special needs.

*Sonya G. Oppenheimer*

# Acknowledgment

As faculty in the Division of Developmental and Behavioral Pediatrics at Cincinnati Children's Hospital Medical Center, this project was supported by Grant No. T73MC00032-16 awarded by the Maternal and Child Health Bureau, Health Resources and Service Administration, DHHS, and Grant No. 90DD0546/05, awarded by Administration on Developmental Disabilities, Administration for Children and Families, DHHS.

I would like to thank Nancy Ice, Administrative Assistant, for all of her help.

# Contents

# Contributors

**Robert T. Ammerman** Division of Behavioral Medicine and Clinical Psychology, Cincinnati Children's Hospital Medical Center, Cincinnati, Ohio, U.S.A.

**Tena Benson** Division of Developmental and Behavioral Pediatrics, Cincinnati Children's Hospital Medical Center, Cincinnati, Ohio, U.S.A.

**Alvin H. Crawford** Division of Pediatric Orthopedic Surgery, Cincinnati Children's Hospital Medical Center, Cincinnati, Ohio, U.S.A.

**Kerry R. Crone** Department of Neurosurgery, Cincinnati Children's Hospital Medical Center, University of Cincinnati College of Medicine, Cincinnati, Ohio, U.S.A.

**Jose Herrera-Soto** Arnold Palmer Hospital for Children, Orlando, Florida, U.S.A.

**Linda S. Lazar** Division of Developmental and Behavioral Pediatrics, Cincinnati Children's Hospital Medical Center, Cincinnati, Ohio, U.S.A.

**Benjamin Ling** Department of Neurosurgery, Cincinnati Children's Hospital Medical Center, University of Cincinnati College of Medicine, Cincinnati, Ohio, U.S.A.

**Gregory S. Liptak** Department of Pediatrics, Upstate Medical University, Syracuse, New York, U.S.A.

**James W. Loomis** Center for Children with Special Needs, Glastonbury, Connecticut, U.S.A.

**Marlene L. Lutkenhoff** Division of Developmental and Behavioral Pediatrics, Cincinnati Children's Hospital Medical Center, Cincinnati, Ohio, U.S.A.

**Kazuyuki Nishinaka** Division of Urology, Cincinnati Children's Hospital Medical Center, Cincinnati, Ohio, U.S.A.

**Marsha J. Nortz** Division of Behavioral Medicine and Clinical Psychology, Cincinnati Children's Hospital Medical Center, Cincinnati, Ohio, U.S.A.

**Godfrey P. Oakley, Jr.** Department of Epidemiology, Rollins School of Public Health of Emory University, Atlanta, Georgia, U.S.A.

**Sonya G. Oppenheimer** Division of Developmental and Behavioral Pediatrics, Cincinnati Children's Hospital Medical Center, Cincinnati, Ohio, U.S.A.

**M. Douglas Ris** Division of Behavioral Medicine and Clinical Psychology, Cincinnati Children's Hospital Medical Center, Cincinnati, Ohio, U.S.A.

**Catherine M. Shaer** The George Washington University Biostatistics Center, Rockville, Maryland, U.S.A.

**Curtis A. Sheldon** Division of Urology, Cincinnati Children's Hospital Medical Center, Cincinnati, Ohio, U.S.A.

**Junichi Tamai** Division of Pediatric Orthopedic Surgery, Cincinnati Children's Hospital Medical Center, Cincinnati, Ohio, U.S.A.

**Nicolay C. Walz** Division of Behavioral Medicine and Clinical Psychology, Cincinnati Children's Hospital Medical Center, Cincinnati, Ohio, U.S.A.

**Thomas S. Webb** Division of Developmental and Behavioral Pediatrics, Cincinnati Children's Hospital Medical Center, Cincinnati, Ohio, U.S.A.

**Donna Cheek Zahra** Nemours Children's Clinic, Jacksonville, Florida, U.S.A.

# 1

# History of Spina Bifida

**Sonya G. Oppenheimer**
*Division of Developmental and Behavioral Pediatrics, Cincinnati Children's Hospital Medical Center, Cincinnati, Ohio, U.S.A.*

## EARLY DESCRIPTION OF SPINA BIFIDA, 10,000 B.C.–1760

The history of neural tube defects begins in prehistoric time with the discovery of skeletons identified as having pathological findings consistent with spinal boney abnormalities (1). These skeletons were carbon dated and felt to exist since 10,000 B.C. and were found in a cave of taforalt in Morocco. Both adults and infant skeletons indicated that this deformity (probably not spina bifida cystica) was compatible with life (2). Spina bifida occulta was found in 90% of 10 adult skeletons from a historic American Indian burial site. The anthropological findings raised questions whether spina bifida was caused by a genetic influence or an environmental influence (3). An article in the Irish Medical Journal in 1986 reviewed archeological sites in Ireland from the Bronze Age 2000 B.C. to Medieval Era 1000 A.D. and the 15th to 18th century. Nonclosure was found in sacral segments. These findings are intriguing in that there was no information concerning children, possibly indicating that higher lesions were fatal. The authors concluded that the high risk noted in recent years, particularly around Dublin, compared with the low risk in the early centuries may indicate the influence of an environmental factor. Detailed data are available in the tables in the Irish Medical Journal. The controversy regarding the etiology continues, despite the discovery of the relationship of folic acid with spina bifida, and continues to allow us to use the term polygenetic multifactored causation.

Descriptions of spina bifida have been suggested in the writings of Hippocrates. Other historical references are seen in the writings of Pieter Van Forest in 1587 and Casper Bauhan in 1964 (4). The most historical connection is the Rembrandt painting "The Anatomy Lesson of Dr. Tulp" in 1632 (5). In it, he described patients with spina bifida as did Ruysch (6), also in a painting by Johan R. Van Neck in 1683. In 1760, Mark Gagne, who is considered the founder of modern pathological anatomy, recognized the link between spina bifida and hydrocephalus. Medical literature continued to describe various aspects of spina bifida including Van Recklinghaus' description of all forms of the condition.

## PARAPLEGIA AND INCONTINENCE

A fascinating description from a papyrus in the 17th century B.C. highlighted quadriplegia and its association with incontinence with urine and sexual function (6). Paraplegia was considered in Edwin Smith's surgical papyrus in the second millennium B.C. as an ailment not to be treated (7). Of interest, bracing and splints, however, have been used since 2400 B.C. Incontinence was also described in the writings of Hippocrates. Galen (8) understood the relationship between disease, spinal cord, and bladder problems. The concept of catheters to achieve continence is not new but has been used since the 17th century, and even catheters made of bronze and lead were used to bypass urinary obstruction. Surgical diversions for continence were attempted in 1852 by developing an ileo conduit with ureters draining into a bowel loop and were refined by Dr. Brickers in 1950.

Surgical repairs of these abnormalities were attempted from 1641 to 1892. Despite the numerous varieties of treatments, they all resulted in death until Dr. Bayer in 1892 recommended using muscular flaps for closure (9). Previous treatments had varied from using excision of the sac to sclerosing the sac with items such as silver nitrate.

## HYDROCEPHALUS

Dr. David Shurtleff, a leader in modern treatment for patients with myelomeningocele, summarizes in his presidential address for the Society of Research in Hydrocephalus and Spina Bifida the history of treatment of spina bifida to the recognition of the associated hydrocephalus and subsequent development of the Holter cerebral shunt which controlled progressive hydrocephalus (10).

In the 17th century, the possible link between hydrocephalus, paraplegia, and incontinence was identified. The Arnold Chiari phenomenon though still not totally understood was recognized in 1894 as a contributing factor to the production of the hydrocephalus (11). The production of cerebral spinal fluid and the circulation of the fluid were further described in 1827 through 1872 and later confirmed by Dandy (12).

## AGGRESSIVE TREATMENT

The treatment for hydrocephalus included trephining, compression, and even continuous drainage (12). Procedures that were done in the time of the ancient Greeks and continued in to the 1880s included injection of sclerosing substances into the ventricles to stop the production of the spinal fluid. Other techniques were used to drain the fluid. The first modern shunt was developed by Nelson, Spitz, and John Holter, an engineer whose son had hydrocephalus in 1952 (1). This led to the beginning of aggressive treatment for infants born with spina bifida.

## OUTCOMES OF TREATMENT

Based on the improvement of all these early techniques, studies analyzing outcomes of treatment began to appear in the literature. Laurence and Tew (13) reviewed 425 cases of children born with spina bifida between 1956 and 1962. Very few had been operated on. Sixteen percent in 1964 were still alive, 111 had been stillborn, 59 died in the first week, 184 died between one week and one year of age, and 5 died over the age of 12 months. The survival rate, therefore, of untreated children with myelomeningocele was 11% or 47 out of 408. Of those 47, 11 had moderate to severe involvement with limited walking ability and impaired bladder control. Twenty-four were wheelchair-bound and incontinent, two-thirds had obvious hydrocephalus; however, the mean intelligence quotient was 86 and more than half were mentally retarded. This would be interpreted that out of every 100 affected children, 25 would be born dead and 5 would die within 24 hours. This would be a group that is considered irreducible minimum mortality. Of the remaining 70, 25 will die in the first month, 20 between two and six months, 10 between 6 and 12 months, another 5 more before school age. Ten children would then be alive at the age of five indicating that one in seven might reach school age but only one in 70 is likely to attend school (14).

The literature then began to cite different examples of various outcomes with treatment. However, overall natural mortality without surgical treatment has been reported by others to be approximately 85%. Of those not treated, only 4% would be considered to have IQs above 85. Once aggressive treatment for all children with spina bifida was undertaken, the question of quality of life began to surface. After aggressive treatment in the early 1950s and 1960s, several large multidisciplinary treatment centers began to review their treatment results. Measures of successful treatment were considered on today's terms. Outcomes were mortality, degrees of morbidity including shunt complications and intelligence (less mental retardation), ambulation, and achievement of continence. The Children's Division of the Institute of the Rehabilitation Medicine at New York University formed an interdisciplinary study group in 1961. This group published a monograph edited by Chester A. Swyniard,

*Comprehensive Care of the Child with Spina Bifida Manifesta* (15). They studied 165 active patients. Care of the patients in the institute primarily consisted of inpatient admissions of approximately 34 days and was followed by periodic outpatient visits. The overall goal of treatment was maximum self-sufficiency, independent living, appropriate educational experiences, and pursuit of vocational endeavors. The premise was that the management of hydrocephalus accounted not only for mortality but also for morbidity of intellect. Of interest, of 75 patients in their nontreated hydrocephalus group, 62% went on to develop hydrocephalus. The natural history of this group became known as non-progressive hydrocephalus. This group would provide information on the natural history of nonpressured hydrocephalus with rapid head growth. These children scored lower in the full scale IQ of the WISC and there were highly significant differences in the untreated group, particularly with lower verbal scores, lower performance scores, and average verbal ability (currently referred to as nonverbal learning disabilities). The group without hydrocephalus was considered to have findings similar to people with spinal cord pathology, whereas those with hydrocephalus presented a group of children with brain damage. Urinary incontinence was achieved by the Crede method which meant pushing on the bladder to empty it. Survival depended on preservation of renal function, elimination of residual urine, and control of the urinary infection. The major form of control of incontinence was a Bricker ureterostomy to prevent renal failure. Eighty-six patients from 7 months to 26 years of age had a measured rehabilitation potential related to the initial degree of neurological deficit. This, however, was influenced by complicating factors including skeletal deformities, bowel and bladder management, decubiti, obesity, IQ, social problems, and parental attitude.

Overall, mortality within the first 21 years of life was between 80% and 85%. The conclusion of Swinyard's report in 1965 stated that the maximum obstacles for those children without hydrocephalus are the lack of community, social, educational, and vocational resources. The second major impact of morbidity was stool incontinence. Despite heroic efforts of parents and interdisciplinary teams, the management of bowel planning remained frustrating. Multiple techniques including suppositories, stool softeners, extra fiber, and enemas did not establish continence. Because of these problems with uncontrollable bowel movements, some patients eventually resorted to a colostomy that, although a major operative procedure, allowed them to have better control of the bowel movements at work, school, and society.

## TREATMENT AMBULATION

The pendulum of aggressively treating ambulation as part of the overall care of children with spina bifida has gone from multiple surgical methods that allowed what was interpreted as normal ambulation to using mobility tools that allow for movement. The concept of paraplegia was known in the middle ages and efforts to heal it have been attempted since the 12th century (16). The use of bracing has been identified in Egyptian tools of the fifth dynasty in 2400 B.C. More advanced splinting was in use since the 17th century. With the advent of lighter plastics, bracing was encouraged. However, to appropriately brace the child, multiple orthopedic surgeries including hip releases and tendon transfers and releases were required. Again, many children who were able to ambulate prior to entrance to school or the beginning of teenage years gradually began to use wheelchairs because they recognized that they could move faster and the fatigue of walking and splints was not there. Surgical techniques were performed by John Sharrard who is best known for his transfer of the psoas tendon and ileac muscles and restoring abductor power to the hips (16). A major deformity, however, that was frequently ignored was the spinal deformity. Harrington (17) developed spinal implementation for surgical correction by using the Harrington rods. Luque and Cardoso (18) developed techniques by incorporating sublaminar wiring of each vertebral body. This subsequently prevented the complication of pulmonary hypertension and progressive spinal deformity. A major more recent orthopedic problem has been the treatment of the kyphotic deformity. A review article by Banta (19) summarizes other orthopedic techniques and wisely questions a better understanding of the importance of long-term outcome and comprehension of evaluation of the motor dynamics involved in paraplegia (1). The years of treatment controversies including surgical techniques and ethical issues raised by the treatment and nontreatment of people born with spina bifida persist until current times and are reviewed in the chapter on bioethical treatment of children with spina bifida.

## FETAL SURGERY

Probably, the newest treatment for infants born with spina bifida is the recommendation of fetal surgery (20). This approach again raises parental and professional hope that in utero surgery will result in the prevention of complications of spina bifida. An NIH study entitled MOMS (Management of Myelomeningocele Study) is in process to determine whether the claims of this surgery (decreased hydrocephalus, changes in the Chiari malformation, and improved ambulation) can be documented by a vigorous research protocol (21).

## ETIOLOGY AND PREVENTION

The history of various hypotheses of possible causes of spina bifida culminated in recognition by Professor Richard Smithells of a possible form of nutrition, particularly folic acid metabolism (22). Folate relationship with this disorder is believed to be related to a genetic predisposition to the metabolism and the MPHFR gene, which is more prevalent in families with neural tube defects and, of interest, is also found in higher incidence in the Irish population. This relates to the prior epidemiological studies that spina bifida was more common in people of Irish/English ancestry. Folic acid used preconceptionally is expected to reduce the incidence of spina bifida by 70%. However, it will not totally eliminate this disorder, just as early prenatal detection by amniocentesis with subsequent choice of pregnancy termination did not eliminate the birth of infants with spina bifida.

A recent issue of the American Journal of Genetics is devoted entirely to causation, better understanding of various aspects of neural tube defects including embryology, epidemiology, genetic causes, and environmental contributions to their etiology (23). Interested readers' attention is brought to this seminar publication and is not summarized in this history.

## PERSONAL EXPERIENCE

As a personal note, the Spina Bifida clinic at the Cincinnati Children's Hospital Medical Center, Division of Developmental Disabilities setting which serves the Southwest area of Ohio and Northern Kentucky (started in 1965) averaged approximately 24 to 25 new children born with spina bifida a year. Despite the folic acid usage, the clinic currently still has 10 to 12 new infants with spina bifida, most of whom are from families who did not take the extra folic acid. This does not include the number of infants that were possibly terminated during this period. The newest phase in the history of spina bifida is the recognition that there are many people who are over 21 and were treated aggressively in the 50s, 60s, and 70s. These people are now adults and present a new continuing challenge for professionals interested in this area. This topic is discussed throughout the book but is also discussed in the chapter on transition.

## REFERENCES

1. Smith GK. The history of spina bifida, hydrocephalus, paraplegia, and incontinence. Pediatr Surg Int 2001; 17:424–432.
2. Kuttner RE. Prehistoric spina bifida occulta. JAMA 1978; 240(24):2631.
3. Saluja PG. Evidence of spina bifida in skeletal remains from Ireland. Irish Med J 1986; 79(6):145–149.
4. (Bauhan) Morgagni JB. The Seats and Causes of Diseases Investigated By Anatomy in 5 Books, Bk. 1, Letter 12. Translated from Latin by Benjamin Alexander. Vol. 1 NY: Hofner, 1960:244–474.
5. Tulip N. Observations medicarum. Ludavics Elzevirius. Vol. 63. Amsterdam: Tulp N. LIB 3, 1641:35.
6. Ruysch F. Practical Observations in Surgery and Midwifery. London: Osborne, 1751:86.
7. Wilkins RH. Neurological Classics. American Association of Neurological Surgeons. Park Ridge: Illinois, 1992:1–5.
8. Galen. Experimental section and hemisection of the spinal cord (from DeLoris affectibus). Ann Med Hist 1917; 1:367.

9. Bayer C. Zur Techoukdu Operation der spina bifida and encephalocoel. Prager Med 1892; 17:317–345.
10. Shurtleff DB. 44 years experience with management of myelomeningocele. Presidential Address, Society for Research into Hydrocephalus and Spina Bifida. Eur J Pediatr Surg 2000; 10(suppl 1):5–8.
11. Ingraham FD, Scott HW. Spina bifida and cranium bifida. The Arnold-Chiari malformation, a study of 20 cases. N Engl J Med 1943; 222:108–114.
12. Dandy WE, Blackfan KD. Internal hydrocephalus; an experimental, clinical, and pathological study. Am J Dis Child 1914; 8:406–482.
13. Laurence KM. Developmental medicine. Child Neurol 1966; (suppl 11):10.
14. Laurence KM, Tew BJ. Follow up of 65 survivors from the 425 cases of spina bifida born in South Wales between 1956 & 1962. Dev Med Child Neurol 1967; (suppl 13):1.
15. Swinyard CA, Ransohoff J, Greenspan L. Comprehensive Care of the Child with Spina Bifida Manifesta. Rehabilitation Monograph XXXI. New York, NY: New York University Spina Bifida Study Group, 1966.
16. Sharrard WJW, Grossfield I. The management of deformity and paralysis of the foot in myelomeningocele. J Bone Joint Surg Br 1968; 50(3):456–465.
17. Harrington P. Treatment of scoliosis. Correction and internal fixation by spine instrumentalation. J Bone Joint Surg Am 1962; 44-A:591–610.
18. Luque E, Cardoso A. Segmental correction of scoliosis with rigid internal fixation. Orthop Trans 1977; 1:136–137.
19. Banta JV. The orthopaedic history of spinal dysraphism. I: The early history. Dev Med Child Neurol 1996; 38:848–854.
20. Tulipan N, Bruner JP, Hernanz-Schulman M, Love LH, Walsh WF, Nickolaus D, Oakes WJ. The effect of intrauterine myelomeningocal repair on the central nervous system structure and neurosurgical function. Pediatr Neurosurg 1999; 31:183–188.
21. Mitchell LE, Adzick S, Melchionne J, Pasquariello PS, Sutton LN, Whitehead AS. Spina bifida. Lancet 2004; 364:1885–1895.
22. Eskes TKB. From anemia to spina bifida—the story of folic acid. A tribute to Professor Richard Smithells. Eur J Obstet Gynecol Reprod Biol 2000; 90(2):119–123.
23. Seminar Med Genet. Am J Med Genet C Semin Med Genet 2005; 135(1).

# 2

# The Global Epidemic of Folic Acid–Preventable Spina Bifida

**Godfrey P. Oakley, Jr.**
*Department of Epidemiology, Rollins School of Public Health of Emory University, Atlanta, Georgia, U.S.A.*

"... euthanasia in newborns ... all involved infants with very severe forms of spina bifida" (1).

"Recommendations alone did not seem to influence trends in neural tube defects .... New cases of neural tube defects preventable by folic acid continue to accumulate. A reasonable strategy would be to quickly integrate food fortification with fuller implementation of recommendations on supplements" (2).

"Rare is the opportunity to implement a sustainable, inexpensive, and effective intervention to prevent major human diseases. Folic acid fortification of flour is one of those rare opportunities. The available evidence argues that governments that do not ensure that flour is fortified with sufficient folic acid are committing public health malpractice" (3).

## INTRODUCTION

The publication of the Medical Research Council (MRC) study, in 1991, proving that folic acid will prevent most cases of spina bifida forever changed the epidemiology and public health aspects of spina bifida (4). We learned, in a single study, the answer to what causes most children to have spina bifida. Spina bifida is a folate deficiency disease. Rather than a focus on seeking clues to etiology, the primary focus of epidemiologists and public health professionals could shift to ending the global epidemic of folic acid–preventable spina bifida (5).

We have the scientific evidence to prevent any new child from having folic acid–preventable spina bifida. We have shown that folic acid fortification of flour is a highly effective public health strategy, not only to prevent spina bifida and anencephaly, but also to virtually eliminate folate deficiency anemia among adults and to lower homocysteine concentrations for adults (6–11). The increased blood folate concentrations and reduced homocysteine concentrations have been associated, as predicted, with very substantial reductions in mortality from strokes and heart attacks (12–15). The Centers for Disease Control and Prevention (CDC) investigators report that folic acid fortification in the United States was associated with 50 times as many deaths from strokes and heart attacks prevented as there were birth defects prevented (16).

Why are there still infants born in every country with folic acid–preventable spina bifida? Why is spina bifida the only indication for euthanasia in infants in the Netherlands? (1). We have simply not created the political will to make the prevention happen. In developed countries, the medical system has in the last 15 years almost eliminated two severe diseases of children—invasive h. influenza diseases and pediatric AIDS. If we create in each country the political will to prevent folic acid–preventable birth defects, it will happen.

Physicians and other health professionals who care for children with spina bifida, parents of children with spina bifida, and adults with spina bifida are the groups that can create the political will for prevention. This chapter is written both to stimulate those in these groups to create the political will for spina bifida prevention and hopefully to give some helpful background to make the job in each country as easy as possible. In addition, I will note some epidemiology that needs yet to be done to assist us in the prevention of all new cases of folic acid–preventable spina bifida.

## CREATE A SENSE OF URGENCY

As a person working to prevent birth defects, I had assumed that the compelling scientific evidence available in the early 1990s would lead, in a matter of months, to full prevention of these life-altering birth defects (17). My colleagues and I at the CDC felt the urgency, getting recommendations for recurrence prevention published within a few days of the MRC paper and getting, in a year, a recommendation that all women should consume 400 μg of synthetic folic acid a day to prevent spina bifida and anencephaly (18–20).

Required/mandatory/universal fortification of a food centrally processed and widely consumed is the least expensive and most sustainable way to prevent spina bifida and anencephaly. In no country has the food fortification culture been able to move within a matter of days. Most countries have food safety regulations that exist to protect the health of the population. These regulations are frequently used to withdraw a dangerous food from the market. Often, the decision to withdraw is based on fairly weak data. Nevertheless, the decision to remove the product is made to give the prevention of human disease the benefit of the doubt.

The United States was the first country to require mandatory fortification of food to prevent spina bifida (21). The Food and Drug Administration (FDA) did not chose to use the emergency power in their regulations to require immediately that "enriched" be fortified with folic acid. Instead, the FDA underwent a long review process that resulted in the publication five years later of regulations permitting folic acid fortification and requiring it 6.5 years after we had randomized controlled trial proof that folic acid would prevent spina bifida. Had it not been for the direct political intervention of the March of Dimes in this process, there may never have been regulations in the United States or Canada requiring folic acid fortification. It was the Canadian millers, who used political influence to get the Canadian government to issue regulations requiring fortification.

Placing something in food that almost everyone will eat is a very serious issue. It should be treated seriously. Being born with folic acid–preventable spina bifida is serious. It is a serious mistake for governments to let it happen. Serious decisions can be made quickly. For example, soon after the United States required fortification the government of Chile decided to require fortification (22).

Given randomized controlled trial proof that folic acid would prevent this birth defect, I cannot understand why it took so long to get fortification required in the countries where it is required, nor can I understand why it is taking so long in other countries. Given the extensive review in the United States and given the success of folic acid fortification in the United States, Canada, and Chile, countries should be able to go from the idea of fortification to making the serious decision to do it within three months. There simply is no need for such long-drawn-out review process that we are currently seeing.

The United Kingdom underwent a two-year review process resulting in the publication of a report recommending fortification of flour in 2002 (23). While this report was being written, there was the "mad cow disease" scare. The public judged that the food safety authorities had not moved fast enough which resulted in the formation of the new Foods Standards Agency to improve decisions on the safety of foods. To its great discredit, its first action was to recommend against folic acid fortification. To this day, the taxpayers who paid for the study that proved that folic acid prevented spina bifida have yet to have the benefit of required folic acid fortification that should flow from such strong data. It is a mystery that concern about hypotheses about "mad cow disease" was viewed as strong enough to get public attention, but that the proof that folic acid would prevent one of the most severe birth defects was not sufficiently strong to get public attention. In retrospect, there have been 137 cases of mad cow disease in total, less than the annual number of cases of spina bifida and anencephaly that folic acid fortification could prevent each year in the United Kingdom. Folic acid fortification is not yet required in the United Kingdom.

Ireland, New Zealand, and Australia are considering whether or not to fortify. Unfortunately, rather than seeing the need to prevent spina bifida as an emergency, these countries have become involved in a long review process that will take years to get to a decision—which may or may not lead to fortification. One might understand the need for such a long process if the information supporting the fortification were new and if no major country had required fortification and evaluated it. There simply is no good reason to have a long process. Three months should be enough.

Folic acid fortification has been required in the United States and Canada since 1998 and in Chile since 2000. We know what happens when you require folic acid for populations. Serum folates immediately increase. The prevention of spina bifida starts immediately. The prevention of folate deficiency anemia starts immediately. The reduction of serum homocysteine begins immediately and reduction of deaths from strokes and heart attacks is not far behind. The quality of the evidence that immediate mandatory fortification of folic acid will improve the health of the population is very strong. What is keeping this prevention from occurring is that the decision makers have grown up in a culture where rapid changes in policy have been considered only when there is risk from a "bad" product. Here the culture understands it is important to move fast on limited amounts of data. This culture does not understand that it is also important to move quickly to add something to food that would improve the lives of the people in the population.

It may not be possible to change this recalcitrant culture. I am an optimist. I have seen the power of parents of children with disabilities to change the culture so that it is friendlier to persons with disabilities. I believe parents, persons with spina bifida, and those who care for persons with disabilities can create the sense of urgency for prevention that will cause food regulators, not only to consider fortification, but also use the emergency powers they have to get fortification implemented on an expedited emergency basis.

Scientists and policy makers met in Ottawa seeking to find ways of increasing the pace at which folic acid–preventable diseases are prevented. They recommended that folic fortification occur as fast as possible in all countries (24). Another group met under the umbrella of the World Health Organization (WHO) Europe and made similar recommendations (25). Apparently, because of a turf issue in the WHO, the WHO refused to accept the report. It is an excellent report showing how many neural tube defect pregnancies would be prevented were all countries in Europe to fortify. It should have become WHO policy. No doubt one day the WHO will make policy as recommended in this report.

## FORTIFICATION IS EASY TO IMPLEMENT QUICKLY

One might think that fortifying flour is difficult to do. That is wrong. It is technically easy to do. It is especially easy to do in countries where flour is already fortified with vitamins and or minerals. It is so easy to do that it can be accomplished in a single day. Vitamins and minerals are added to flour at the end of the milling process by a dosimeter called a feeder. The dosimeter has a container that the vitamin/mineral "premix" is placed so that the dosimeter can put the vitamin/minerals in at the concentration desired. To change a flour mill into a spina bifida prevention factory requires only adding the vitamin/mineral premix that contains folic acid. In countries where there is no fortification, it is necessary to equip the mills with feeders and premix and train staff how to use and monitor. In most countries, this can be accomplished within six months if there are the resources and commitment to get fortification done. What has delayed folic acid fortification in so many countries has been the antagonism to fortification by food regulators and the unwillingness of the food regulators to invoke emergency powers to get fortification done expeditiously.

## PROVIDE THE EVIDENCE FOR FORTIFICATION

Policy makers need to be informed with the best available information. There is a need to provide them with information that is current. The Committee on Medical Aspects of Food and Nutrition Policy report in 2000 (23) was such a technical update for policy makers. Our group and Dr. Bower (26,27) recently provided such an update for New Zealand and Australia. This review shows the strong evidence proving that folic acid will prevent most of spina bifida. It also shows the improvements to health that have actually occurred where folic acid fortification is required. In addition, it pointed out that a postfortification study found no evidence to support the hypothesis that consuming more folic acid might make it more difficult to diagnose vitamin B12 deficiency (28). While directed at New Zealand and Australia, much of the review can be helpful in any country.

Since the publication of the paper, there have been some new studies of note. Casas has produced evidence that makes it almost certain that decreasing homocysteine concentrations with folic acid will result in the prevention of heart attacks and strokes (15). Ray has shown that programs to teach women to consume vitamin supplements reach less than half the women of reproductive age (29). Thus, supplement programs must be seen as a complement to, not a substitution for, required folic acid fortification programs. Botto and colleagues showed that merely having a recommendation for women to consume more folic acid is not effective in preventing spina bifida (2).

Thus the way to best improve prevention is to require folic acid fortification complemented by an active health education/social marketing campaign that is well funded and that eliminates cost as a barrier to women consuming supplements.

## FOLIC ACID BENEFITS THE ELDERLY

One obstacle to getting governments to require folic acid fortification has been the suggestion by some that yes folic acid will benefit children, but will not benefit adults, so why expose all adults to folic acid. This framing of the issue is not data driven.

For many years, there have been discussions about whether or not the elderly consume enough folic acid. In fact in the mid-1970s, there was a major policy review in the United States that assumed the elderly did not have enough folic acid. The Food and Nutrition Board recommended that flour be fortified with folic acid and a few other vitamins. The FDA decided not to follow the advice. Instead, the FDA permitted companies to voluntarily add more folic acid to vitamin pills and to breakfast cereals. As a result of the FDAs actions, most multivitamins subsequently sold in the United States had 400 μg of synthetic folic acid and most breakfast cereals had 100 μg of folic acid. A few breakfast cereals began to contain 400 μg of synthetic folic acid per servings.

The American public, since the mid-1970s has been a large consumer of synthetic folic acid. Around 25% of adults consume multivitamins. Older Americans consume vitamins most frequently. In multiple studies, the consumers of multivitamins have been judged have improved health outcomes and no adverse effects have been reported. Because multivitamin consumption is so common, studies like the Harvard's Nurse's Study have been able to evaluate both the possible benefits and harm from such widespread exposure. No harm has been identified in these studies, but multivitamin consumption has been associated with a lower risk of heart attacks, strokes, birth defects, and colon cancer (30).

Those who hypothesize risk for the elderly deny the large exposure to folic acid to Americans for more than 20 years before folic acid fortification. To deny the exposure is not to be data driven. One must look at the data, not deny it, for rational decision making.

## PREVIOUS HIGH EXPOSURE OF EMBRYOS AND FETUSES

Some discussions of folic acid fortification have suggested that this would be a new experiment; that human fetuses have never been exposed to synthetic folic acid. Again this is simply an error. Most pregnant women in the United States have for decades before fortification was instituted consume a "prenatal" vitamin with 800 to 1000 μg of synthetic folic acid. If consumption of folic acid in a bolus of 300 μg results in absorption and circulation of free synthetic folic acid as is likely, then American fetuses have almost all been exposed to free folic acid for many weeks of their prenatal life. During these years, the infant mortality steadily declined. If there is harm, it has not been found after decades of exposure to large numbers of American fetuses. It is simply an error in fact to say that human fetuses have not in large numbers been exposed to synthetic folic acid before fortification. It simply is not true.

Given that folate is needed DNA synthesis and cell division, it would not be a surprise if nature developed a system to give developing fetuses an adequate supply of folate. At term, cord blood had three times the serum folate that mother's blood had. This three-fold difference applied across wide differences in folate consumption—from women who consumed no synthetic folic acid a day to women who consumed 6000 μg a day (31). This paper not only documents how high synthetic folic acid consumption can be among American women who are pregnant, but shows that biology favors the fetuses being exposed to concentrations of folate that are three times the mother's level.

## FOLIC ACID DOES NOT HARM PEOPLE WITH VITAMIN B12 DEFICIENCY—THE LACK OF VITAMIN B12 HARMS PEOPLE WITH VITAMIN B12 DEFICIENCY

Unfortunately, the hypothesis that folic acid might harm persons with vitamin B12 deficiency has been one of the arguments that have complicated policy discussions on folic acid fortification and delayed or prohibited a decision to fortify. There are little data to support this hypothesis (32). It is important to understand the facts for they led to the conclusion that people with vitamin B12 deficiency need vitamin B12 and they will not improve with folic acid, penicillin, or any other drug that is not vitamin B12.

Confusion is considerable. Concern about the adverse clinical effects derives primarily from what we know about the effects of symptomatic pernicious anemia. Untreated symptomatic pernicious anemia and other forms of severe vitamin B12 deficiency will get worse leading ultimately to paralysis and death. Symptomatic, severe vitamin B12 deficiency should be treated with vitamin B12.

Very high doses of folic acid, 5000 μg a day or more, can cure the anemia of severe vitamin B12 deficiency. We first learned this in a series of studies in the 1940s and 1950s (33). These studies were of individuals diagnosed as having pernicious anemia by the then current diagnostic studies and who were successfully treated with liver extract. All of the patients in these studies were taken off the successful therapy and put on a drug that we now know is not effective against the neuropathy of severe vitamin B12 deficiency. That drug was folic acid. As a result of taking these patients off effective therapy and putting them on an ineffective therapy, many became sick. It is well known today that patients with symptomatic, pernicious anemia in remission on adequate injections or oral consumption of high doses of vitamin B12, will become symptomatic again if they stop their effective vitamin B12 therapy. They get sick again, not because they are taking some other medicine, but because they stop taking the effective medicine.

The older studies that withdrew liver extract treatment and substituted the ineffective folic acid found, as expected in hindsight, that many patients got sick again. Some of them get rapidly sick which is where the misunderstanding about folic acid accelerating the course of B12 deficiency came. Surely, it is much more likely that the natural history of the disease has sufficient variance to include "rapid" courses as was found even before folic acid was synthesized.

The clinical course, in about equal parts, had patients who never got sick again. Perhaps they had folate deficiency anemia as folate is in the liver extract, too. About 25% had a recurrence of anemia, and about 25% had a recurrence of neuropathy and anemia. The final 25% had only neuropathy. From this observation derived the notion of masking. The notion of masking, as nondata driven as it is, served for years as a way to teach medical students that if one sees a patient with macrocytic anemia, that one should not treat the patient with folic acid to see if they would get better. It was recommended that there should be a proper diagnosis and the patient then be treated with folic acid, vitamin B12, or both as the diagnosis indicated. Even here the message is treat vitamin B12 deficiency with vitamin B12. There is no need to continue the idea that folic acid will harm people with vitamin B12 deficiency. The evidence does not support it. The evidence is that lack of B12 causes the diseases.

More recently there is in the literature a "new" vitamin B12 deficiency. It is fairly common—maybe 20% of people over 50 have it. It has been discovered by population studies such as the Framingham and National Health and Nutrition Examination Survey (NHANES) (11,34). It is a lab-based diagnosis. It is not clear how much, if any, disease is caused by this rather common, but apparently mostly subclinical B12 deficiency. The Institute of Medicine has suggested that, even though a benefit has not been established, everyone 50 and over should consume 2.4 μg of synthetic vitamin B12 a day to prevent this "new" vitamin B12 deficiency. Were everyone over 50 to consume such vitamin B12, this new vitamin B12 would disappear. Fortifying food with B12 would be the most effective way to eliminate the new vitamin B12 deficiency.

Given that the "new" pre-clinical vitamin B12 still affects 20% of those over 50, this group confuses policy makers. They make the nondata driven inference that a little folic acid, 100 to 200 μg a day, from fortification may make 20% of the population seriously ill from newly symptomatic vitamin B12 deficiency. The current evidence does not support this inference. It is time for policy discussions to become unencumbered by such speculation.

## THE ELDERLY ARE FOLATE DEFICIENT

The elderly were perceived to be folate deficient in the 1970s. NHANES and a recent study suggest that in the United Kingdom that many of the elderly are folate deficient (11). Thus, folic acid fortification would improve folate nutrition for the elderly. It is time for policy discussions to acknowledge that folic acid fortification will benefit the elderly. It is time for the policy papers to compare the risks and benefits of folic acid fortification for the elderly rather than saying there can only be risk for the elderly.

## MONITORING THE DISAPPEARANCE OF FOLIC ACID–PREVENTABLE SPINA BIFIDA

One job for future epidemiologists is to accurately track the progress, or lack of it, in the prevention of spina bifida and anencephaly. Botto has used most of the existing surveillance systems to show that the job has barely begun (2). Because of prenatal diagnosis and abortion of affected fetuses, getting an accurate count of pregnancies affected by spina bifida will require diligence and extra resources. In addition, we do not know the prevalence of nonfolic acid–preventable spina bifida. In the China study, the treated rates for spina bifida and anencephaly were approximately 5 per 10,000 (35). Until there are better data, I suggest that we consider countries with good spina bifida and anencephaly surveillance to have folic acid–preventable spina bifida and anencephaly continuing to occur if the rate of spina bifida and anencephaly pregnancies exceed 5 per 10,000. Thus a rate of 10 per 10,000 would be a two-fold epidemic and a rate of 20 per 10,000 would be a four-fold epidemic. Thus rates of spina bifida and anencephaly above 5 per 10,000 indicate population folate deficiency requiring folic acid intervention programs.

## MONITORING SERUM FOLATE AS A BIOMARKER FOR RISK OF FOLIC ACID–PREVENTABLE SPINA BIFIDA

It is unlikely that we will have accurate spina bifida surveillance in every country. Furthermore, the spina bifida rates cannot be as timely as serum folate concentrations as an indicator of progress or lack of it towards preventing folic acid–preventable spina bifida. There is epidemiological and laboratory research to be done. We are not certain at what maternal serum concentration above which there is no or almost no folic acid–preventable spina bifida occurring. We know that setting the low cut-point for serum folate based on preventing folate deficiency anemia as is the current standard is inappropriate indicator of folate deficiency. That cut-point must be higher (36). It must be as least 10 ng/mL as measured in the Dr. Scott's lab in Ireland (37). Because almost all persons over 50 have elevated serum homocysteine because they do not have high enough concentrations of folate, there is a discussion to base the low folate serum cut-point on a homocysteine standard (11,36). This would be an improvement over continuing to use the red cell standard. It is not best. It is likely that the best indicator of folate adequacy would be the folate serum concentrations above which there in little if any folic acid–preventable spina bifida.

The polio eradication program needed a measure of prevention that would assure that there was no polio being transmitted in a country. Their criterion is that a country must have a surveillance system that identified a rate of "nonpolio polio"—called acute flaccid paralysis at a rate of 1 per 100,000. They have it a bit easy, because this non-polio polio can be confirmed by laboratory testing.

Determining whether or not a population is vitamin A deficient no longer waits for the deficiency to become so severe that children become blind. Instead, vitamin A scientists have determined a blood vitamin A level above which blindness does not occur. If they find the blood level lower, they institute vitamin A programs even though there is no vitamin A deficiency caused blindness.

I suggest that epidemiologists and other scientist soon set a default serum concentration of folate above which folic acid–preventable spina bifida rarely is ever occurs. Nutritional evaluations should include a serum folate concentration. The subjects will be determined to be folate deficient if more than 5% are below the cut-point experts think will prevent almost all, if not all, folic acid–preventable birth defects. I suggest that this default cut-point should be 15 ng/mL until there are data to change the default.

## CAPILLARY BLOOD FOLATE METHOD FOR FIELD STUDIES

Venous blood is often not collected in field studies evaluating nutrition status. The lack of a widely validated and accepted field method to access blood folate status on capillary blood hampers assessment of folate status in many current field studies. Monitoring the progress towards total prevention of folic acid–preventable spina bifida would be improved by the availability of folate concentrations from capillary blood with an understanding of where to put the cut-point that would be consistent with the serum folate cut-point.

## REFERENCES


1. Verhagen E, Sauer PJ. The Groningen protocol—euthanasia in severely ill newborns. N Engl J Med 2005; 352(10):959–962.
2. Botto LD, Lisi A, Robert-Gnansia E, et al. International retrospective cohort study of neural tube defects in relation to folic acid recommendations: are the recommendations working? BMJ 2005; 330(7491):57.
3. Oakley GP Jr. Inertia on folic acid fortification: public health malpractice. Teratology 2002; 66(1):44–54.
4. MRC Vitamin Study Research Group. Prevention of neural tube defects: results of the Medical Research Council Vitamin Study. MRC Vitamin Study Research Group. Lancet 1991; 338(8760):131–137.
5. Oakley G. Global prevention of all folic acid–preventable spina bifida and anencephaly by 2010. Community Genet 2002; 5:70–77.
6. Mersereau P, Kilker K, Carter H, et al. Spina bifida and anencephaly before and after folic acid mandate—United States, 1995–1996 and 1999–2000. MMWR-Morb Mortal Wkly Rep 2004; 53(17):362–365.
7. De Wals P, Rusen ID, Lee NS, Morin P, and Niyonsenga T. Trend in prevalence of neural tube defects in Quebec. Birth Defects Res 2003; 67(11):919–923.
8. Persad VL, Van den Hof MC, Dube JM, and Zimmer P. Incidence of open neural tube defects in Nova Scotia after folic acid fortification. CMAJ 2002; 167(3):241–245.
9. Erickson JD. Folic acid and prevention of spina bifida and anencephaly. 10 years after the U.S. Public Health Service recommendation. Morb Mortal Wkly Rep. Recomm Rep 2002; 51(RR-13):1–3.
10. Erickson D, Mulinare J, Yang Q, et al. Folate status in women of childbearing age, by race/ethnicity—United States, 1999–2000. MMWR Morb Mortal Wkly Rep 2002; 51(36):808–810.
11. Selhub J, Jacques PF, Rosenberg IH, et al. Serum total homocysteine concentrations in the third National Health and Nutrition Examination Survey (1991–1994): population reference ranges and contribution of vitamin status to high serum concentrations. Ann Intern Med 1999; 131(5):331–339.
12. Boushey CJ, Beresford SA, Omenn GS, and Motulsky AG. A quantitative assessment of plasma homocysteine as a risk factor for vascular disease. Probable benefits of increasing folic acid intakes. JAMA 1995; 274(13):1049–1057.

13. Mark SD, Wang W, Fraumeni JF, et al. Lowered risks of hypertension and cerebrovascular disease after vitamin/mineral supplementation: the Linxian nutrition intervention trial. Am J Epidemiol 1996; 143(7):658–664.
14. Wald DS, Law M, Morris JK. Homocysteine and cardiovascular disease: evidence on causality from a meta-analysis. BMJ 2002; 325:7374.
15. Casas JP, Bautista LE, Smeeth L, Sharma P, and Hingorani AD. Homocysteine and stroke: evidence on a causal link from mendelian randomisation. Lancet 2005; 365(9455):224–232.
16. Anonymous. Folic acid fortification may have lowered stroke deaths. http://www.americanheart.org/presenter.jhtml?identifier=3019554. 2004.
17. Oakley GP Jr. Folic acid-preventable spina bifida and anencephaly. JAMA 1993; 269(10):1292–1293.
18. Centers for Disease Control and Prevention. Use of folic acid for prevention of spina bifida and other neural tube defects—1983–1991. MMWR Morb Mortal Wkly Rep 1991; 40(30):513–516.
19. Centers for Disease Control and Prevention. Recommendations for the use of folic acid to reduce the number of cases of spina bifida and other neural tube defects. MMWR Morb Mortal Wkly Rep 1992; 41(RR-14):1–7.
20. Oakley GP, Erickson JD, James LM, Mulinare J, and Cordero JF. Prevention of folic acid-preventable spina bifida and anencephaly. Ciba Foundation Symposium, 1993.
21. Food and Drug Administration. Food standards: amendment of standards of identity for enriched grain products to require addition of folic acid. Fed Regist 1996; 61: 8781–8807.
22. Freire WB, Hertrampf E, Cortes F. Effect of folic acid fortification in Chile: preliminary results. Eur J Pediatr Surg 2000; 10(suppl 1):42–43.
23. Committee on Medical Aspects of Food and Nutrition Policy (COMA) of the Department of Health (U.K.). Folic acid and the prevention of disease. Report of the committee on medical aspects of food and nutrition policy. Reports on Health and Social Subjects. London: The Stationery Office, 2000:i–xv, 1–101.
24. Oakley GP Jr, Bell KN, Weber MB. Recommendations for accelerating global action to prevent folic acid-preventable birth defects and other folate-deficiency diseases: meeting of experts on preventing folic acid-preventable neural tube defects. Birth Defects Res 2004; 70(11):835–837.
25. Istituto Superiore di Sanità. Folic acid: from research to public health practice. In: D. Taruscio, ed. Istituto Superiore di Sanità, 2004:36.
26. Oakley GP Jr., Weber MB, Bell KN, and Colditz P. Scientific evidence supporting folic acid fortification of flour in Australia and New Zealand. Birth Defects Res 2004; 70(11):838–841.
27. Bower C, Stanley FJ. Case for mandatory fortification of food with folate in Australia, for the prevention of neural tube defects. Birth Defects Res 2004; 70(11):842–843.
28. Mills JL, von Kohorn I, Conley MR, et al. Low vitamin B-12 concentrations in patients without anemia: the effect of folic acid fortification of grain. Am J Clin Nutr 2003; 77(6):1474–1477.
29. Ray JG. Poor use of folic acid tablet supplements periconceptionally explains much. BMJ Rapid Response to Botto LD, Lisi A, Robert-Gnansia E, et al. International retrospective cohort study of neural tube defects in relation to folic acid recommendations: are the recommendations working? BMJ 2005; 330(7491):12.

30. Giovannucci E, Stampfer MJ, Colditz GA, et al. Multivitamin use, folate, and colon cancer in women in the Nurses' Health Study. Ann Int Med 1998; 129(7):517–524.
31. Huber A, Wallins L, DeRusso P. Folate nutriture in pregnancy. J Am Diet Assoc 1988; 88:791–795.
32. Dickinson CJ. Does folic acid harm people with vitamin B12 deficiency? QJM 1995; 88(5):357–364.
33. Vilter CF, Vilter RW, Spies TD. The treatment of pernicious and related anemias with synthetic folic acid: observations on maintenance of normal hematologic status and on occurrence of combined system disease at the end of one year. J Lab Clin Med 1947; 32:262–273.
34. Selhub J, Jacques PF, Wilson PW, Rush D, and Rosenberg IH. Vitamin status and intake as primary determinants of homocysteinemia in an elderly population. JAMA 1993; 270(22):2693–2698.
35. Berry RJ, Li Z, Erickson JD, et al. Prevention of neural-tube defects with folic acid in China. China-U.S. Collaborative Project for Neural Tube Defect Prevention [corrected; erratum to be published]. N Eng J Med 1999; 341(20):1485–1490.
36. Brouwer DA, Welten HT, Reijingoud DJ, von Doormal JJ, and Muskiet FA. Plasma folic acid cutoff value, derived from its relationship with homocyst(e)ine. Clin Chem 1998; 44(7):1545–1550.
37. Daly LE, Kirke PN, Molloy A, Weir DG, and Scott JM. Folate levels and neural tube defects. Implications for prevention. JAMA 1995; 274(21):1698–1702.

# 3

# Multidisciplinary Management Including Prenatal Care

**Catherine M. Shaer**

*The George Washington University Biostatistics Center, Rockville, Maryland, U.S.A.*

## INTRODUCTION

With the advent of maternal serum alpha-fetoprotein testing and advances in diagnostic ultrasound, it is increasingly likely that an open neural tube defect will be detected prenatally. Therefore, it is almost always the obstetrician, perinatologist, or genetics counselor who first counsels the family about myelomeningocele in this early, critical, decision-making time. Most of these professio-nals have little to no knowledge of what spina bifida means for an individual child or for the family beyond what they have read in textbooks or learned at medical conferences. Regardless of whether the family is considering termination as an option or has decided to continue the pregnancy, they are much better served by referral to a center experienced in the treatment of individuals with spina bifida and whose staff of providers has a wealth of first-hand experience with this complex disability (1,2). Most such centers have a multidisciplinary team consisting of physicians, nurses, social workers, physical, occupational and speech therapists, and dieticians who work together to care for patients with myelomeningocele and their families. This multidisciplinary team format is widely recognized as the best model for providing comprehensive, coordinated care to this population (3–8). When families are presented with the diagnosis of an open neural tube defect in their fetus, meeting with members of this team will provide them with an opportunity to discuss, with health-care professionals who actually are familiar with this disability, all aspects of the condition including the medical, surgical, social, psychological, and educational issues which they and their child will likely face over the coming years. It is most effective if two complementary members of the spina bifida team, such as a physician and social worker or clinical nurse specialist, participate in the initial meeting. In this way, not only will the family have an opportunity to interact with several members of the team that may ultimately care for their child, but each team member can also provide information about and discuss those areas in which he or she has the most expertise. The primary focus of this meeting should be to clearly and openly present comprehensive, up-to-date information about open neural tube defects including the basic pathophysiology as well as the educational, social, and psychological factors associated with myelomeningocele. This information should be offered without bias and with an understanding that some families will elect to terminate the pregnancy. Whenever possible, written materials that present this information in lay terms should also be given to the family. This will allow them to review the material presented at their own pace and to formulate questions that they can then go over with team members. For families who have decided to continue with the pregnancy, a therapeutic relationship begins to form with these multidisciplinary team members during this initial meeting. This affords the team an early opportunity to establish trust, clarify the way in which they operate, discuss how treatment recommendations are arrived at, and explain to whom the family should turn when they have questions and concerns.

## THE PERINATAL PERIOD

It is especially important to talk about what is most likely to occur soon after the child's birth: explaining the need for evaluations by multiple specialists and the role of the team leader or attending physician in coordinating examinations and diagnostic tests and in communicating the results to the parents as well as to the rest of the team. This is imperative if the child will be cared for in a hospital which has medical and/or surgical training programs, as the number of attending physicians, nurses, residents, fellows, and other health-care professionals involved in the treatment of a hospitalized child can be staggering. In addition, by educating themselves about the facts of spina bifida and the early management plan, the family will often gain a measure of control. For example, they may be able to choose their neurosurgeon and have some input as to where the baby will be delivered.

The decision as to where to deliver can have a number of implications. It is not unusual, for example, for the delivery institution to send the neonate to a separate facility for treatment where neurosurgery and other necessary specialized medical and surgical resources are available. This would be true, for example, in cities with excellent pediatric facilities such as freestanding children's hospitals, which do not have maternity services. In many hospitals, the birth of a child with an open neural defect is a rare occurrence and can be traumatic and confusing for the staff. Since most children with spina bifida are very stable at birth, all that is usually required in the first few hours after delivery is to cover the lesion with a moist sterile dressing, protect the exposed spinal cord from trauma, and, perhaps, administer intravenous antibiotics. The reaction of many community obstetric and pediatric units, however, is to whisk the child away from the mother, often before she even has a chance to hold her baby. When the plan for delivery is considered early on, one member of the spina bifida team can contact the mother's obstetrician or the head of the nursery at the delivery institution and initiate a frank discussion of what is safe for the baby, how to protect the open defect, and how maternal–infant contact can be facilitated. Hopefully, by dealing with the concerns of the staff in an anticipatory fashion, a lot of the anxiety surrounding the care of the baby can be dispelled and the mother will be allowed to see and hold her infant before it is taken to the neonatal intensive care unit or transferred to the treating institution. This type of early intervention goes a long way toward allaying the family's concerns about their child being gravely ill, facilitates maternal–infant bonding, and lays the groundwork for their viewing the baby as having medical needs but not being defined by those needs. Whenever possible, a tour of the neonatal intensive care nursery should be arranged so that the parents can familiarize themselves with the nursery staff, discuss how preferences such as breast feeding are accommodated, and be appropriately informed of any important institutional regulations such as those governing visitation.

It is routine in most areas of the United States for infants with spina bifida to be delivered by cesarean section. If this is the case, the parents will also have to consider what the father and other significant individuals will do after the delivery: stay with the mother or go immediately to the institution where the baby will be treated. Because the mother will most likely be hospitalized for at least a few days and the father will need to travel to the treating facility in order to meet with the management team and sign necessary paperwork, it is very helpful if the family has already met with the physician who will have primary responsibility for directing their child's care, the treating neurosurgeon if different from the attending, as well as the spina bifida program director and nurse coordinator if applicable.

Another important resource available to a spina bifida clinic or program that would not necessarily be available to obstetricians or genetics counselors is a familiarity with local spina bifida support groups, families who have children with spina bifida, and older individuals with spina bifida. When families are expecting a child with an open neural tube defect, there are pros and cons to their meeting others who have a child with this condition or affected children and adults themselves. When people are just beginning to face the reality of having a child who almost assuredly will have special needs, it can be invaluable for them to meet with others who have been in their position and who are not only coping but have found pleasure and fulfillment in parenting their child (9,10). Meeting a child with a motor deficit similar to what is anticipated in their child can diffuse a lot of the anxiety associated with the unknown. Talking to the child, watching them ambulate, and seeing how that child is normal in so many ways can mitigate the great fear most expectant parents feel: fear that their child will look very abnormal or unusual, fear that the handicap will be so severe their child will not be able to participate as a meaningful member of the family, and fear that none of the hopes and dreams they have for this child could possibly come true.

However, it can be difficult, even threatening, for people in crisis to meet with strangers and discuss their situation, share the roller coaster of emotions they are experiencing, and ask about the very uncertain future. When facilitating such a contact, it is incumbent upon the health-care provider to carefully consider the personal style and views on spina bifida of the contact family as well as any hidden agendas they may have. It is completely unacceptable for the contact family to burden the expectant family with their problems or draw them into any conflicts they may have with treating institutions, schools, or the disability community. It is paramount that the variability and complexity of spina bifida not be minimized. Although it can be difficult, one must strive for a careful balance when presenting realistic information about the condition and introducing parents to other families or affected children (11).

## THE NEONATAL PERIOD

When a family has had the opportunity to meet with members of the treatment team and tour the facility where their baby will be cared for, the immediate post-delivery period rarely brings big surprises. The situation is usually very different if the birth of the baby with spina bifida comes as a surprise in the delivery room or the presence of the birth defect was known but the family has not met with the treating medical professionals beforehand. In these situations, it is unlikely that they will have a clear and accurate understanding of the complexities of spina bifida or an accurate idea of what the management after delivery will most likely entail. Ideally, key members of the spina bifida team will meet with, or at least speak to, the parents within hours of the delivery. Although it is much less desirable than meeting earlier in the pregnancy, the team should explain the basics of spina bifida in order to be sure that the parents have an accurate understanding of the fundamentals of the condition, present the plan for transferring the baby if necessary, discuss the initial treatment needs, and provide contact information for the attending physician, neurosurgeon, and the unit to which the child will be admitted. Again, if possible, written materials such as booklets explaining spina bifida and pamphlets containing basic information about the treating institution should be provided to the family. It is also quite important to discuss who will be involved in their child's care. As mentioned earlier, if the facility is a teaching institution, the number of individuals involved in the care, diagnosis, and treatment of the child will be quite large and the parents should be prepared for this as well as for the fact that there are clear lines of responsibility and that there is, indeed, an experienced clinician responsible for the care of their child.

Regardless of when the family meets the team, once the child is born and care begins, either in the birth hospital or in another facility, it is essential that the team leader be clearly identified. Because of the plethora of specialties involved in the management of these children, it is most efficient and effective if one person is responsible for making sure that all of the necessary specialists evaluate the child and that any required diagnostic testing is done in a timely and sensible fashion. Actually, making a chart of what evaluations and tests are scheduled, posting it by the child's bedside, and updating the status of each entry on a daily basis are very effective ways of keeping all of the health-care professionals informed about the treatment plan and what has and has not been accomplished. It is very important for the team leader to be familiar with the entire plan, communicate it to the family, and be accountable for keeping them up-to-date on what has been done, informing them of test results and getting answers to questions as they are raised.

## COMMUNITY CARE

A comprehensive, institutionally based multidisciplinary team alone is only one of the components necessary for the successful management of these children, however. Having a committed primary-care provider is required if the myriad of medical, psychological, educational, and social challenges that face children with spina bifida and their families are to be adequately addressed (11). There are several important reasons to separate the child's primary care from the specialty care offered by the multidisciplinary team. The primary care provider is usually located closer to the family, making it easier to get to appointments. Having a "regular" doctor or nurse practitioner involved in their child's care minimizes, to some extent, any tendency the parents may have to see their child as medically special and, perhaps, fragile. It is also important to remember that although multidisciplinary teams have expertise in many areas, they may not have the time to devote sufficient attention to the critical areas of behavior, discipline, and preventive medicine which form the backbone of excellent general pediatric care.

Although it is unusual to find a community provider who has extensive experience treating children with spina bifida, it is more than sufficient to identify one who is both comfortable with and accomplished in caring for children with special health-care needs. Once found, it is crucial that the community provider be viewed and welcomed as a member of the team. A complete discharge summary of the child's hospital course as well as a copy of the assessment of the child's status as it relates to their spina bifida and the plan for managing all identified medical and surgical needs should be sent to the community provider. That provider should also be advised as to how to contact the various multidisciplinary team members and provided with guidelines about whom to call should they have a question about the child's medical condition. It is often helpful for the team leader to serve as the main contact for the primary-care provider as he or she can help determine who should evaluate the child when specific problems arise. Likewise, the parents should be given some guidance as to when they should contact the primary-care provider and when they should call the spina bifida team when their child is ill. Again, it is extremely helpful if the team leader can be available as the person to whom the parents can turn whenever they are in doubt about how to proceed when they think their child needs medical attention.

In addition to a committed primary-care provider, other integral members of the child's multidisciplinary team are based in the community. All of the needs of the child should be carefully considered prior to discharge and the types of providers required should be identified so that referrals for assessments can be made, as soon as possible, to the appropriate early intervention programs. Arrangements for continuing important therapies during the evaluation process must also be made.

Access to adequate therapeutic and educational services is also a priority in the first three years of life. A single program that meets both of these needs is best, but the setting in which services are provided to the young children varies widely from community to community. Home-based programs are usually most convenient for parents and more comfortable for the child, but center-based programs frequently offer a greater breadth of services. The team member most familiar with the options available in a given area should discuss these choices with the family before the initial discharge from the hospital. When necessary, the spina bifida team leader should work with the primary-care provider to advocate for appropriate services for the child and its family.

## ONGOING ROLE OF THE MULTIDISCIPLINARY TEAM

### The Early Years

If the search for a primary-care provider truly willing to take on the care of a special needs child has been successful, it will, to some extent, cut down on the number of visits to the spina bifida specialists. It will still be vital, however, for the team to be intimately involved in the management of that child's health. Although the parents will gradually become more comfortable with their child's temperament and personality and, as a result, be more able to recognize the signs of a potential medical problem such as shunt failure or a urinary tract infection, all infants change rapidly in the first year of life and special needs infants are no exception. Regular assessments by the multidisciplinary team are integral to maximizing function and minimizing the impact of the complications experienced by these children. If the child is stable at the time of discharge from the hospital and there are no significant pending medical issues such as whether or not a shunt is required, they will most often need to be seen by the multidisciplinary team at one to two months of age and every three to four months thereafter for the first year.

At the beginning of each multidisciplinary appointment, the family should meet with the team's designated "generalist," a role most often assumed by a general or developmental pediatrician. That team member should sit with the family at the beginning of each appointment and talk about how things have been going since the last visit. It is important to discuss which community resources are currently being utilized and to clarify whether or not they are meeting the child's needs as well as the parents' expectations. This team member should also identify any concerns the parents have and do a physical examination to evaluate the child's current medical condition and to identify any problems. Specific areas of concern can then be brought to the attention of the subspecialists who should all see the child in turn, each concentrating on their individual areas of expertise. This pattern will, hopefully, continue through the years, as long as the child is followed by the multidisciplinary team.

Specifically, a neurosurgeon will assess the child's shunt, look for early signs of a symptomatic Arnold Chiari II malformation and of a tethered cord, and continue to educate the family about symptoms that may indicate developing neurosurgical complications. Muscle function may be easier to determine and confirm than it is in the early neonatal period, and a determination of the child's functional motor level is often more accurately made in later infancy.

Given a more certain assignment of motor level, the orthopedic surgeon can begin to discuss what aids the child may require for good ambulation. Abnormalities of positioning and alignment unresponsive to casting, stretching, and strength training will become apparent over time and the plan for management will need to be refined by orthopedics. It is important to broach the topic of ambulatory aids with the family early on as this issue often becomes a focus for the parents' overall anxiety about their child's disability (12). If it is anticipated that surgical intervention may be necessary to facilitate ambulation or improve alignment, the team leader should initiate, or at least participate in, any discussion of what developmental and family issues should be considered when planning a hospitalization.

The urologist will often investigate bladder and sphincter function with urodynamic studies within the first few months after discharge as some degree of spinal shock, very often present for the first 10 to 14 days after closure of the open neural tube defect, can undermine their ability to obtain accurate information from a study performed during the initial hospitalization. The results of the urodynamics will guide the management of the child's urinary tract and help predict what may be necessary for the child to achieve continence down the road.

If available to the team either as core members or as consultants, infants should also be monitored by a physiatrist, physical, occupational, and speech therapists, a nutritionist, a social worker, and a nurse specialist during each multidisciplinary clinic visit. Each of these providers should assess the child's current status and function in their area of expertise and review, with the family, the issues which will most likely need to be considered in the coming months. If all of these specialists are not available to the team, provisions must be made to identify and meet the broad needs of the child. Most commonly, team members will function in a cross-disciplinary fashion, the nurse assuming the responsibility for nutritional issues, for example. It is especially important for there to be designated team members whose charge includes discussing bowel management and the avoidance of constipation, nutrition, and strategies for maintaining a healthy diet, and weight, skin care, the early identification of pressure points, and general developmental concerns with the family. It is never too early for the parents to develop an awareness of those considerations which may not be obvious to them but which will have a tremendous impact on their child's ability to maintain health and function successfully among their peers (13).

Preferably, the team leader will meet again with the family at the end of the appointment to discuss how the visit has gone, make sure that all parental concerns have been satisfactorily addressed, and probe for any reservations the family may have about the recommendations made by each provider. By reviewing the written instructions given to the family by each specialist, it often becomes clear whether the parents understand the plan, how they feel about what has been discussed, and whether or not they intend to comply with the proposed care plan. It is not always imperative for the family to agree with the treatment recommendations, but the team and the family should reach a final agreement as to what plan will actually be implemented.

In the best of circumstances, the team will meet together at the end of each clinic session to discuss the status and needs of the patients seen that day and to go over the diagnostic and treatment plans. A meeting such as this enables all team members to get a holistic view of each child's status and affords an opportunity for any disagreements in approach or timing of interventions to be discussed and resolved. If it is not possible for the team to meet together, the team leader should go over the notes made by each specialist, bring any differences of opinion to the attention of the principals, and, if any potential conflicts are identified, make sure that some resolution is reached. If this is not done, the family will inevitably be confused about the plan of management and will be put in the position of having to decide which recommendations to follow without the benefit of understanding the intricacies of balancing what may be conflicting goals. Of course, it is possible that there will be no plan that is clearly correct, and in that circumstance, the team leader can present the options to the family for open discussion and arrange a group meeting with the family if necessary.

In any event, for each multidisciplinary clinic visit, a comprehensive report should be generated which reviews the child's general status, contains a synopsis of each of the specialists' evaluations, and includes a detailed plan for management as well as for any testing which is anticipated over both the short and long term. Copies of this visit summary should be sent to the institution's medical records department and, with the family's permission, additional copies should be sent to any appropriate community health-care providers and educators. This facilitates communication between institutional and community care givers and provides an easily reviewed record of what occurred during each visit as well as a chronological record of what the specialists see as important issues which will have to be dealt with over time. Compiling this report also forces the team leader to carefully consider the recommendations of each specialist, identify conflicts, and formulate a follow-up schedule which minimizes the number of visits needed to accomplish all of the recommended evaluations and tests. Generating a comprehensive clinic summary of the patient's visit is something that should continue as long as that individual is followed by the spina bifida team.

After the first year of life, the interval between multidisciplinary team evaluations will vary significantly from patient to patient. Those who are doing well, who have few medical concerns, and whose parents have exhibited a good understanding of symptoms which may indicate the need to consult with a medical professional can be seen less often than those dealing with more complex medical matters or whose parents are still very anxious. The specific timing and structure of the visits should be tailored to the needs of each child, but all should continue to have regular evaluations by the core specialists discussed above. The key to successful medical management of these children is anticipating problems that may develop and early recognition and treatment of those which do.

Within the first year, it usually becomes apparent whether physical therapy and positioners are adequately addressing contractures and other problems of joint alignment. A more accurate determination of the need for corrective surgery can therefore be more readily made than is possible in the first few months of life. Also, it is in the first few years of life that the orthopedist begins to formulate a clearer picture of how a given child will best ambulate and what will be needed in terms of therapy, ambulatory aids, and surgery to accomplish that goal. In addition, at this point in time, the child's inner drive to ambulate and readiness to utilize equipment can more easily be assessed and considered along with the functional motor level. Although it may be months or years before any surgery could or should be done, various treatment options can be presented to the family, affording them the opportunity to participate in any decisions that need to be made. For instance, there may be several surgical alternatives and the timing of an intervention may be flexible as well.

For most children, it is rare for new neurosurgical issues to develop in their first few years. Some, of course, will have a host of problems and complications with their shunts and may have multiple revisions. Problems secondary to the Chiari II can become more pronounced and, although it is relatively rare, symptomatic tethered cord or syringomyelia can present in the first three years of life. For those who do not have a particularly complex neurosurgical course early on, the neurosurgeon's job primarily involves periodic assessment of shunt function and screening for signs and symptoms of treatable brainstem and spinal cord problems. It is also very important to continue to educate the child's caretakers about symptoms which may indicate a developing neurosurgical problem and to be sure that they know whom to contact between scheduled multidisciplinary clinic visits should the need arise.

The team urologist has a vital role that begins in the nursery and continues throughout the child's life. Bladder and sphincter dynamics can be defined within the first three to six months after birth but it is not at all unusual for them to change over time. The urologist is charged with the task of preserving renal function in the majority of children in whom it is normal at birth and of preventing further damage in those with early changes in the upper tracts. Although some pediatric urologists routinely recommend beginning a clean intermittent catheterization program at birth, it is more common to put a child on such a program closer to the time they will need to be out of diapers for social reasons such as entry into preschool or when urological problems such as reflux or a high pressure bladder develop. The timing of when to institute a catheterization program should be discussed with the parents early on and their input in terms of whether the family is ready to take on this responsibility must be carefully considered.

Like bladder management, bowel management ought be addressed well before the age it is hoped the child will be continent. Actually, the need for a bowel program to manage fecal incontinence and the importance an appropriate diet plays in the eventual success of that program must be discussed with the parents from the very first. It is clear that the success of any bowel management program depends heavily on parental commitment. Frequent communication with open discussion of what is working and what is not must take place if there is to be any chance of success. Because it can be quite time consuming and does not fall naturally into the province of any of the surgical specialists, it is usually the program pediatrician or nurse coordinator who is responsible for designing a child's bowel management program and for assisting the family with implementation.

## The Early School Years

As the child moves from the toddler stage into the early school years, their needs will, of course, continue to change. From a medical perspective, the early school-aged child should be seen at intervals dictated by their health-care needs, although most will do well with an annual multidisciplinary spina bifida visit as long as they are receiving comprehensive general pediatric care in the interim. During these clinic visits, each subspecialist will continue to address their areas of concentration, always keeping paramount the goal of preventing complications when possible and detecting early those which do occur. They should also continue to share with the family their assessment of the child's current status as well as their long- and short-term vision of the child's medical needs. These goals are accomplished by discussing the overall management plan with the family at each visit and making modifications that acknowledge changes in the child's condition as well as medical and surgical advances. It is key that the family continue to be informed about what the plan is, what pieces they are responsible for, and to whom they should turn if they have any questions between visits. Specific team members should continue to take responsibility for guiding the management plan in all areas that do not clearly fall into one of the medical or surgical subspecialties.

Beginning in early childhood, it is not sufficient to be sure that the family understands the issues and is on board with the plan of care. All members of the multidisciplinary team have the responsibility of going beyond discussing these issues with the adult caretakers and of recognizing the need to educate the child about the basics of their medical condition. They and the family should work diligently to aid the child in developing some ownership of their health-care management from as early an age as possible. The child should be involved in discussions of what medications they are taking and why they take them, details of their bladder and bowel management programs including their degree of independence in these areas, issues of diet, exercise, and surveillance for pressure areas on the skin. The role good hygiene plays in making and keeping friends and in being able to integrate as fully as possible in peer activities cannot be overstated (14). It is of the utmost importance that the child begins, as early as possible, to assume responsibility for their well being and understand the importance of effective health maintenance in allowing them to live the fullest life possible.

Entry into school is a major milestone for all children, and for those with a chronic condition, their illness presents an additional source of significant stress and is best addressed in an anticipatory fashion (15). The type of educational program that will best meet the needs of the child is something to be carefully considered and reviewed at least annually. At a minimum, one member of the team should be well versed in the options available in the communities from which the program draws its patients. It is usually at about the age of three that a cognitive evaluation along with specific neuropsychological and developmental tests can be performed and used to get a fairly accurate idea of a child's intellectual level. Coupled with an understanding of the child's personality, temperament, and physical requirements, these test results can be used to determine the optimal educational setting. Some children will need to be in special, contained classrooms from a very early age, others will function well in a completely integrated setting, and a number will do best in a program that combines elements of both. It is important that the family and the multidisciplinary team keep the abilities, medical needs, and personality of the child foremost in their minds when considering these alternatives. At each multidisciplinary visit, the team member most knowledgeable about educational issues should meet with the family to discuss the current school setting, review the related services required by the child, and help the family evaluate whether changes need to be made, either in setting or in content. If it is determined that the school setting is satisfactory from an educational perspective but other needs are not being met, the team should be prepared to help the family define what the unmet needs are and have a list of available alternatives from petitioning the school for additional resources to other public and private programs which can meet those needs.

It is also essential to promote involvement in peer activities outside of the school. Children with spina bifida often have very limited social circles with few peers within those circles (15). Thus, giving the child the opportunity to develop relationships and explore their strengths and weaknesses is as invaluable as it would be for any child. After school programs, organized groups such as Cub Scouts, church clubs, sports teams, and local spina bifida associations all present good opportunities for social integration.

The child's role in the family also must be carefully attended to during these critical early years. The adults with spina bifida who achieve the most independence are those who were allowed to go through the normal stages of maturation and individuation. The team social worker, nurse, or pediatrician should discuss these matters with the family at each visit, and based on the child's age, physical abilities and intellectual level make concrete suggestions for ways to increase the child's responsibilities in the home, foster independence, and improve socialization. Although abilities vary widely, all children can assist, to some degree, with simple tasks such as setting the table, keeping their room neat, dusting, and so on. As much as possible, the demands placed upon the child with spina bifida should be commensurate with what is asked of other children in the family.

As the child moves from early to middle and late childhood, many medical issues will have stabilized, but others often change in ways that may require new adaptations on the part of the child and its family. Those who have done well with crutches and braces may find that a wheelchair, used for part of the day or even exclusively, better meets their needs. The decision as to when this change should be made is easier when the orthopedist has discussed the possibility in a matter-of-fact fashion with the child and its family over the years, thus hopefully avoiding the misconception that such a change represents some sort of failure.

It is also during these years that it may become obvious that an acceptable level of bowel and/or bladder continence will not be achieved without surgical intervention. Again, it is the responsibility of the team to have discussed the possibility of such measures with the family over time. The importance of clear and open communication about what has worked and what has not, how compliant the family and the child have been with the programs that were tried in the pasts, and what options are available cannot be overstated. If this does not occur, it will not be possible to make appropriate changes to the current management plan or to determine when medical management is not going to work and surgery should be considered.

## Adolescence

As children with spina bifida enter adolescence, they, their families, and their health-care providers face a host of new challenges. Although most of the primary medical issues would have been well managed for years and major planned procedures such as hip and spine corrections may have already been accomplished, these individuals still need to be seen annually by the spina bifida team. Each specialist should continue to thoroughly review the patient's status and go over key management issues. Health-care providers bear the responsibility of attending to the fact that the child is on the threshold of adulthood and the parents can no longer be solely or even primarily responsible for managing their child's health care or making treatment decisions. The patient's wishes should, whenever possible, be the primary factor taken into consideration when refining or changing the management plan. If, for example, continence has not been successfully achieved and there are surgical options available for bowel and/or bladder management, it is folly to proceed in this direction because the family wants to pursue surgery but the patient is opposed or has been noncompliant with the treatment plan in the past. A key factor which will indicate how much responsibility a specific individual will ultimately be able to assume is their level of intellectual functioning, the primary issue being whether or not they can integrate and process the complex factors which go into successful management of all of their medical problems.

Actually early adolescence is often a good time to repeat, or perform for the first time if not previously done, a cognitive evaluation in order to firmly establish the child's intellectual strengths and weaknesses. This will enable the health-care team and the family to realistically plan for the future. Not only will the family need to know how much of the responsibility for their child's health care they can gradually turn over to that child, but such testing will also yield information that will allow a judgment to be made as to how likely it is that that child will eventually be self-supporting and live independently. A formal evaluation at a vocational/rehabilitation center can also provide important information about what type of educational path is most realistic. With the results of the cognitive and vocational/rehabilitation evaluations available to them, the multidisciplinary team can better help the family and the patient consider their options and plan pragmatically for the long term.

Adolescence is also a time when it is important to address issues of dating and sexuality. Medical concerns such as gynecological issues, fertility, birth control, and sexually transmitted diseases should be openly and honestly addressed. Although it would have been done in the past, a frank discussion about the role personal hygiene and social skills play in forming peer relationships often needs to take place at this stage of development.

It is also important to note that the level of psychological stress experienced by the individuals with spina bifida as they grow and mature does not necessarily correlate with their level of disability. Patients in whom the dysraphic defect is low and whose level of disability is concomitantly mild to moderate often need as much or more support as those who are more physically impaired. It is the supports available to them through their family, schools, and greater community, not their motor level, which ultimately determines their ability to cope with any limitations placed on them by their disability (16,17).

## Adulthood

The need for coordinated follow-up by a team of health-care providers does not disappear as those with spina bifida move into adulthood. On the contrary, they not only remain at risk for a whole host of medical and surgical problems that stem directly from their condition, but also face many new problems (18–21). It is unfortunate that no real system within the medical community has yet been developed to follow individuals with birth defects into adulthood. Most multidisciplinary spina bifida teams are based in tertiary care children's hospitals, within the pediatric departments of general hospitals, or in other facilities that serve children such as the Shriners Hospitals for Children. Some of these programs have created specific services for the adult with spina bifida, but the need for more specialists versed in the medical needs of this population and for programs that have the needed services is growing because of improved long-term survival (22).

Physicians and other health-care providers specializing in the care of adults rarely have experience with the multidisciplinary model which works so well or even with special health care needs of this population. Although it is theoretically possible for the patient or their family to piece together the needed services, experience has shown that without the multidisciplinary framework compliance with the treatment plan, periodic assessments by key specialists and necessary diagnostic tests all too frequently just do not happen, resulting in more complications and a poorer outcome (23). Even when a concerted effort is made to continue with necessary periodic evaluations, it is difficult for individuals to coordinate appointments and an inordinate amount of time may be spent going for tests and making a multitude of visits to individual health-care providers. Additionally, communication between specialists who do not work together is difficult and rarely takes place. It is extraordinarily complicated for the family or patient to assume the role of coordinator and ensure that what needs to happen does indeed happen.

With the improved long-term survival of those with spina bifida, physicians and other health-care providers must be prepared to participate in the treatment of adults with special needs. Introducing the topic of the care of the handicapped and the role of the multidisciplinary team in maximizing health and improving long-term outcome into undergraduate, medical, and postgraduate education and training programs will go a long way toward preparing physicians and other health-care providers to participate in the care of these individuals with complex and challenging medical needs.

## REFERENCES

1. Michie S, Smith D, Marteau TM. Prenatal tests: how are women deciding? Prenat Diagn 1999; 19(8):743–748.
2. Barr O, Millar R. Parents of children with intellectual disabilities: their expectations and experience of genetic counseling. J Appl Res Intellect Disabil 2003; 16(3):189–204.

3. Kinsman SL, Levey E, Ruffing V, Stone J, Warren L. Beyond multidisciplinary care: a new conceptual model for spina bifida services. Eur J Pediatr Surg 2000; 10(suppl 1):35–38.
4. McLaurin RL, Warkany J. Management of spina bifida and associated anomalies. Compr Ther 1986; 12(2):60–65.
5. McDonald CM. Rehabilitation of children with spinal dysraphism. Neurosurg Clin N Am 1995; 6(2):393–412.
6. Chambers GK, Cochrane DD, Irwin B, Arnold W, Thiessen PN. Assessment of the appropriateness of services provided by a multidisciplinary meningomyelocele clinic. Pediatr Neurosurg 1996; 24(2):92–97.
7. Spina bifida. Key primary issues. Aust Fam Physician 2002; 31(1):66–69.
8. Hoeman SP. Primary care for children with spina bifida. Nurse Pract 1997; 22(9):60–62.
9. Soloman M, Pistrang N, Barker C. The benefits of mutual support groups for parents of children with disabilities. Am J Community Psychol 2001; 29(1):113–132.
10. Law M, King S, Stewart D, King G. The perceived effects of parent-led support groups for parents of children with disabilities. Phys Occup Ther Pediatr 2001; 21(2–3): 29–48.
11. Ayyangar R. Health maintenance and management in childhood disability. Phys Med Rehabil Clin N Am 2002; 12(4):793–821.
12. McCormick MC, Charney EB, Stemmler MM. Assessing the impact of a child with spina bifida on the family. Dev Med Child Neurol 1986; 28(1):53–61.
13. Peterson PM, Rauen KK, Brown J, Cole J. Spina bifida: the transition into adulthood begins in infancy. Rehabil Nurs 1994; 19(4):229–238.
14. Blum RW, Resnick MD, Nelson R, St Germaine A. Family and peer issues among adolescents with spina bifida and cerebral palsy. Pediatrics 1991; 88(2):280–285.
15. Ellerton ML, Stewart MJ, Ritchie JA, Hirth AM. Social support in children with a chronic condition. Can J Nurs Res 1996; 28(4):15–36.
16. Padua L, Rendeli C, Rabini A, Girardi E, Tonali P, Salvaggio E. Health-related quality of life and disability in young patients with spina bifida. Arch Phys Med Rehabil 2002; 83(10):1384–1388.
17. McAndrew L. Adolescents and young people with spina bifida. Dev Med Child Neurol 1979; 21(5):619–629.
18. McDonnell GV, McCann JP. Issues of medical management in adults with spina bifida. Childs Nerv Syst 2000; 16:222–227.
19. Epstein F. Meningomyelocele: "pitfalls" in early and late management. Clin Neurosurg 1983; 30:366–384.
20. Hunt GM, Oakeshott P. Outcome in people with open spina bifida at age 35: prospective community based cohort study. BMJ 2003; 326:1365–1366.
21. Bates K, Bartoshesky L, Friedland A. As the child with chronic disease grows up: transitioning adolescents with special health care needs to adult-centered care. Del Med J 2003; 75(6):217–220.
22. McDonnell GV, McCann JP. Why do adults with spina bifida and hydrocephalus die? A clinic-based study. Eur J Pediatr Surg 2000; 10(suppl 1):31–32.
23. Kaufman BA, Terbrock A, Winters N, Ito J, Klosterman A, Park TS. Disbanding a multidisciplinary clinic: effects on the health care of myelomeningocele patients. Pediatr Neurosurg 1994; 21(1):36–44.

# 4

# School-Age Child: Academic Issues

**James W. Loomis**
*Center for Children with Special Needs, Glastonbury, Connecticut, U.S.A.*

## INTRODUCTION

Children with neural tube defects (NTDs) experience a range of psychosocial challenges throughout their development. Research has consistently found difficulties with academic learning, social functioning, and functional behavior related to NTDs (1–3). Because of this, effective elementary school programming is extremely important to this group of children. Strong school programs are seen to facilitate the development of children with NTDs in powerful ways and to enable them to overcome many of their primary and secondary disabilities so that many may attain a high quality of life in adulthood (4,5). Effective schools create an accessible environment that allows for full inclusion. They provide an individualized instructional program to ensure academic learning and prevocational skills. They structure the social environment and provide social skills training to promote age-appropriate social behavior and the formation of peer relationships. They actively teach self-care and functional skills. Ultimately, the school (along with the family; see Chapter 12) plays a pivotal role in creating independence and a high quality of life in adulthood.

The elementary school environment is generally designed for typical children. Since the enactment of the Individuals with Disabilities Education Act (IDEA) (6), there are systems in place to adapt the school program so that it is appropriate for children with disabilities such as NTDs. However, schools vary greatly in their ability to anticipate the unique challenges associated with NTDs, their access to resources to make appropriate program adaptations, and even their support for the goal of full integration of special needs children. Consequently, there may be components missing, which impedes the child's efforts to take full advantage of the school program. There may be a lack of physical accessibility to the entire school and all of its activities. Instruction may not be modified so that it matches the child's learning profile. Adequate training in the areas of social skills and adaptive functioning may not be provided. The developmental cost of less-effective school programs can be high, as they do not give the child the skills needed to succeed in middle and high school. This may open the door to secondary disabilities (5) and curtail the potential for a full, independent life as an adult.

Studies of children with NTDs have consistently found a range of cognitive processing challenges related to visual-perceptual/visual-motor functioning, attention regulation, memory, language processing, organizational skills, and problem solving (see Chapter 5) (2,7,8). A large percentage of children with NTDs are seen to fit the diagnosis of nonverbal learning disability (NLD) [a neuropsychological syndrome seen to be associated with spina bifida and shunted hydrocephalus among other conditions (9)] but there is such a high level of variance in the cognitive profile that the pattern is seen to be a "cognitive phenotype" with a great deal of individual variation (10). Problems with social development have also been consistently documented and found to be associated with the aforementioned cognitive processing difficulties as well as mobility/accessibility challenges and bowel and bladder functioning (11–13). Similarly, individuals with NTDs present poor outcomes with regard to self-care and adaptive functioning (3,5) and this, too, is seen to result from the combination of problems with cognitive functioning and the physical and medical challenges of NTDs. This constellation of challenges is seen to persist in adulthood (3) and investigators point to the primary disabilities of NTDs (e.g., lack of muscle control in the lower extremities, disrupted bladder functioning, and cognitive processing problems) leading to secondary or acquired disabilities (e.g., poor academic learning, social isolation, and depression) (5). However, although there has been consistent identification of the challenges associated with NTDs, there has been relatively little study of the factors that cause these challenges or of effective treatment and interventions.

Research focusing on school-related issues has consistently found that children with NTDs perform at a lower level than typical peers in school, especially in math (2,14,15). However, there has been limited examination of the factors that underlie academic problems as well as of the efficacy of educational interventions. Much of the literature on school strategies has come from educational experience and anecdotal evidence. In 1993, Rowley-Kelly and Reigel (4) compiled a comprehensive set of educational recommendations into an edited volume addressing the education of children with spina bifida. More recently, interest generated by Rourke's model of NLDs (9,16) has led to a number of volumes addressing educational programming for these children (17–19). However, although there is a consistent model of providing effective school programs for children with NTDs, there has yet to be empirical evaluation of specific interventions or strategies.

This chapter first reviews the educational challenges associated with NTDs and then examine the assessment and intervention strategies that promote full participation in elementary school, mastery of academic, social, and functional learning objectives, and preparation for subsequent challenges in school and adult life.

Before starting, it is important to note that children with an NTD vary greatly in the impact their condition has on their functioning. For some, there is minimal impact and they manage the developmental challenges of elementary school in the same manner as typical children. For others, the level of medical, physical, and cognitive challenges prevents the participation in mainstream schools. In between (and these are the children we are primarily addressing in this chapter), there is a wide range of challenges with diverse profiles of strengths and weaknesses relative to learning, social functioning, self-care, and medical management. In this chapter, much of the discussion focuses on the modal presentation of challenges for children with NTDs. However, there is such a degree level of variability within this group that ultimately all school programs need to be tailored to the profile of the individual.

## SCHOOL-BASED CHALLENGES ASSOCIATED WITH NEURAL TUBE DEFECTS

NTDs present a range of challenges that can undermine a child's success in school. These fall into five categories: (*i*) accessibility, (*ii*) academic functioning, (*iii*) social functioning, (*iv*) self-care and adaptive behavior, and (*v*) behavioral functioning.

### Accessibility

A child must have access to the activities of school in order to take advantage of its educational programs. This means that not only physical accessibility throughout the school building, but also access to the playground and its equipment, the cafeteria line and tables, school hallways, bathrooms, and class field trips. Although the Americans with Disabilities Act (ADA) and IDEA (20) have helped to ensure optimal levels of accessibility, there are subtle challenges to access associated with NTDs that are difficult and at times impossible to address.

NTDs present a range of challenges to accessibility (21). First is the issue of mobility. With disrupted neural connections to lower extremities, many children with NTDs rely on wheelchairs and/or bracing systems to move about. This requires a physically accessible environment, appropriate equipment, and some staff assistance. Even with the best resources and team support, there are situations where accessibility is denied.

Bowel and bladder programs present a second challenge to accessibility (22). Many children with NTDs require specialized techniques for managing their elimination such as clean intermittent catheterization. It is essential that the school has appropriately fitted bathrooms near the classroom, assistance from a nurse (when necessary), and routines that ensure privacy. However, even with excellent facilities and staff involvement, catheterization can still take the child out of academic or social activities for prolonged periods because of the time needed to get to the bathroom, set up, void, and clean up.

A third impediment to accessibility is the medical need for surgery, hospitalization, or bed rest, making uninterrupted attendance at school impossible (23). During these times, the child loses out on some academic instruction and social participation. It also requires two challenging transitions, from school to the relative isolation and boredom of home and hospital, and then back from home to school where the children must re-integrate themselves with the peer group, catch up on missed assignments, and get back into the routine of the class. We know that transitions in general are difficult for children with NTDs because of the cognitive challenges (19), so these times of extended school absences can be stressful.

It is important to note that there are different levels of accessibility to consider. In the most basic terms, accessibility means the child must be able to be present in all parts of the physical environment (21). This basic level of accessibility requires appropriate installation of elevators, door openers, ramps, and wide doorways. The more the child can reach all places independently and without delay, the greater the accessibility. At a higher level, accessibility means full participation in all of the academic and functional activities that occur throughout the school day. Children may be able to reach all parts of the classroom, but can they go to the board to do an example, reach up to feed the class pet, serve themselves, and make full choices of food selections in the cafeteria? Social accessibility is the highest level and the most difficult to fully reach. Here the question is, even if children can go to all parts of the building and participate in learning activities, can they fully engage in social interactions? Can they move about in their seat to pass notes or whisper with peers, choose any open seat in the room, approach any peer that they seek, or sit in the back of the bus? On the playground, can they keep up with peers in a game of tag or kickball?

For most children with NTDs, complete accessibility is not possible. However, creative planning, flexible problem solving, effective resource management, and supportive peers and staff can minimize the impact of even the more subtle barriers. Still, every situation that does not allow complete, independent participation potentially reduces the child's academic and social progress.

## Academic Functioning

In general, the primary focus of school programs is academic learning. Children with NTDs present a range of cognitive processing challenges, and there is substantial diversity among the learning profiles presented by children with NTDs (2,7,8,24–26). Some experience no significant learning challenges. These are generally students with lower-level lesions and an absence of hydrocephalus and other neurological anomalies. Far more common is the presence of learning disabilities with visual-spatial and visual-motor functions being compromised or with all the components of an NLD (9,10,16). A small group of children with NTDs experience comprehensive challenges that leave their overall functioning in the range of intellectually deficient/mental retardation. For the purposes of this chapter, the focus will be on children with learning disabilities who are able to participate in mainstream education. This group comprises the majority of students with NTDs.

Keeping in mind the degree of variation across individuals, a modal progression of academic development can be discerned. Children with NTDs typically do well accomplishing preacademic skills in preschool and kindergarten. Often they are seen as verbally advanced, as they are extremely fluent in their speech and enjoy engaging in conversation (2,27). Students with NTDs continue to do well through the early elementary years as their strong verbal memory, speech, and rote learning skills are effective in mastering the goals of the early elementary curriculum, such as letter and word identification, simple addition and subtraction, spelling, and writing simple sentences with concrete referents. They also do well with retention of basic facts in the areas of science and social studies. The visual-motor challenges of handwriting can present some challenges, but with repetitive practice, many students utilize their strong rote learning abilities to overcome this and develop good graphomotor skills (9).

Significant learning difficulties are seen to emerge in middle to late elementary school, as educational objectives require the student to master more complex and more abstract bodies of information. At this point, there are continued academic demands for simple memorization of facts and concrete symbols, but also increasing demands for problem solving (being able to determine what a problem is asking and identifying the information and operations needed to solve it) and making inferences (drawing conclusions from limited information and using deductive and inductive reasoning). These types of tasks require the children to utilize learning skills beyond their area of strength (rote verbal learning) and their difficulties with attentional regulation, memory, and organizational skills further undermine academic progress (28–31).

Problems are most often seen in three areas: math, reading comprehension, and compositional writing (2,4,19). In early and middle elementary school, math learning moves from basic memorization of numbers, counting, and applying simple operations (e.g., addition and subtraction) to dealing with more conceptual challenges (fractions, place value, multiplication, and division) and increasing visual-motor demands (lining up numbers for computation, identifying geometric shapes, and using visual schema to understand math concepts). Further, demands for computation are put into word problems, requiring comprehension of language as well as determination of what information is relevant and needed, what operations should be applied, and what steps are necessary to reach a final solution. These new demands tax several key areas of challenge, including visual-spatial processing, higher-order conceptual reasoning, and problem-solving skills (30,32).

The development of letter and word recognition skills usually proceeds well for students with NTDs, whereas reading comprehension is frequently a challenge. Letter identification, learning grapheme–phoneme relationships, and recognizing single words can be strengths, as these tasks draw heavily on rote verbal learning. However, reading comprehension soon requires understanding word meanings as they occur in context, making inferences from the information that is presented, and tracking more extended sequences of words at the level of sentence and paragraph. The latter processes draw on areas of learning weakness for children with NTDs including memory, reasoning, and comprehension of more complex language (28–30,32). Consequently, as the curriculum moves from "learning to read" to "reading to learn," difficulties with reading comprehension emerge and increasingly limit academic gains. Determining the main point of a passage, identifying supporting details, and understanding implied meanings can be very challenging for students with NTDs.

The third area of academic challenge is compositional writing (17,33). Similar to math and reading, basic skill acquisition goes well and children with NTDs can generally master spelling and basic sentence construction. However, as the tasks become more advanced and there is a need to arrange words through grammatical construction into lengthier and more complex sentences and then to order sentences into paragraphs, the child's organizational skills, language processing, and reasoning can be overwhelmed, leading to disorganized or impoverished writing production.

The challenges with reading comprehension and compositional writing are sometimes overlooked by educators, as language is usually seen to be an early strength of children with NTDs. In this context, it is important to differentiate between the production of verbal speech and rote verbal memory, which are strengths, and the processing and organization of more advanced language concepts, which are weaknesses. This disjunction is often most clearly reflected in the child's speech which, although fluent and copious in amount, is often superficial, containing repetitive, stereotypical phrases, and relatively simplistic content (27,34). It is also important to note that the cognitive diagnostic label often applied to these children, NLD, can be misleading. The NLD pattern of learning disability impacts nonverbal functioning at a more basic level, but it also impedes higher-order verbal processing as well (9,16).

In general, the success seen with early learning objectives can make it more difficult for school teams to recognize the full extent of the learning challenges seen in children with NTDs. Often, problems are first seen in the middle elementary years. Typically, children with higher overall intelligence evidence difficulties in later years because they can use their learning abilities to better adapt to the processing challenges they encounter. For some students with high intelligence, problems may not emerge until high school. Problems may first be misinterpreted to be motivational ("laziness") or behavioral ("manipulative"), as the success of the early elementary years and the verbal fluency skills make it hard to recognize the cognitive challenges.

Homework completion presents a set of challenges that can be particularly difficult for children with NTDs, as it demands the use of organizational skills, autonomous learning/problem solving, and the generalization of skills learned in the classroom to a different setting (18,19). Consequently, homework completion is often an academic bellwether, as struggles escalate and are reflected in taking long periods of time to finish homework, requiring a high level of monitoring and assistance from parents, completing homework inconsistently, or failing to bring needed materials home and back to school.

## Social Functioning

In many respects, challenges in the social realm for children with NTDs parallel those seen with academic learning. Problems begin to be evident in the early to middle elementary years and then escalate if not addressed. During the preschool years, children with NTDs are generally able to manage the requirements of social interaction with peers, including approach skills, sharing, turn-taking, basic conversation, and age-appropriate humor. Sometimes, because of physical challenges as well as verbal strengths, children with NTDs show an early preference for verbal activities over the more typical physical and visual-motor play of toddlers and preschoolers. For this reason, a child with an NTD may appear to be precocious and seek out contact with older peers and adults rather than to engage in the "rough and tumble" physical activities, imaginary play, and art activities of the peer group.

However, although social skills in this early stage may allow age-appropriate interactions, medical issues can impede social activities. Some parents and children will avoid contact with a peer who appears "different." Play dates are difficult to arrange outside the home because of difficulties with gaining access to other residences with braces or a wheelchair or making arrangements for catheterization outside the home.

With development, the demands of peer interaction become more challenging to most children with NTDs. Over the elementary years, peer interaction requires the child to develop skills associated with self-observation, perspective taking, empathy, and the understanding of emotions (35). These skills can be very challenging for children with significant cognitive processing difficulties, especially those with NLD. Communication also becomes more complex and demanding. Reading nonverbal gestures and body language can be very difficult in the face of visual-spatial processing difficulties (36). Conversation skills demand greater proficiency with listening, knowing when to break in to the flow of the conversation, and appropriately managing changes in topic (37).

Problems with the development of conversation skills are often seen in interruptions, abrupt changes in topic, and talking at length, while not giving the other person a chance to talk (38). Furthermore, over the course of development, social functioning requires greater problem solving and understanding more complex social rituals, conventions, and patterns (e.g., game rules, the use of jargon and colloquial language, greetings, and tailoring behavior to specific social situations) and this too can overwhelm the child's ability to process social information and manage social situations.

Further undermining social development are the barriers to accessibility experienced by children with significant orthopedic challenges who require the use of braces or a wheelchair. Over the course of development through the elementary years, mobility takes on more importance for children as they travel throughout neighborhoods, malls, and the schoolyard. For many, the use of bicycles becomes central to their play activities. At this point, the child with an NTD can be left behind as they cannot keep up with the movements of the peer group or cannot access homes or stores the group is visiting or may experience fatigue that curtails his level of physical activity.

In the face of growing social challenges, a number of behavior patterns are seen. Many children rely on their verbal production skills to connect with others and are seen to be excessively talkative while avoiding physical activities or other types of interaction. Some children are seen to gravitate toward older peers (who are more tolerant of their communication challenges) or younger peers (who communicate at a more basic level). A pattern of dependency can also develop whereby the child uses its unique status to get attention and help from others without having to engage in age-appropriate communication or reciprocal interaction. In some cases, the child may be "adopted" by the class as a type of mascot or "special" child. Although this type of prosocial response is well intended, it can also prevent the development of more reciprocal and age-appropriate peer interactions.

As development progresses, children with NTDs who struggle with social demands can demonstrate growing behavioral challenges (e.g., oppositional behavior and tantrums), stress reactions (e.g., anxiety attacks), and withdrawal from social contact (19,39). Often, the child develops a heavy involvement with television, videogames, and other solitary, passive pursuits where some control may be experienced. This isolates the child from social contacts, however, and further undermines social development. This pattern can ultimately lead to poor social outcomes in adulthood with great isolation and few significant relationships (1,3).

## Self-Care and Adaptive Behavior

NTDs create challenging requirements for self-care and the skills of daily living (40,41). In most cases, the child must learn self-catheterization, bowel management, caring for bracing/wheelchair, skin checks, taking medication, and dietary adjustments. Dressing, feeding, hygiene, household chores, and safe transportation may also be compromised. The daily regimen presents a high level of challenge.

Mastering these tasks is complicated by the child's cognitive processing difficulties (e.g., memory and visual-motor coordination), undermining successful completion. For example, a task such as self-catheterization requires fine motor coordination (in many cases without being able to see what you are doing), memorizing a lengthy list of steps, and considerable problem solving, which can be difficult for children with NTDs (42).

Further, social factors can reduce the motivation to master these challenges. In some cases, the child feels unable to be successful in the peer group and so withdraws from solitary activity, making hygiene, appearance, and continence less important. Alternately, some individuals develop tendencies to be more dependent on others. In these cases, well-intended family members and school staff impede the children's development by performing some of these functions for the children rather than insisting that they master it themselves.

Ultimately, difficulties with managing one's own body and learning how to autonomously engage with the school and community environments can be the most daunting obstacle to independence, vocational advancement, social functioning, and quality of life as an adult (43). Being able to manage one's health (so as to stay out of the hospital), establish socially appropriate continence, maintain expected levels of hygiene and dress, and move about the community are all requirements of independent adult functioning and present challenges for most individuals with NTDs. The early establishment of these key skills is seen to be essential for success and reducing secondary disabilities (43). Consequently, consistent with the mandates of IDEA and the ADA, school programs must be designed to promote the mastery of these skills and competencies through active teaching and providing an environment that supports their development.

## Behavioral Functioning

A significant number of school-age children with NTDs present behavioral challenges (39). The same as any other child, they may present the range of childhood psychiatric conditions. Furthermore, they are vulnerable to behavioral problems that result from the challenges of the NTD. Many of these behaviors can be seen to be responses to overwhelming academic or social challenges. Avoidant, withdrawn, or manipulative conduct can be seen to occur in the face of situations that are difficult for the child to master. Other problem behaviors can be seen to be the result of stress reactions to all the challenges that are associated with NTDs. These latter behaviors include depression, anxiety symptoms (anxiety or panic episodes, general nervousness, and worry), and angry, frustrated outbursts, usually directed at parents and family members (19,39).

## ASSESSMENT ISSUES

Effective assessment of challenges in all five of these areas is critical for providing an appropriate school program. The earlier a problem is detected, the easier it is to address and overcome. Typically, when teams wait for problems to be more disruptive, the child's motivation is impacted. Once lost, motivation can be difficult to resuscitate. With most neurotypical students, a "wait and see" attitude works well, as many problems are overcome through development without any intervention needed. For children with NTDs, a more aggressive approach to assessment (and intervention) is necessary. Even children with minimal medical challenges should be considered as "at risk" for learning and social difficulties. In this regard, their progress should be systematically monitored. When seemingly minor problems emerge, they should be fully assessed and addressed through intervention (when needed). This more proactive approach helps to best facilitate development and to prevent the most serious challenges to learning and social functioning.

## FORMAL ASSESSMENT

Children with NTDs require comprehensive multidisciplinary school evaluations including participation by professionals from special education, psychology, speech and language, occupational therapy, physical therapy, assistive technology, and (when necessary) augmentative communication. The school-based assessment should then be integrated with medical evaluations in order to best understand what interventions are needed, which challenges can be changed and which cannot, what medical conditions can be anticipated, and how to best carry out medical treatment regimens in the school environment so as to promote inclusion and social integration.

The usual model of conducting evaluations on a triennial basis is sufficient for most children with NTDs. However, at key points such as the middle of elementary school, the transition to middle school and high school, and in the face of learning, social or behavioral difficulties, more frequent evaluations (even yearly) may be needed.

Special education evaluation should provide a measure of current achievement levels and the presence of learning challenges. As indicated above, particular areas of focus should include reading comprehension, math, and writing skills. Evaluators should pay particular attention to inconsistencies within skill areas as well as realms where the child is falling behind grade expectations.

Psychological evaluation provides an assessment of basic cognitive processes including attention, memory, retention of factual information, and visual-motor functioning (see Chapter 5). Behavior ratings of parents and school staff can also be helpful in identifying difficulties with attention, avoidant behaviors, and social functioning. Because of the subtle nature of the cognitive challenges, in many cases, neuropsychological evaluation is needed to gain a complete picture of the child's cognitive functioning. For any child with an

NTD, evidencing cognitive processing difficulties or showing significant scatter on an intelligence battery, neuropsychological evaluation is recommended for the early elementary years. The findings of such an assessment are essential for fully understanding the learning profile, gaining a baseline measure of cognitive functioning, and anticipating and intervening with learning challenges (44).

Occupational therapy evaluation addresses visual-motor functioning and fine motor coordination of the upper extremities. This is a key area for children with NTDs, as this type of challenge is frequently present and can exert a negative impact on academic learning (e.g., handwriting) as well as on the development of self-care skills (e.g., self-catheterization). A full understanding of fine motor coordination and assessment of the need for occupational therapy services is essential for program planning. Further, the occupational therapist can design accommodations, specialized devices, and environmental adjustments to allow greater independence for the child.

Speech and language evaluation provides a more detailed look at language functioning and can identify the types of language processing challenges that were noted above. Key areas for this part of the evaluation include understanding abstract and complex language, pragmatic skills, and conversation skills.

Physical therapy and orthotic/prosthetic evaluations are typically conducted at the hospital or healthcare facility, but are an important part of the school evaluation. Assessing the current status of muscle functioning, gross motor coordination, and muscle fatigue, as well as designing the best possible mobility system, is necessary in order to optimize accessibility and activity at school.

### Informal Assessment

Beyond the periodic formal evaluations, it is important to incorporate an ongoing system of monitoring consistent with a preventive model. Staff should be trained to recognize indicators of potential problems and there should be regular meetings where progress is reviewed and adjustments to the program considered. As noted above, indicators of unmet challenges may be subtle and hard to read. These include decreased academic motivation, inconsistency in task performance ("she gets it one minute and then loses it the next"), problems with homework completion, avoidance of academic tasks, difficulties with bringing the right materials or assignments to class, and social withdrawal. In cases where oppositional trends, manipulative behavior, or a drop in motivation occur, it is important to look carefully for learning or social challenges that are overwhelming the child and require intervention or support. Functional behavioral assessment is often necessary in these cases to fully understand the factors that underlie the behavior.

## SCHOOL-BASED INTERVENTIONS

Educating children with NTDs requires a team approach including regular and special education teaching staff as well as specialists from psychology, speech and language, occupational therapy, and physical therapy (19). Effective team functioning allows for the most coordinated services and the integration of observations across discipline to design the most creative solutions to challenges. In order to ensure optimal team collaboration, a case manager should be appointed and regular meetings held every two weeks to once a month. The school team should work to maintain regular communication with the hospital or healthcare team to best understand the medical condition and how it affects school performance.

## Instructional Adaptations

There are a number of instructional adaptations and strategies that are recommended for children with NTDs (4,17–19,45–49).

### General Instructional Approach

The optimal instructional approach focuses on engaging the child in active learning and building on strengths and skills that the child possesses. Effective instructional programs carefully assess the areas of challenge and determine which skills can be improved through remediation and which skills will not improve. The former areas are addressed through remedial instruction and practice, whereas the latter through devising compensatory strategies for the child that utilizes other skills.

Most children with NTDs benefit from a linear, sequential format of teaching with tasks broken into small components to be mastered before building them together into higher-order skills. Children with NTDs generally learn best through a rote, verbal approach that presents information through the verbal channel with repetition. Because learning through discovery or through higher-order reasoning is more difficult, these demands should be reduced. Learning activities that require primarily visual-spatial processing or rapid completion should be eliminated, as children with NTDs struggle with this type of challenge and learning progress is minimal. Basic recommendations for different subject areas are found in Table 1.

### Communication in the Classroom

Children with NTDs generally struggle with attention regulation and understanding nonverbal or visual communication. Consequently, teachers should utilize verbal direction (along with appropriate visual information) and encourage verbal feedback and questions from the student. With the challenges to higher-order language processing, instructors should not assume that the child understands the information and directions that are being presented; checking in with the child on an ongoing basis to ensure comprehension is a good practice. With the attentional challenges, establishing eye contact before speaking can also be helpful to ensure that the child is taking in the information. Teachers can also develop a special cue to indicate when the child is off-task. This can be done in a subtle way to minimize peers' awareness of the child's difficulties.

**Table 1** Basic Recommendations for Subject Areas

| | |
|---|---|
| Mathematics | |
| | Use a concrete, structured approach with earlier objectives being mastered before moving on to more advanced objectives. |
| | Use an interesting math text with simple, clear visual format. Provide a copy of the text that the student can write in. |
| | Use manipulatives, visual diagrams, and verbal instruction together in explaining new or difficult concepts. |
| | Have the student use graph paper to help line up numbers for computation. |
| | Provide a calculator if computation presents difficulty. |
| | Minimize the use of timed tasks, quizzes, or tests. |
| | Simplify word problems in order to facilitate comprehension. |
| | Teach estimating and predicting outcomes to help the student master the conceptual basis of a problem. |
| | Teach a concrete sequence of steps for problem solving that can be applied to math problems. |
| Reading | |
| | Use a guided, sequential, phonetic/linguistic approach to reading rather than a visual, word recognition approach. |
| | To aid reading comprehension, provide outlines/notes/summaries or use texts with the key information highlighted. |
| | Monitor the volume of reading to be assigned and reduce the expectation when necessary. Allow extra time for reading assignments and build in breaks when reading to minimize fatigue. |
| | Use texts that allow the student to write in the book. |
| | Build comprehension through systematic questioning of what they read. |
| Writing | |
| | Break writing assignments into small components with modulated levels of challenge. |
| | Provide support with the initiation of writing. Help the student get started by asking questions or providing a series of steps to follow. |
| | Allow extra time for the completion of writing tasks. |
| | Use graphic organizers with verbal coaching to help the student compose writing assignments. |
| | Provide word processor for students with severe handwriting challenges. |

## Facilitating Conceptual Learning

Developing an understanding of abstract and complex concepts and relationships can be particularly difficult for children with NTDs. Teachers can address this by describing conceptual relationships (and not assuming that the child has mastered them), by presenting a variety of examples with key factors exaggerated or flagged. Examples should be concrete and related to real-life experiences that the child encounters. Using visual diagrams along with a verbal message can also enhance conceptual learning.

**Special Teaching Objectives**: Beyond the usual curricular objectives, it is important that instructors actively teach students with NTDs the learning strategies and study skills that typical children usually learn automatically without requiring instruction from teachers. This includes organizational strategies (keeping books and papers organized, tracking and completing homework assignments), note taking skills, memory techniques (using rehearsal and mnemonics such as pairing, acronyms, and visualization), problem solving, and self-monitoring. Further, explicit teaching of spatial concepts (e.g., up, down, right, left, over, and under) and metaphorical and figurative language can be extremely beneficial.

## Learning Tasks

To optimize learning, tasks should be short, with a clear beginning and end and with a level of challenge that promotes a high percentage of success. The volume of work should be adjusted to minimize redundancy. If mastery is reached with five problems, then a 20-item work sheet should be pared back. Tasks with time pressures should be eliminated, as motor, attention, fatigue, and rate of processing factors undermine the speed of completion of children with NTDs. Similarly, tasks with heavy demands for visual-spatial processing should be eliminated or restructured so that they include verbal-based supports.

## Evaluating Student Progress

All evaluations should be adapted to a format that will best capture what the child knows and what skills it has mastered. Timed tests and tasks with heavy visual-motor demands will produce inaccurately low estimates of student skills because of challenges with rate of processing and visual-motor integration. Rather, tests should provide information in ways that the children can understand and adapt the mode of response to the ways the children best expresses themselves. In general terms, this means combining verbal and visual information in the presentation of items and allowing verbal responses with a minimal of motor demands.

On a more general level, standardized scores and comparisons to normative groups are not useful for children with significant learning problems. Many children with NTDs present subtle learning disabilities that are not picked up by standardized tests. Alternately, difficulties in processing the visual inputs of standardized tests as well as the timed and visual-motor response demands can lead to gross underestimation of a child's competencies. Generally, it is preferable to use criterion-based evaluations, which look at what skills are being mastered and which areas need more attention.

## Teaching Materials

Certain materials are valuable to facilitate the learning of children with NTDs. These include thick pencil grips to aid graphomotor coordination, color-coded notebooks and storage bins to help with the organization of books and papers, a ruler to mark the line that is being read, and a visual timer to help them monitor time periods. Some children benefit from reference charts being attached to the desk top (e.g., the alphabet and math tables) or from having a copy of what is written on the blackboard at the desk to minimize having to shift their attention from their desk to the board and back again. All response sheets should be adapted with key information highlighted, response spaces clearly marked, and additional space provided to write in. Math assignments should be done on graph paper to help with lining up numbers in calculation. Checklists can also be helpful in managing homework or tracking the steps of complicated tasks. Study aids should be provided whenever possible. This includes outlines or summaries of information to be presented, lecture notes, and reading materials with the main idea and supporting details clearly marked.

Technological supports should always be considered. These include word processors for the child with extreme challenges with handwriting, calculators for students struggling with computation, tape recorders to tape lectures or to make notes to oneself, watches with alarms to help with monitoring deadlines, and PDAs to help with schedules and task lists. There is also a growing choice of learning software programs that can be uniquely effective.

### Managing Transitions

Children with NTDs can experience unique difficulties transitioning between tasks, classes, or activities. A predictable, clear schedule in writing that is reviewed verbally is extremely helpful. Further, cues related to upcoming transitions should be provided or a timer placed on the desk to help children anticipate changes. The physical challenges of NTDs make class changes more difficult than for typical children. A plan for safe and timely procession from class to class should be established in advance. Extra time may need to be allowed, or in some cases, the child may have to change classes before or after the end of the period to avoid the crowds in the halls. A clear map should be provided to help the child learn its way around the building. Class assignments that minimize the amount of mobility required should be made to combat the possible impact of fatigue.

On a different level, there should be transition plans for times when the student is out of school for health reasons. There should be ongoing communication between the teacher and the home- or hospital-based tutor. Assignments should be provided during periods when the child can complete work. There should be opportunities for peer contact through visits, cards, phone, or e-mail. Prior to the return to school, key transitional difficulties should be anticipated and a welcome planned in the classroom.

### Classroom Environment

Children with NTDs do best in well-organized and structured classrooms without too much visual or auditory stimulation. Placement of their seat should be made to ensure easy viewing of the blackboard, minimize distractions, and provide easy access to the teacher. Use of a carrel is recommended in some unusual cases in order to minimize distraction. Arrangement of the classroom should be designed to allow access throughout the room by the child. The seat and desk should be carefully assessed to ensure proper positioning and support. Postural aides should be utilized when needed.

## Social Skills Facilitation

There are four important components to social skills programs for children with NTDs. First, it is important to teach the key social skills that may be missing. There are many skills that seem to be automatically learned by neurotypical children (e.g., perspective taking and reading nonverbal communication), which cause children with NTDs to struggle. However, many of these skills can be taught if effective instruction is provided. Second, research into social skills training has found that generalization and maintenance of skills are difficult to establish (50). For this reason, it is essential to provide opportunities for the children to apply the social skills they are learning and to give enough support that the children can be successful in using his skills. Third, it is important that social skills training and social activities in general are provided in a way that is enjoyable to the children. With the threats to their social motivation, it is essential that they see social interaction as potentially fun and something they want to do. Finally, throughout development, it is important to keep the child involved in peer activities through clubs, teams, or other organized events. The more socially active the children are, the more they can practice social skills and the less likely they are to fall behind the peer group with regard to social functioning.

### Social Skills Groups

Generally, social skills training interventions are most effectively provided in group settings. Children with NTDs evidencing any social difficulties should receive weekly social skills group interventions. There are a number of social skills curriculums that identify objectives and provide learning activities. These include skillstreaming (51), the Walker curriculum (52), and others. Groups include structured discussion, role-playing difficult social situations, exercises to develop key skills, and social games. The types of objectives that are most relevant for children with NTDs include initiating contact, joining a group discussion, conversation skills, and understanding nonverbal communication.

### Peer Integration Techniques

As noted above, outcome studies of social skills training programs generally show that key skills can be taught, but that generalization and maintenance are difficult to establish (50). For this reason, it is essential to provide opportunities for the students to practice social skills and apply what they are learning in their group. This is addressed through interventions that bring together a diverse group of typical and special needs students into structured social situations where they are given cues when needed and where there is enough structure (clear expectations, limited noise and stimulation, and activities with clear turn-taking patterns) that the child with an NTD can have a successful social experience (53).

A common example of peer integration is a "Lunch Bunch." In this type of intervention, a group of children have lunch outside of the hustle and bustle of the cafeteria with a staff member who structures the conversation and activities and provides needed cues or coaching to the student(s) with an NTD. Another variant is the "Peer Mentorship" model where the student is paired with a typical child and given a project or activity to do. As with a Lunch Bunch, the staff provides enough support and cueing to ensure the child's successful participation. There are many other types of peer integration techniques. During recess, staff can recruit appropriate peers and organize structured games. During work breaks or between classes, teachers can cue the child to initiate interaction with a peer or can structure a conversation among a group of students. In all of these situations, the objective is to create opportunities for successful, satisfying social interaction between special needs and typical children. The essential ingredient is the staff-provided structure, which allows the child to be successful. As the child's social skills develop, the structure should be faded.

### Scripting Techniques

Another useful set of techniques to facilitate social development utilizes script-based learning. These interventions emphasize the child's strength with rote, verbal learning by creating a script, a set of instructions, or a list of things to say for the child to use in difficult situations. The information is repeatedly read with the child to maximize learning and retention and then cues can be provided in the actual situation if needed. Social Stories (54) are the most commonly used technique of this type. Carol Gray has developed a versatile model where staff collaborates with the child to write a brief story about difficult situations. The story describes a challenging situation, indicates the perspectives of different participants, and spells out how to act. Other techniques in this regard include creating a rule card, directions list, or scripted dialog for the child to carry with. Reviewing this key information multiple times helps the child master the instructions and follow them in the actual situation.

### Social Cognitive Approaches

Children with NTDs often present deficits in knowledge related to social functioning, such as nonverbal communication, perspective taking, identifying social conventions or rules, and adopting appropriate situation-based roles (19,38,55). Learning in this area occurs "automatically" for typical children, whereas children with NTDs often require explicit instruction. Group or individual teaching can be very effective in facilitating social development by presenting social learning exercises that emphasize rote verbal learning. Objectives to address can include nonverbal communication (36), listening (35), social inference and reasoning (35), or recognizing and coping with emotions (56).

### Promoting Social Participation

Social skills develop through practice. As a result, ongoing participation with social peer activities is very important for children with NTDs. There is the risk of a negative cycle, where social challenges lead to withdrawal, which reduces practice and leads to further social challenges. For some children with NTDs, social activities can be difficult and frustrating, causing them to avoid social activities and develop a preference for solitary activities (e.g., reading, playing video games, and watching television). Consequently, it is important to keep them socially active (even when they try to avoid it) by providing social activities with enough support and structure that they can be successful and experience some satisfaction. Arranging play dates, providing modified peer activities for children with orthopedic disabilities, and joining clubs, teams, and peer organizations (e.g., Scouts, Boys and Girls Club) at school and in the community is essential for social development. For children with NTDs, this can be difficult because of challenges to accessibility and the inconsistent social motivation. Aggressively addressing these challenges is, therefore, essential.

## School-Based Special Services

The skills of a range of professionals are needed to provide a successful and appropriate school program for children with NTDs.

### Special Education

Instructors with special education training are a central component to the programs of most children with NTDs. These educators design the adaptations and modifications to instruction and materials and coordinate their delivery by mainstream and special education teachers and instructional aides/paraprofessionals. Sometimes these services are best provided within a special education classroom, sometimes in a resource room/learning center, and sometimes in the mainstream classroom. The objective is to maximize integration with the mainstream while providing instruction in a setting that allows for successful learning.

### Speech and Language Therapy

Despite their strength with verbal production and basic verbal learning, many children with NTDs experience difficulties with processing abstract, complex, and higher order language concepts (32). As a result, speech and language therapy is an important component to the school program. The speech clinician should be assessing language processing on an ongoing basis and identifying subtle difficulties for the rest of the team. Regular speech therapy is needed by many children with NTDs in order to address semantic processing of higher-order language and pragmatic language skills. Further, speech clinicians are typically involved in providing the social skills training.

## Occupational Therapy

Occupational therapists play a central role in the school team for children with NTDs. Assessment and treatment of upper extremity coordination and oral-motor coordination issues are extremely important. Further, occupational therapists can help with the assessment of sensory processing atypicalities when they occur. They are also often called on to assess adaptive behaviors, including self-care, and to provide adapted equipment and treatment, which allow greater independence.

## Physical Therapy/Orthotics and Prosthetics

Although these professionals are usually based in hospitals or healthcare settings, their participation with the school team is critical. Mobility and other physical activity require ongoing assessment of motor functioning, provision of appropriate treatments, ensuring appropriate positioning in the classroom, and design of optimal bracing and wheelchair systems. This is necessary for all of the children with orthopedic challenges in order to maximize activity and minimize motor fatigue.

## Counseling/Behavioral Services

A range of counseling services provided by school psychologists, school social workers, and other counselors is essential for effective school programs for children with NTDs. These children are generally poor candidates for psychodynamic therapy, but respond well to supportive counseling addressing disability awareness issues, body image, self-esteem, problem solving, and social skills development. Furthermore, family-based counseling can provide needed support to the family's efforts at managing resources, coping with stress, and facilitating the child's development.

Behavioral interventions may also be needed to address oppositional conduct, social withdrawal, depression, anxiety/stress responses, or angry outbursts and are usually provided by the school psychologist or behavioral consultant. With the complexity of medical, cognitive, motivational, and social factors that can be involved in these behavioral challenges, functional behavioral assessment of all problem behaviors is important in order to be able to differentiate among behavioral functions such as avoiding demands, seeking attention, dealing with transitions, or getting one's way. Following assessment, positive, reinforcer-based programs should be utilized to teach more adaptive behaviors and limit behaviors that undermine development.

Behavioral specialists in the team should also consider situations where there is a clinical need for psychotropic medication. Medications addressing depression or attention regulation are regularly considered for children with NTDs. Referral to medical practitioners on the healthcare team or to psychiatrists in the community may be helpful.

### School Nurse

The school nurse fills an essential role for the child with NTDs (57). The presence of nursing expertise at the school allows for more effective bowel and bladder management programs, dispensing medication during the school day, and immediate evaluation of symptoms (e.g., fever and headaches). Further, the school nurse often is called upon to be the liaison to the medical team.

## Functional Skills Development

Children with NTDs also present unique learning challenges in the area of adaptive and functional skills. This includes self-care (e.g., hygiene, skin checks, toileting, dressing, and brace/wheelchair management), mobility, domestic functions (e.g., cooking and cleaning), using technology (e.g., phones and computers), transportation in the community, interacting with waiters, retail clerks, etc., and managing money. These skills are necessary not only to school success but ultimately to independence and quality of life as an adult. Although these skills are outside of the traditional academic focus of schools, for many children with NTDs, they are more important to ultimate success in adulthood than academic objectives and so should be well integrated into the school program.

The school program can best address these skills in several important ways. First, all situations presenting functional challenges where the child is not independent should be carefully assessed. Children should be encouraged (and rewarded) for being as independent as possible. In these situations, accommodations and special equipment should be used to maximize independent functioning. Staff should be trained not to "do for the child" but to encourage greater independence through providing necessary support and then fading the assistance over time as the child learns to function independently.

Second, teaching functional skills should be included in the curriculum when indicated. Time in the school day should be designated for active instruction and practice of key functional skills that need work. Coteaching by the special education teacher, the occupational therapist, and the physical therapist can help the child establish independent functioning in many difficult situations. Additionally, consultation with the psychologist can provide appropriate reinforcers to further motivate the child.

Third, community-based activities should be provided to give learning experiences and practice in managing full participation in the community. Regular community field trips provide opportunities to identify key skill deficits and to practice new skills. The ultimate objective is to enable the child to use public transportation to get around the community, to communicate with merchants and service providers in the community, and to access recreational and entertainment activities.

### School Culture and Environment

The context in which the adapted instruction, interventions, and special services are offered has a powerful impact on the overall effectiveness of the program. The school culture should value diversity and inclusion and be sensitive to issues of disability. The physical environment should be completely accessible. Ongoing efforts should be made to improve the ease of movement for children with orthopedic challenges. There should be an easy-to-reach private bathroom and school nurse available to allow private self-catheterization, with minimal time away from class activities. The use of technology to support students with disabilities should be actively pursued. Disability awareness discussions should be conducted on a regular basis to help all staff and students become comfortable with disability and learn ways to be supportive (e.g., how to offer help and how to ensure inclusion in social activities) (58). As individuals with disabilities are disproportionately the target of antisocial behavior, there should also be an active antibullying and teasing program with strong administrative response to all episodes of antisocial behavior.

## CONCLUSION

Children with NTDs are at risk for a range of difficulties with academic learning, social development, functional skills, and vocational competencies (1–3). Schools play a crucial role in facilitating the development of children with NTDs and minimizing the occurrence of these secondary disabilities. This starts with establishing an environment that is accessible and supportive to individuals with disabilities. It means carefully assessing the child's learning profile and then adjusting instruction and providing services to optimize academic learning. Further, schools need to actively address social functioning and the development of adaptive and functional skills. Although these areas are beyond the traditional focus of education, they are consistent with the mandates of IDEA and the ADA and are necessary to promote independence, full participation in the community, and a good quality of life in adulthood.

## REFERENCES

1. McAndrew I. Adolescents and young people with spina bifida. Dev Med Child Neurol 1979; 21:619–629.
2. Tew B. The effects of spina bifida upon learning and behaviour. In: Bannister CM, Tew B, eds. Current Concepts in Spina Bifida and Hydrocephalus. Oxford: MacKeith Press, 1991:158–179.
3. Thomas AP, Bax MCO, Smyth DPL. The Health and Social Needs of Young Adults with Physical Disabilities. Oxford: MacKeith Press, 1989.
4. Rowley-Kelly FL, Reigel DH, eds. Teaching the Student with Spina Bifida. Baltimore: Paul H. Brookes, 1993.

5. Lollar D, ed. Preventing Secondary Conditions Associated with Spina Bifida or Cerebral Palsy: Proceedings and Recommendations of a Symposium. Washington, D.C.: Spina Bifida Association of America, 1994.
6. Individuals with Disabilities Education Act Amendments of 1997. (P.L. 105-17). 20 U.S.C. 1400 et seq. (Congressional Record 1997).
7. Jacobs R, Northam E, Anderson V. Cognitive outcome in children with myelomeningocele and perinatal hydrocephalus: a longitudinal perspective. J Dev Phys Disabil 2001; 13(4):389–405.
8. Wills KE. Neuropsychological functioning in children with spina bifida and/or hydrocephalus. J Clin Child Psychol 1993; 22:247–265.
9. Rourke BP, ed. Syndrome of Nonverbal Learning Disabilities. New York: Guilford Press, 1995.
10. Yeates KO, Loss N, Colvin AN, Enrile BG. Do chidren with myelomeningocele and hydrocephalus display nonverbal learning disabilities? An empirical approach to classification. J Int Neuropsychol Soc 2003; 9(4):653–662.
11. Ammerman RT, Van Hasselt VB, Hersen M, Moore LE. Assessment of social skills in visually impaired adolescents and their parents. Behav Assess 1989; 11:327–351.
12. Breslau N. Psychiatric disorder in children with physical disabilities. J Am Acad Child Psychiatry 1985; 24(1):87–94.
13. Tin GL, Teasdale GR. An observational study of the social adjustment of spina bifida children in integrated settings. Br J Educ Psychol 1985; 55:81–83.
14. McMillen JS, Simeonsson RJ. Evidence of educational effects and outcomes for children and youth with spina bifida. Proceedings of Evidenced Based Practice in Spina Bifida: Developing a Research Agenda, Washington, 2003.
15. Friedrich WN, Lovejoy MC, Shaffer J, Shurtleff DB, Beilke RL. Cognitive abilities and achievement status of children with myelomeningocele: a contemporary sample. J Pediatr Psychol 1991; 16(4):423–428.
16. Rourke BP. Nonverbal Learning Disabilities: The Syndrome and the Model. New York: Guilford, 1989.
17. Molenaar-Klumper M. Non-Verbal Learning Disabilities: Characteristics, Diagnosis, and Treatment within an Educational Setting. London: Jessica Kingsley, 2002.
18. Tanguay P. Nonverbal Learning Disabilities at School: Educating Students with NLD, Asperger Syndrome, and Related Conditions. London: Jessica Kingsley, 2002.
19. Thompson S. The Source for Nonverbal Learning Disorders. East Moline, IL: Linguisystems, 1997.
20. Americans with Disabilities Act of 1990, Public Law 101-336, 104 Stat. 327-378, 1990.
21. Baker SB, Rogosky-Grassi MA. Access to the school. In: Rowley-Kelly FL, Reigel DH, eds. Teaching the Student with Spina Bifida. Baltimore: Paul H. Brookes, 1993:31–70.
22. Stauffer DT. Catheterization—a health procedure schools must be prepared to provide. J School Health 1984; 54:37–38.
23. Reigel DH. Spina bifida from infancy through the school years. In: Rowley-Kelly FL, Reigel DH, eds. Teaching the Student with Spina Bifida. Baltimore: Paul H. Brookes, 1993:3–30.
24. Shaffer J, Wolfe L, Friedrich W, Shurtleff H, Shurtleff D, Fay G. Developmental expectations: intelligence and fine motor skills. In: Shurtleff D, ed. Myelodysplasias and Exstophies: Significance, Prevention, and Treatment, New York: Grune and Stratton, 1986:359–372.

25. Snow J, Prince M, Souheaver G, Ashcraft E, Stefans V, Edmonds J. Neuropsychological patterns of adolescents and young adults with spina bifida. Arch Clin Neuropsychol 1994; 9(3):277–287.
26. Wills K, Holmbeck GN, Dillon K, McLone D. Intelligence and achievement in children with myelomeningocele. J Pediatr Psychol 1990; 15(2):161–176.
27. Hurley AD, Dorman C, Laatsch L, Bell S, D'Avignon J. Cognitive functioning in patients with spina bifida, hydrocephalus, and the "cocktail party" syndrome. Dev Neuropsychol 1990; 6(2):151–172.
28. Cull C, Wyke MA. Memory function of children with spina bifida and shunted hydrocephalus. Dev Med Child Neurol 1984; 26:177–183.
29. Horn DG, Lorch EP, Lorch RF, Culatta B. Distractibility and vocabulary deficits in children with spina bifida and hydrocephalus. Dev Med Child Neurol 1985; 27:713–720.
30. Snow JH. Executive processes for children with spina bifida. Child Health Care 1999; 28(3):241–253.
31. Fletcher JM, Brookshire BL, Bohan TP, Brandt ME, Davidson KC. Early hydrocephalus. In: Rourke BP, ed. Syndrome of Nonverbal Learning Disabilities. New York: Guilford Press, 1995:206–238.
32. Culatta B, Young C. Linguistic performance as a function of abstract task demands in children with spina bifida. Dev Med Child Neurol 1992; 34(5):434–440.
33. Culatta B. Intervening for language-learning disabilities. In: Rowley-Kelly FL, Reigel DH, eds. Teaching the Student with Spina Bifida. Baltimore: Paul H. Brookes, 1993:171–192.
34. Hurley AD. Conducting Psychological Assessments. In: Rowley-Kelly FL, Reigel DH, eds. Teaching the Student with Spina Bifida. Baltimore: Paul H. Brookes, 1993:107–124.
35. Garcia-Winner M. Thinking About You, Thinking About Me: Philosophy and Strategies to Further Develop Perspective Taking and Communicative Abilities for Persons with Social Cognitive Deficits. San Jose, California: M. Garcia Winner, 2002.
36. Duke MP, Nowicki S, Martin EA. Teaching Your Child the Language of Social Success. Atlanta: Peachtree Publishing, 1996.
37. Stewart K. Helping a Child with Nonverbal Learning Disorder or Asperger's Syndrome. Oakland: New Harbinger Publications, 2002.
38. Rowley Kelly F. Social and emotional developments. In: Rowley-Kelly FL, Reigel DH, eds. Teaching the Student with Spina Bifida. Baltimore: Paul H. Brookes, 1993:213–244.
39. Ammerman RT, Kane VR, Slomka GT, Reigel DH, Franzen MD, Gadow KD. Psychiatric symptomatology and family functioning in children and adolescents with spina bifida. J Clin Psychol Med Settings 1998; 5(4):449–465.
40. Andren E, Grimby G. Dependence and perceived difficulty in activities of daily living in adults with cerebral palsy and spina bifida. Disabil Rehabil 2000; 22:299–307.
41. Bodzioch J, Roach JW, Schkade J. Promoting independence in adolescent paraplegics:A 2-week camping experience. J Pediatr Orthoped 1986; 6:198–201.
42. Neef NA, Parrish JM, Hannigan KF, Page TJ. Teaching self-catheterization skills to children with neurogenic bladder complications. J Appl Behav Anal 1989; 22(3):237–243.
43. Patrick DL, Richardson M, Starks HE, Rose MA. A framework for promoting the health of people with disabilities. In: Lollar D, ed. Preventing Secondary Conditions Associated with Spina Bifida or Cerebral Palsy: Proceedings and Recommendations

of a Symposium. Washington, D.C.: Spina Bifida Association of America, 1994:3–16.
44. Rourke BP, van der Vlugt H, Rourke SB. Practice of Child-Centered Neuropsychology: An Introduction. Exton, PA: Swets and Zeitlinger Publishers, 2002.
45. Culatta B. Developing abstract concepts. In: Rowley-Kelly FL, Reigel DH, eds. Teaching the Student with Spina Bifida. Baltimore: Paul H. Brookes, 1993:125–144.
46. Culatta B. Building mathematics skills. In: Rowley-Kelly FL, Reigel DH, eds. Teaching the Student with Spina Bifida. Baltimore: Paul H. Brookes, 1993:145–170.
47. Rogosky-Grassi MA. Working with perceptual-motor skills. In: Rowley-Kelly Fl, Reigel DH, eds. Teaching the Student with Spina Bifida. Baltimore: Paul H. Brookes, 1993:193–212.
48. Lollar DJ. Educational issues among children with spina bifida. Spotlight. Washington: Spina Bifida Association of America, 1993.
49. Lollar DJ. Learning issues among children with spina bifida. Spotlight. Washington: Spina Bifida Association of America, 1993.
50. Elksnin LK, Elksnin N. Introduction to the special issue. Exceptionality 2001; 9(1–2):19–32.
51. McGinnis E, Goldstein AP. Skillstreaming the Elementary School Child: New Strategies and Perspectives for Teaching Prosocial Skills. Champaign, IL: Research Press, 1997.
52. Walker HM, McConnell S, Holmes D, Todis B, Walker J, Golden N. The Walker Social Skills Curriculum: ACCEPTS. Austin, TX: Pro-Ed, 1983.
53. Frederickson N, Turner J. Utilizing the classroom peer group to address children's social needs: an evaluation of the Circle of Friends intervention approach. J Spec Educ 2002; 36(4):234–245.
54. Gray C. The New Social Stories Book. Arlington, TX: Future Horizons, 2000.
55. Warchausky S, Argento AG, Hurvitz E, Berg M. Neuropsychological status and social problem solving in children with congenital or acquired brain dysfunction. Rehabil Psychol 2003; 48(4):250–254.
56. McAfee J. Navigating the Social World. Arlington, TX: Future Horizons, 2002.
57. Leo RE. Accommodations for students via school nursing. In: Rowley-Kelly FL, Reigel DH, eds. Teaching the Student with Spina Bifida. Baltimore: Paul H. Brookes, 1993:71–104.
58. Rowley-Kelley FL. Social acceptance and disability awareness. In: Rowley-Kelly FL, Reigel DH, eds. Teaching the Student with Spina Bifida. Baltimore: Paul H. Brookes, 1993:245–280.

# 5

# Psychological Functioning in Children and Adolescents with Spina Bifida

**Robert T. Ammerman, Marsha J. Nortz, M. Douglas Ris, and Nicolay C. Walz**

*Division of Behavioral Medicine and Clinical Psychology, Cincinnati Children's Hospital Medical Center, Cincinnati, Ohio, U.S.A.*

## INTRODUCTION

Numerous advances developed in the 1960s and 1970s have greatly improved the medical care of children with spina bifida, from birth through their transition into adulthood. Significant strides have been made in neurosurgery, orthopedics, urology, and physical therapy. Yet, while such improvements have enhanced the health of children with spina bifida, psychological and social maladjustment have emerged as major challenges for this population. This chapter reviews the literature on psychological functioning in children and adolescents with spina bifida. First, neuropsychological features are examined. Second, behavioral and psychiatric adjustment, social functioning, and family issues are addressed. Third, methodological limitations of the scientific literature are considered. Fourth, implications of research findings for treatment are discussed. Finally, recommendations for future research are presented.

## NEUROPSYCHOLOGICAL FUNCTIONING IN SPINA BIFIDA

Neuropsychological impairments in spina bifida result from congenital brain abnormalities emanating from the syndrome and additional damage caused by hydrocephalus. Infections secondary to shunt revision can further impair cognitive functioning and can lead to devastating consequences for intellectual ability. In spina bifida, brain abnormalities have been identified in the midbrain/tectum, corpus callosum, cerebellum, cortical abnormalities have also been identified, particularly in posterior relative to anterior brain regions. In a subset of the largest cohort of children with spina bifida systematically studied to date ($n = 302$ school-aged children), Fletcher et al. (1) described the range of brain dysmorphologies observed using magnetic resonance imaging. Abnormalities were more often found in children with upper versus lower lesions, although both groups exhibited a number of dysmorphologies. These included the Arnold-Chiari II malformation (found in 96% of upper level lesion children and 90% of their lower level lesion counterparts), small or maldeveloped pons and medulla, and abnormalities (hypoplasia, dysgenesis) in the corpus callosum (96% of the sample). Taken together, these abnormalities have been linked to the core neuropsychological impairments typically found in children with spina bifida.

## Core Neuropsychological Features

Fletcher et al. (1) have articulated the modal neuropsychological profile of children with spina bifida, noting that there is considerable variability in the population and there are numerous external influences (e.g., socioeconomic status) that moderate expression and impact of cognitive impairments. The neuropsychological profile involves deficits in attention, short-term memory, language comprehension and discourse, visual-spatial abilities, and motor functioning. Additional features of the profile include impairments in intellectual and academic functioning, particularly in reading, mathematics, and writing.

Attentional dysfunction has long been recognized as common sequelae of spina bifida and hydrocephalus. Parent-reported attention problems are common in samples of children and adolescents with spina bifida (2,3). In a sample of 205 children aged 7 to 16 years, of which 164 had spina bifida, Burmeister et al. (3) found that 31% of the spina bifida group met diagnostic criteria for attention deficit hyperactivity disorder (ADHD). The inattentive subtype was most represented, comprising 23% of the sample. In a subsample of children with spina bifida who were also mentally retarded, Fletcher et al. (1) found that 27% met criteria for ADHD. Once again, the inattention subtype was most frequently observed (14%), followed by the combined inattentive/impulsive subtype (8%) and the hyperactive-impulsive subtype (6%). Fletcher et al. (4) found deficits in executive function measures and select aspects of attention in a mixed group of children with hydrocephalus, and these deficits were distinct from children with documented frontal lobe injuries. In a larger study, Dennis et al. (5) documented deficits in covert and overt attention shifting, which were related to tectal dysmorphology and reductions in white matter volume, respectively. Difficulties in attention shifting were particularly evident in children with higher-level lesions.

Few studies are available that specifically assess new learning and memory in children with spina bifida. A number of studies assess the effects of hydrocephalus, in which subjects with spina bifida represent the majority. Yeates et al. (6), for example, found deficits in children with hydrocephalus on a verbal memory measure. Scott et al. (7) found deficits in new learning in children with spina bifida and hydrocephalus. Frequent complaints concerning "memory problems" in this population may actually reflect attentional or executive function deficits.

Although children with spina bifida exhibit relative strengths in verbal abilities when compared with nonverbal abilities, this population displays distinct language processing deficits. Children and adolescents with spina bifida develop a generally sophisticated vocabulary, but there are deficiencies in a variety of higher-level linguistic skills and narrative discourse (8). Hyperverbosity and contamination of discourse with contextually irrelevant or perseverative statements is often seen. Dennis and Barnes (9) found deficits in narrative discourse and cohesiveness of expression, paucity of content, and problems interpreting ambiguous material. Impairments in discourse have also been implicated in reading comprehension difficulties observed in the population (10).

Deficits in perceptual integration skills, processing of spatial information, and visual motor abilities have been consistently documented in this population (11). Brookshire et al. (8) found that the lower performance IQ (PIQ) and deficits on spatial-constructional tasks in children with spina bifida are core impairments that cannot be attributed to the motor demands of the tasks. Dennis et al. (12) administered an assessment battery comprised of tests measuring multiple aspects of visual-perception abilities to a sample of children with spina bifida and controls. Deficits were most evident in tasks measuring action-based visual perception (i.e., which permits visually guided, goal-direction actions) than object-based visual perception (i.e., which detects visual–perceptual features such as contour, shape, size, and orientation). In a study of perceptual timing, Dennis et al. (13) presented to children with spina bifida and to a control group a series of paired tones that differed in frequency and time interval between tones. Results revealed that children with spina bifida and controls were similar in their ability to discriminate frequencies, although those with spina bifida were less accurate than their counterparts in discriminating time intervals, and this is relevant to observations such as the temporal regulation of speech (ataxic dysarthria) and eye–hand coordination requiring the constant modulation of motor timing.

Impairments in somato-sensory and motor functioning have been found in children and adolescents with spina bifida and are likely related to cerebellar abnormalities associated with the Arnold-Chiari II malformation, disruption of the pyramidal systems secondary to hydrocephalus, and/or abnormalities in the spinal cord above the level of the lesion (11). Children and adults with spina bifida have been found to evidence more motor speech deficits, including dysfluency, ataxic dysarthria, and slower speech rate, relative to age-matched controls (14). Additional fine, gross, and visuomotor impairments associated with spina bifida are well documented (15). However, despite hypotheses of impaired procedural motor learning or motor adaptation (i.e., acquisition and retention of a skill with repeated practice or exposure independent of conscious recall of the exposure) based upon knowledge of the role of the cerebellum in mediating this skill (16), studies have found no deficits relative to controls (17,18).

## Intellectual and Academic Functioning

Measures of general intellectual ability have consistently shown lower mean IQ scores in children and adolescents with spina bifida (19,20), typically clustering in the low normal range [mean full scale IQ (FSIQ) of approximately 90]. An inverse relationship between IQ and level of lesion has been established (21,22). IQ also varies by ethnicity and economic disadvantage (1). While the number of shunt revisions has not in itself been found to be a factor contributing to diminished general cognitive performance (23,24), infection does appear to be related to lower IQ (11). Significant discrepancies between verbal IQ (VIQ) and PIQ have also been identified (25,26) with as many as one-half of participants with SB having lower PIQ than VIQ. Fletcher et al. (1) found that 21% of a large cohort of children with spina bifida met criteria for mental retardation.

Children with spina bifida are at increased risk for academic problems. For example, Wills et al. (20) found weaknesses in math, written expression, and reading comprehension. The deficit in math was worse with increasing age. Reading decoding skills, however, were found to be intact. This pattern is consistent with the larger literature on children with hydrocephalus (9). Fletcher et al. (1) documented the wide variability of intellectual and academic functioning in children with spina bifida. In their sample, 22% manifested average functioning in intelligence and academic performance. The remaining subjects evinced a wide array of difficulties in reading and math. Using the 25th percentile as a cutoff, it was found that 55% of the full sample exhibited deficits in reading and/or math, and 26% had deficits in both domains.

## Nonverbal Learning Disability and Spina Bifida

The pattern of neuropsychological strengths and weaknesses in spina bifida corresponds closely to the syndrome of nonverbal learning disability (NLD). This neuropsychological phenotype was first described in relation to children with learning disabilities and subsequently applied to children with various medical disorders such as hydrocephalus, cancers treated with cranial radiation, and certain metabolic disorders. Rourke (27,28) has argued that the underlying pathophysiology in these conditions is disruption of right hemispheral systems that may be a consequence of either lateralized brain injury or widespread disruption of white matter pathways (typical of spina bifida and hydrocephalus).

NLD is characterized by a series of intact (assets) and impaired (deficits) cognitive processes (29). Primary assets include relative strengths in auditory perception, simple motor tasks, and rote material. Primary deficits consist of impaired tactile perception, visual perception, complex psychomotor tasks, and response to novel material. Additional cognitive strengths include auditory and verbal attention and memory, with corresponding weaknesses in tactile and visual attention and memory, and deficits in problem solving and concept formation. Despite strengths in phononology and verbal reception, children and adolescents with NLD have several verbal weaknesses such as hyperverbosity, poor verbal comprehension, and shallow speech content. Social impairments are key characteristics of NLD and are believed to emanate from the patterns of cognitive assets and deficits listed above. In addition to superficial content, those with NLD have difficulty engaging in smooth, bidirectional social interactions; often fail to respect boundaries associated with social distance; may fail to appreciate nonverbal cues in social discourse; and have problems identifying the emotional state of others gleaned from simultaneous integration of facial expression, vocal tone, and posture/gesture. In addition, they typically fail to appreciate humor and have limited insight into the nature of their behavior.

Examination of these features reveals a striking overlap with common vulnerabilities in persons with spina bifida. The prevalence of NLD in spina bifida has not been extensively studied. However, Ammerman et al. (30) found that, among children and adults with spina bifida referred for neuropsychological evaluation, 40% to 50% had profiles consistent with NLD. Yeates et al. (31) found that 50% of a sample of children with spina bifida met research criteria for NLD, and among those who did not, there was considerable variability in the array of cognitive assets and deficits observed. It is evident that a sizable portion of children with spina bifida exhibit the NLD profile, and this subgroup is potentially important to the extent that psychosocial impairments associated with NLD may also be present in those with spina bifida.

Methodological shortcomings and limitations in the literature documenting neuropsychological functioning in children with spina bifida bears mention, and these have been presented previously by Fletcher et al. (1). Existing studies largely report group means to summarize outcome domains, but a greater understanding of the neuropsychological functioning of children with spina bifida will require additional attention to the variability in the overall level of functioning and the factors (both medical and environmental) that may mediate that variability. However, an additional limitation in spina bifida research has been that of relatively small sample sizes, and larger samples will be needed in order to more fully explore the variability in outcomes. In addition, outcome studies have largely focused on school-aged children, and greater attention to the neuropsychology of spina bifida during both early childhood and adulthood will be important in order to understand both the origins of neuropsychological difficulties and the long-term outcomes of impaired neuropsychological functioning.

## Psychosocial Functioning in Children and Adolescents with Spina Bifida

From the earliest descriptive reports on psychosocial functioning in children with spina bifida (32), it was suggested that this population manifested clinically significant impairments in emotional, behavioral, and social domains. This was thought to emerge from cognitive impairments associated with the condition, mobility limitations restricting access to age-appropriate normal social activities essential to normal psychosocial development, social rejection by able-bodied peers, and family dysfunction secondary to maladaptive adjustment to raising a child with a disability. As with other areas in spina bifida, research on psychosocial adjustment has yielded a modestly sized literature that is limited by methodological shortcomings and sometimes conflicting results (33). However, taken together, these studies have revealed that many children and adolescents with spina bifida are at risk for psychological maladjustment, particularly social impairments. In addition, it has been found that psychological maladjustment can be moderated by lesion level, cognitive impairment, family functioning, and sociodemographics. In this section, we first examine broad perspectives of the relationships between disability and psychosocial functioning, and their relevance to spina bifida. We then review findings on emotional/behavioral and social adjustment in spina bifida, and the impact of family influences on psychosocial functioning. Given the sizable quantity of uncontrolled research in these areas, our review is selective and focuses primarily on studies that incorporate control groups and use standardized measures. Finally, we summarize and synthesize key findings and reflect on the current state of knowledge of psychosocial functioning in this population.

## Models of Disability and Psychosocial Functioning

Three broad conceptualizations have been put forth to account for why children and adolescents with disabilities are at increased risk for behavioral and social dysfunction. The first approach emphasizes the social and cultural barriers that individuals with disabilities face in participating in mainstream society. The resulting social isolation, marginalization, and disempowerment deny children and adolescents with disabilities opportunities to fully engage in normative social activities that promote and are essential to optimal social, emotional, and behavioral development (34). Moreover, social rejection damages self-esteem and self-efficacy, contributes to learned helplessness in social domains, and increases the risk for depression. Given the sizable literature on social reactions to disability, including stereotyping and prejudice, it is surprising that this perspective is almost completely absent from research on psychosocial functioning in children and youth with spina bifida. This limitation is due, in large part, to the fact that research has relied exclusively on the ascertainment and measurement of clinical samples and their families, to the exclusion of social contexts and the peer groups in which social rejection occurs. Although the field would benefit from incorporation of this perspective in research designs, it is important to note that the social and cultural barrier formulation fails to account for the wide variability in outcomes observed both within and between different disabilities.

A second model proposes that behavioral and social development is determined, in part, by the impact of and limitations resulting from specific features of the disability. According to this view, specific features of a disability can contribute etiologically to psychosocial maladaptation in children and adolescents. Of course, the types and ranges of disabilities will differentially affect psychosocial adaptation and functioning, and there will be significant heterogeneity both within and between disabilities. An important implication of the disability-specific model is that, although there may be similarities in psychosocial outcome from one disability to another (e.g., social isolation), the causal pathways leading to that outcome may be different between disabilities (e.g., orthopedic vs. cognitive impairments). Examples of this approach in spina bifida include studies in which shunt status or lesion level are examined as correlates of psychosocial functioning.

The third conceptualization is the ecological model (35), which stipulates that psychosocial development emanates from multiple influences. Specifically, these influences originate from four nested levels: child, family, community, and society. Development proceeds from the synergistic interaction of forces that promote or undermine positive outcomes. Some variables interfere with optimal development, such as poverty, inadequate stimulation, and violence in the family. Other factors promote positive outcomes and serve as buffers against negative influences, such as social support and effective coping. The ecological model has been the dominant perspective of recent research on psychosocial development in children and adolescents with disabilities and chronic illnesses in general (36), and spina bifida in particular (37).

## EMOTIONAL, BEHAVIORAL, AND PSYCHIATRIC ADJUSTMENT

Difficulties in emotional and behavioral adjustment have been observed in a number of disabilities and chronic medical conditions, and spina bifida is no exception. In the case of spina bifida, there are several potential contributing factors to such difficulties, including cognitive impairments (both lower IQ and neuropsychological profiles associated with behavioral and emotional disturbance, such as NLD), limited socialization experiences and peer rejection, and inadequate development of coping and self-regulatory capabilities. Although research conducted to date has rarely examined mechanisms by which children and youth with spina bifida develop emotional and behavioral problems, it is clear that this population is at elevated risk.

In a series of studies, Wallander and colleagues (36,38) examined emotional and behavioral functioning in children with chronic illnesses and disabilities, including spina bifida. Relying primarily on maternal reports using the Child Behavior Checklist (CBCL), these studies found elevated scores on scales reflecting internalizing (e.g., depression, anxiety) and externalizing (e.g., conduct problems, hyperactivity) adjustment problems. It was noted that scores were higher than the general population, but generally not in the range of highly significant mental health problems.

Fletcher et al. (39) administered the CBCL to 32 mothers of children aged five to seven years with spina bifida, of which 23 had hydrocephalus. Results indicated that 26% of children with spina bifida and hydrocephalus (and 11% without hydrocephalus) obtained elevated *T* scores ($T > 63$ a score greater than 90% of that obtained by the community normative sample) on behavior problem summary scales, with greater frequency of disturbance occurring with internalizing rather than externalizing disorders.

Ammerman et al. (40) found that children and youth with spina bifida display higher levels of psychopathology than peers without disabilities and relative to empirically derived normative standards. Specifically, the authors administered the CBCL to 25 mothers and fathers of adolescents (aged 10–17 years) with spina bifida. In addition, adolescents completed the youth self-report form (YSRF), a parallel version of the CBCL. Using the $T > 63$ criterion for clinical significance, mean scores for adolescents with spina bifida based on parental reports exceeded this level on withdrawal (mother only), immature (mother and father), and uncommunicative (father only). A comparison with 25 control adolescents without a disability revealed statistically significant differences in that adolescents with spina bifida obtained higher scores on schizoid (father only), withdrawal (mother only), somatic complaints (father only), uncommunicative (mother and father), and internalizing (mother only). An additional comparison with adolescents with visual impairments found that this group differed from their peers with spina bifida on the uncommunicative subscale (both mother and father). Divergence between mothers and fathers in reports of psychological functioning underscore the importance of multi-informant assessments in obtaining a broad clinical picture of children and adolescents with spina bifida. Interestingly, no group differences were found on the YSRF. This finding may be accounted for in part by the clinical observations that adolescents with spina bifida are likely to under-report psychopathology (41).

In a second study, Ammerman et al. (2) administered the Stony Brook Child Symptom Inventory (SBCSI), a screening measure for psychiatric symptomatology and psychiatric disorder, to mothers and fathers of 59 children and adolescents (mean age = 12.92 years) with spina bifida. Findings revealed that 43% of the sample met criteria [as established by the Diagnostic and Statistical Manual of Mental Disorders, Fourth Edition (DSM-IV)] for at least one psychiatric diagnosis and 17% received two or more diagnoses. In general, the sample exhibited a high rate of overall symptomatology, as evidenced by the fact that mothers endorsed a mean of 9.64 clinically significant symptoms (out of 95 items) per subject. Internalizing symptoms were reported more than externalizing symptoms. Attention problems were widely reported in this sample. For those receiving the diagnosis of ADHD, symptoms involving attention were more frequently endorsed than those having to do with impulsiveness and hyperactivity (in contrast to the ADHD population as a whole).

Holmbeck et al. (37) used the CBCL to examine emotional and behavioral adjustment in 68 children with spina bifida and 68 controls, aged eight to nine years. In examining mother, father, and teacher reports, group differences were found on attention problems, although there were no significant findings for other internalizing and externalizing problems (self-reported depression using another measure yielded significant differences, although this finding dropped out after controlling for verbal intelligence). Aggression was higher in lower socioeconomic status (SES) subjects in contrast to their higher SES peers, independent of disability status.

Appleton et al. (42) compared 72 children with spina bifida to case controls using self-reported measures of depression and self-esteem. Increased levels of depression and lower self-esteem were reported in the spina bifida group. Self-perceptions of physical appearance were associated with self-esteem ratings, and girls exhibited more depression than boys.

Vachha and Adams (43) administered the Carey Temperament Scales to primary caregivers of 46 children aged 5 to 12 years with spina bifida, and contrasted scores with population norms for the measure. Temperament reflects core personality features that are thought to emerge very early in life, and typically are stable throughout childhood. Results indicated that, relative to population norms, children with spina bifida were found less adaptable, wary of approaching and more likely to withdraw from novel situations, more distractible, less attentive and persistent, less predictable in biological rhythms. A positive correlation was found between maternal mood and negative endorsements of temperament. It was noted that the cluster of temperament characteristics was atypical and did not readily fit into widely observed categories (e.g., easy vs. difficult).

## Social Adjustment

Given the documented cognitive impairments in many children and adolescents with spina bifida, it is clear that they are at risk for impaired social information processing and subsequent social dysfunction. These impairments, in turn, undermine full development and utilization of more complex cognitive processes as the child matures. The impact of this is cumulative and compounding. In mid-to-late adolescence, as interpersonal interactions and social relationship rely increasingly on more complex cognitive processes, those with spina bifida are believed to be particularly vulnerable to social dysfunction. As with behavioral and psychiatric functioning, there is limited empirical data on social adjustment in children and youth with spina bifida. Extant research, however, documents the vulnerability of this population to social dysfunction.

Several descriptive studies have documented social maladjustment in children and adolescents with spina bifida. These include findings of having no or few friends, restricted social experiences that are often passive in nature, and increased loneliness (44). The CBCL has been the most often used index of social competence in this population. The CBCL yields four scores reflecting social competence: activity, social, school, and total social. Van Hasselt et al. (45), in a study of young children (age 7–9 years, $N = 26$) with spina bifida, found that these children obtained lower scores relative to controls without disabilities on the school and total social scales as reported by fathers.

In their study of 68 children with spina bifida (age 8–9 years old) and controls, Holmbeck et al. (37) documented extensive social difficulties in those with spina bifida. Using the CBCL, mothers and fathers reported lower scores on the activity involvement and social competence scales. The children, parents, and teachers also completed the Self-Perception Profile for Children (SPPC). Results indicated that children with spina bifida obtained lower scores on scales reflecting views of physical appearance, athletic competence, and social competence. Additional measures revealed traits and behaviors that would be expected to adversely affect socialization. For example, relative to controls, children with spina bifida evidenced less intrinsic motivation, greater reliance on adults, increased passivity, and greater social immaturity. Findings from this study are noteworthy in that the clinical hallmarks of social dysfunction in those with spina bifida, observable in adolescence and into adulthood, are detectable at such an early age.

Ammerman et al. (40) found significant social maladjustment in adolescents (aged 10–17) with spina bifida. Mothers and fathers reported impaired social competence on all four of the CBCL social functioning scales. In general, adolescents with spina bifida obtained lower scores than both adolescents without disabilities and those with visual impairments. On the YSRF, completed by the adolescents, those in the spina bifida group obtained lower scores than their peers without disabilities on the activities and total competence scales. Nonambulatory status was associated with increased maladjustment.

Only one study has examined social skills in adolescents with spina bifida. Ammerman et al. (40) used a role-play test (RPT) to examine social skills in 75 adolescents aged 10 to 17 years, divided equally between groups of adolescents with spina bifida, visual impairments, and no disability. Cluster analysis was conducted on the social skill components and overall rating in an effort to determine whether or not the three groups differed on aspects of social skill. Results revealed two distinct clusters reflecting adolescents with enhanced and diminished social skills. In other words, disability-specific profiles of social skill deficits did not emerge (with the exception of gaze, which was highly discrepant in the visually impaired group). Twelve percent of adolescents with spina bifida belonged to the cluster reflecting diminished social skills. This latter finding is surprising, although closer examination of RPTs suggest that this may be an insensitive measure of social functioning in spina bifida. Many individuals with spina bifida are thought to be proficient at memorizing simple (rote) information, including relatively simple and stereotyped aspects of interpersonal interactions. The three prompt format of the RPT may not be as challenging to adolescents with spina bifida in contrast to the more flexible response repertoire essential to ongoing social relationships. Also germane to this point is the observation that children and adolescents with spina bifida make "good first impressions" because of their chatty, albeit shallow, conversational style (46). Such a response style may elicit negative reactions from others, but would be undetectable using typical RPT procedures.

## Family Functioning

There is a sizable literature documenting that many families of children with disabilities struggle to adapt to the challenges of raising a child with special needs (47). There is considerable variability between disabilities and families, and it is generally believed that most families eventually adjust adequately as they evolve and adapt to new roles and responsibilities. For some of those families that do not, premorbid family dysfunction has been implicated in maladjustment observed after the birth of a child with a disability, which may exacerbate already established negative patterns of relating. The research literature on families of children with spina bifida is considerably smaller, although findings have essentially mirrored that found in families of children with other types of disabilities.

Holmbeck et al. (48) conducted a comprehensive review of research on the impact of spina bifida on family functioning. These authors identified 32 studies that reported results form 25 data sets. The studies had a number of methodological limitations, including small sample sizes, no or inadequate control groups, and restricted sources of data. Importantly, as with other domains in spina bifida, results were divergent, variability was the rule rather than exception, and findings were sometimes contradictory.

Holmbeck et al. (48) concluded that between 12% and 25% of families exhibited clinically elevated levels of distress, suggesting that normal adaptation to spina bifida is the modal outcome. For example, Ammerman et al. (2) found that 13% of families exhibited high levels of problematic functioning using the Family Assessment Device. The most significant negative impact was in the area of family roles and responsibilities, reflecting the difficulties some families have in constructing systems to accommodate the needs of a child with spina bifida (such as mobility issues, frequent medical appointments, acute medical needs). Problematic family functioning was correlated with child and adolescent behavior problems. This type of relationship, in which stress related to caring for the child is exacerbated by intrafamilial or extrafamilial stressors, has been found in other studies as well (49). Holmbeck et al. (50) found that families of young children with spina bifida exhibited less cohesion and the children were passive in their interactions with family members, relative to able-bodied controls. These relationships were mediated by IQ, such that lower IQ (which was more represented in the spina bifida group) was associated with less family cohesion. Similar to Ammerman et al. (40), this study found that the majority of families functioned in the average range.

Findings have been more consistent in research on parental adjustment. Specifically, a sizable proportion of mothers and fathers report increased stress, marital dissatisfaction, parenting dissatisfaction, and psychological distress (48). Illustrative is a study by Holmbeck et al. (51) in which mothers and fathers of children with spina bifida were contrasted with parents of children without disabilities. Results indicated that parents of children with spina bifida reported less parenting satisfaction, more psychological symptoms, and use of less effective coping strategies than their counterparts of children without disabilities. Once again, however, the majority of parents (75%) reported average adjustment.

## METHODOLOGICAL LIMITATIONS OF PSYCHOSOCIAL RESEARCH IN SPINA BIFIDA

There are several methodological shortcomings and limitations in the extant literature. First, sample sizes typically are small. Small sample sizes cast doubt on the representativeness of the sample and the generalizability of obtained results. Moreover, small sample sizes provide inadequate statistical power to detect actual differences. Another methodological concern, especially given that the empirical literature on spina bifida is relatively sparse, is that some of the papers reviewed in this section are based on the same samples. As a result, biases in sample selection are repeated across studies, and generalizability of results becomes suspect.

Second, much of the research conducted on spina bifida and psychosocial functioning is descriptive in nature and lacks a theoretical base. Although description is an important first step in the development of a scientific literature, explication of causative relationships and testing of theoretical models is essential to the identification of at-risk children and the subsequent design of interventions. This need becomes particularly relevant given the variability in outcome exhibited by children and adolescents with spina bifida. Accounting for this variability is an essential next step in the literature. Research guided by the ecological model (37) is an important first step leading to theoretically driven research. However, the ecological model provides more of an organizing conceptual framework than a specific theoretical formulation. The latter are essential to developing testable hypotheses, identifying mechanisms by which spina bifida leads to negative psychosocial outcomes, and eventually designing effective treatments.

Third, the over-reliance on mothers as sources of information for their children and adolescents is a problem in the child development and child psychology literatures in general, although it is particularly problematic in research on spina bifida. Evidence suggests that, for children with or without disabilities, there is often a divergence of opinion between mothers, fathers, children, and other caregivers (e.g., teachers). This is especially true for internalizing disorders, such as anxiety, depression, and low self-esteem. Accuracy of parental reports seems to decrease in adolescence, and several authors have noted that mothers of adolescents with spina bifida may under-report psychopathology (41). Given that adolescents with spina bifida may also present themselves as functioning at healthier levels that may actually be true (40), it becomes imperative that multiple sources of information be obtained to arrive at a more accurate picture of the adolescent's psychosocial adjustment. Although the self-report of adolescents with spina bifida must be interpreted cautiously, it is surprising that so few studies have asked children and adolescents directly about their own feelings, behaviors, and beliefs. Given that adolescents with spina bifida are viewed as relatively uncommunicative by their parents (40), certain domains (e.g., internalizing symptoms) are unlikely to be known by mothers and fathers, and can only be ascertained by querying the adolescent directly. [As noted, these reports, too, may be biased. The only acceptable approach is to gather information from multiple sources, a strategy used quite successfully by Holmbeck et al. (37).]

## CLINICAL IMPLICATIONS

Development of psychosocial treatments to address psychopathology, social maladjustment, and family maladaptation has lagged behind the basic research in these areas. This is due, in large part, to the relatively small literatures that have emerged on psychosocial functioning in spina bifida, methodological limitations that preclude drawing firm conclusions and impede design of targeted interventions, conflicting findings on the extent and severity of specific psychosocial impairments, and the wide variability in behavioral and social functioning observed in children and adolescents with spina bifida. An additional concern is the virtual absence of research on mechanisms by which features of spina bifida contribute to psychosocial difficulties. Because interventions should emerge from an understanding of such mechanisms, the dearth of research to guide such efforts is a significant impediment.

Although the empirical literature offers limited guidance in selection and implementation of psychosocial interventions, psychologists and other mental health professionals are often called upon to provide treatment to children and adolescents with spina bifida and their families. Prout and Strohmer (52) suggest that psychotherapeutic approaches be adapted for use with cognitively impaired persons through simplification of language, working on more modest goals, and using strategies that are more effective for this with intellectual limitations. Hurley (53) recommended six adaptations to psychotherapy that are designed to enhance effectiveness and relevance: (*i*) use a directive approach, (*ii*) involve both family members and other caregivers, (*iii*) deliver the intervention to the person's cognitive and developmental level, (*iv*) identify and acknowledge the person's interpersonal distortions and biases, (*v*) be flexible in choosing and implementing treatments, and (*vi*) help the person in their journey toward accepting their disability.

Behavior therapy strategies, which are less reliant on intact cognitive processes than cognitive therapy or other forms of verbally-based therapies, have the potential to helpful for children and adolescents with spina bifida and their families. Such approaches have a strong empirical foundation (54) and are both flexible and adaptable to the individual needs of patients. These include social skills training to enhance social competence, contingency contracting to shape adaptive behaviors, and exposure to reduce anxiety. However, given the unique learning challenges associated with spina bifida, there is little guidance about how to alter such treatments to optimize their effectiveness with this population. There is a similar dearth of empirical data on the use of psychotropic medications for psychiatric disorders in persons with spina bifida. Psychosocial and psychopharmacological treatment design and testing should be a major focus of future clinical research in spina bifida.

## FUTURE DIRECTIONS

The nascent stage of research in psychosocial development in children and adolescents with spina bifida provides a unique opportunity for framing the future evolution of the field. The complexity of the disorder, and the enormous variability observed in outcomes, requires that future scientific efforts use methodologically rigorous designs, draw upon theoretical models that are multivariate and developmental in nature, and utilize measurement strategies that are psychometrically sound.

To this end, recommendations from the conference proceedings, "Evidence-Based Practice in Spina Bifida: Developing a Research Agenda" (55), provides a roadmap for carrying out programmatic research that informs the field and guides clinical practice. The paucity of high quality and integrated research was noted in this conference. It was suggested that basic issues, such as prevalence of problems, developmental risk factors, and interventions to address more common clinical concerns, be a priority for future empirical studies. It was further noted that future research needs to be guided by strong theoretical conceptualizations, test competing theories, use objective and standardized measurements, use appropriate control groups, use longitudinal designs, and adhere to tight experimental methodologies (e.g., randomized clinical trial). Studies of children and adolescents with spina bifida are typically underpowered because of small sample sizes, which create a formidable challenge for a low base rate syndrome such as spina bifida. Multisite studies are essential to addressing the power issue through increasing sample sizes and have the added benefit of enhancing external validity and generalizability by incorporating diverse populations in terms of race and ethnicity, socioeconomic status, and geographic residence.

## ACKNOWLEDGMENT

This chapter was written with the support of Grant No. H133G000134 from the National Institute in Disability and Rehabilitation Research, U.S. Department of Education, and by USPHS GCRC Grant No. M01 RR 08084 from the National Center for Research Resources, NIH.

## REFERENCES

1. Fletcher JM, Dennis M, Northrup H, et al. Spina bifida: genes, brain, and development. In: L Glidden, ed. International Review of Research in Mental Retardation. San Diego: Academic Press, 2004:63–117.

2. Ammerman RT, Kane V, Slomka GT, Reigel DH, Franzen M. Psychiatric disorder and family functioning in children and adolescents with spina bifida. J Clin Psychol Med Setting 1998; 5:449–465.
3. Burmeister R, Hannay HJ, Fletcher JM, Boudousquie A, Dennis M. Attention problems and executive functions in children with spina bifida meningomyelocele. Child Neuropsychol 2005; 11:265–283.
4. Fletcher JM, Brookshire BL, Landry SH, et al. Attentional skills and executive function in children with early hydrocephalus. Dev Neuropsychol 1996; 12:52–76.
5. Dennis M, Edelstein K, Frederick J, et al. Peripersonal spatial attention in children with spina bifida: associations between horizontal and vertical line bisection and congenital malformation of the corpus collosum. Neuropsychologia 2005; 4:2000–2010.
6. Yeates KO, Enrile BG, Loss N, Blumenstein E, Delis DC. Verbal learning and memory of children with myelomeningocele. J Ped Psychol 1995; 20:801–815.
7. Scott MA, Fletcher JM, Brookshire BL, et al. Memory functions in children with early hydrocephalus. Neuropsychology 1998; 4:578–589.
8. Brookshire BL, Fletcher JM, Bohan TP, Landry SH, Davidson KC, Francis DJ. Verbal and nonverbal skill discrepancies in children with hydrocephalus: a five-year longitudinal follow-up. J Ped Psychol 1995; 20:785–800.
9. Dennis M, Barnes MA. Oral discourse after early onset hydrocephalus: Linguistic ambiguity, figurative language, speech, acts, and script-based inferences. J Ped Psychol 1993;18:639–652.
10. Barnes MA, Dennis M. Discourse after early-onset hydrocephalus: core deficits in children of average intelligence. Brain Lang 1998; 61:309–334.
11. Wills KE. Neuropsychological functioning in children with spina bifida and/or hydrocephalus. J Clin Child Psychol 1993; 22:247–265.
12. Dennis M, Fletcher JM, Rogers T, Hetherington R, Francis D. Object-based and action-based visual perception in children with spina bifida and hydrocephalus. J Intern Neuropsychol Soc 2002; 8:95–106.
13. Dennis M, Edelstein K, Hetherington R, et al. Neurobiology of timing in children with SB: short duration perceptual timing and isochronous rhythmic tapping in relation to cerebellar volumes. Brain 2004; 127:1–10.
14. Huber-Okrainec J, Dennis M, Brettschneider J, Spiegler BJ. Neuromotor speech deficits in children and adults with spina bifida and hydrocephalus. Brain Lang 2002; 80:592–602.
15. Hetherington R, Dennis M. Motor function profile in children with hydrocephalus. Dev Neuropsychol 1999;15:25–52.
16. Thach W. A role for the cerebellum in learning movement coordination. Neurobiol Learn Mem 1998; 70:177–188.
17. Colvin AN, Yeates KO, Enrile BG, Coury DL. Motor adaptation in children with myelomeningocele: comparison to children with ADHD and healthy siblings. J Internat Neuropsychol Soc 2003; 9:642–652.
18. Edelstein K, Dennis M, Copeland K, et al. Motor learning in children with spina bifida: dissociation between performance level and acquisition rate. J Internat Neuropsychol Soc 2004; 10:877–887.
19. Shaffer J, Wolfe L, Friedrich W, Shurtleff J, Shurtleff D, Fay G. Developmental expectations: Intelligence and fine motor skills. In: Shurtleff D, ed. Myelodysplasias and Exstrophies: Significance, Prevention, and Treatment. New York: Grune & Stratton, 1986.

20. Wills KE, Holmbeck GN, Dillon K, McLone D. Intelligence and achievement in children with myelomeningocele. J Ped Psychol 1990; 15:161–176.
21. Mapstone T, Rekate H, Nulsen F, Dison M Jr, Glaser N, Jaffe M. Relationship of CSF shunting and IQ in children with myelomeningocele: a retrospective analysis. Childs Brain 1984; 11:112–118.
22. Shaffer J, Freidrich W, Shurtleff D, Wolf L. Cognitive and achievement status of children with myelomeningocele. J Ped Psychol 1988; 10:325–335.
23. Billard C, Santini JJ, Gilbert P, Nargeot MC, Adrien JL. Long term intellectual prognosis of hydrocephalus with reference to 77 children. Ped Neurosc 1986; 12:219–225.
24. Fletcher JM, Brookshire BL, Bohan TP, Brandt ME, Davidson KC. Early hydrocephalus. In: Rourke BP, ed. Syndrome of Nonverbal Learning Disabilities. New York: Guilford Press, 1995:206–238.
25. Ammerman RT, Reigel DH, Slomka GT, Zapadka ME. Neurosurgical and neurological correlates of neuropsychological functioning in spina bifida. Annual meeting of the American Academy for Cerebral Palsy and Developmental Medicine, San Antonio, 1998.
26. Donders J, Rourke BP, Canady AI. Neuropsychological functioning of hydrocephalic children. J Clin Experim Neuropsychol 1991; 13:407–413.
27. Rourke BP. Socioemotional disturbances of learning disabled children. J Consult Clin Psychol 1988; 56:801–810.
28. Rourke BP, ed. Syndrome of Nonverbal Learning Disabilities: Neurodevelopmental Manifestations. New York: Guilford Press, 1995.
29. Ris MD, Nortz MJ. Nonverbal learning disorders. In: Morgan JE, Ricker JH, eds. Handbook of Clinical Neuropsychology. Lisse, The Netherlands: Swets & Zeitlinger Publishers. In press.
30. Ammerman RT, Slomka GT, Reigel DH. Achievement and NLD features in spina bifida. Annual convention of the American Psychological Association, Chicago, 1997.
31. Yeates KO, Loss N, Colvin AN, Enrile BG. Do children with myelomeningocele and hydrocephalus display nonverbal learning disabilities? An empirical approach to classification. J Int Neuropsych Soc 2003; 9:653–662.
32. Dorner S. Adolescents with spina bifida. How they view their situation. Arch Dis Childhood 1976; 51:439–444.
33. Adams RC, Brei TJ, Sawin KJ. Behavioral health/mental health in spins bifida: an evidence-based medicine review of the literature. In: Liptak GS ed. Evidence-Based Practice in Spina Bifida: Developing a Research Agenda, May 9–10, 2003, Washington, DC. Washington, DC: Spina Bifida Association of America, 2003.
34. Yuker HE. Variables that influence attitudes toward people with disabilities: conclusions from the data. J Soc Beh Personality 1994; 9:3–22.
35. Bronfenbrenner U, ed. The Ecology of Human Development: Experiments by Nature and Design. Cambridge, MA: Harvard University Press, 1979.
36. Wallander JL, Varni JW. Social support and adjustment in chronically ill and handicapped children. Am J Community Psychol 1989; 17:185–201.
37. Holmbeck GN, Westhoven VC, Phillips WS, et al. A multimethod, multi-informant, and multidimensional perspective on psychosocial adjustment in preadolescents with spina bifida. J Consult Clin Psychol 2003; 71:782–796.
38. Wallander JL, Hubert NC, Varni JW. Child and maternal temperament characteristics, goodness of fit, and adjustment in physically handicapped children. J Clin Child Psychol 1988; 17:336–344.

39. Fletcher JM, Brookshire BL, Landry SH, et al. Behavioral adjustment of children with hydrocephalus: relationships with etiology, neurological, and family status. J Ped Psychol 1995; 20:109–125.
40. Ammerman RT, Van Hasselt VB, Hersen M, Moore LE. Assessment of social skills in visually impaired adolescents and their parents. Behav Assess 1989; 11:327–351.
41. Anderson EM, Clarke L. Disability in Adolescence. London: Methuen, 1982.
42. Appleton PL, Ellis NC, Minchom PE, Lawson V, Boll V, Jones P. Depressive symptoms and self-concept in young people with spina bifida. J Ped Psychol 1997; 22:707–722.
43. Vachha B, Adams R. Myelomeningocele, temperament patterns, and parental perceptions. Pediatrics 2005; 115:e58–e63.
44. Ellerton ML, Stewart MJ, Ritchie JA, Hirth AM. Social support in children with a chronic condition. Can J Nurs Res 1996; 28:15–36.
45. Van Hasselt VB, Ammerman RT, Hersen M, Reigel DH, Rowley FL. Assessment of social skills and problem behaviors in young children with spina bifida. J Dev Phys Disabilities 1991; 3:69–80.
46. Hurley AD, Dorman C, Laatsch L, Bell S, D'Avignon J. Cognitive functioning in patients with spina bifida, hydrocephalus, and the "cocktail party" syndrome. Dev Neuropsychol 1990; 6:151–172.
47. Quittner AL, DiGirolamo AM. Family adaptation to childhood disability and illness. In: Ammerman RT, Campo JV, eds. Handbook of Pediatric Psychology and Psychiatry, Vol. 2. Boston: Allyn & Bacon, 1998:70–102.
48. Holmbeck GN, Greenley RN, Coakley RM. Family functioning in children and adolescents with spina bifida: an evidence-based review. In: Liptak GS, ed. Evidence-Based Practice in Spina Bifida: Developing a Research Agenda, May 9–10, 2003, Washington, DC. Washington, DC: Spina Bifida Association of America, 2003.
49. Barakat LP, Linney JA. Optimism, appraisals, and coping in the adjustment of mothers and their children with spina bifida. J Child Fam Studies 1995; 4:303–320.
50. Holmbeck GN, Johnson SZ, Wills KE, et al. Observed and perceived parental overprotection in relation to psychosocial adjustment in preadolescents with a physical disability: the mediational role of behavioral autonomy. J Consult Clin Psychol 2002; 70:96–110.
51. Holmbeck GN, Gorey-Ferguson L, Hudson T, et al. Maternal, paternal, and marital functioning in families of preadolescents with spina bifida. J Ped Psychol 1997; 22:167–181.
52. Prout HT, Nowak-Drabik KM. Psychotherapy with persons who have mental retardation: an evaluation of effectiveness. Am J Ment Retard 2003; 108:82–93.
53. Hurley AD. Individual psychotherapy with mentally retarded individuals: a review and call for research. Res Dev Disabil 1989; 10:261–275.
54. Ammerman RT, Coe ME. Psychological and behavioral interventions. In: Coffey CE, Brumback RA, eds. Textbook of Pediatric Neuropsychiatry, 2nd ed. Washington, D.C.: American Psychiatric Press. In press.
55. Liptak GS, ed. Evidence-Based Practice in Spina Bifida: Developing a Research Agenda, May 9–10, 2003. Washington, D.C.: Spina Bifida Association America, 2003.

# 6

# Teenage Emphasis Achieving Independence

**Donna Cheek Zahra**
*Nemours Children's Clinic, Jacksonville, Florida, U.S.A.*

## INTRODUCTION

The teen years are a time of tremendous change in the lives of all young people and their families. This period of adolescence marks the time between childhood and adulthood and is recognized as a critical phase in the preparation for adult life. Although teens with spina bifida share the typical adolescent issues with all other teens, some aspects of adolescence can be complicated by the challenges of living with spina bifida. The purpose of this chapter is to examine the process of achieving independence as the focus of adolescence for individuals with spina bifida. This will include identifying factors that impact the ability of individuals with spina bifida to develop skills necessary to achieve independence, describing barriers to independence for teens with spina bifida, assessing progress in achieving independence, examining mechanisms for fostering independence, and evaluating outcomes related to achieving independence.

Adolescence is a dynamic period of biological change associated with physical and sexual maturity, changing relationships with parents and peers, and increasing autonomy and independence (1). It is an important crossroad in which the skills and abilities developed from childhood experiences are integrated and tested as the teen prepares for adult life. By the teenage years, young people are typically eager to test their independence. The process of achieving independence can be compromised by chronic conditions like spina bifida, when circumstances create obstacles that impede the acquisition of life experiences. These obstacles and the way in which individuals with spina bifida and their families manage them have a major effect on the process of achieving independence during adolescence.

## EMERGENCE OF INDEPENDENCE AS A PRIORITY FOR YOUTH WITH SPINA BIFIDA

As advances in medical technology made it possible for most children with spina bifida to live well into adulthood, the potential for these children to become productive, successful adults became evident (2). Issues related to independence emerged as expectations for the lives of individuals with spina bifida changed. The risk of sustained long-term dependence on parents and family was recognized as a major threat to their potential for success as adults (3). Promoting independence for individuals with spina bifida has been a priority for youth with spina bifida since the early 1980s.

The detailed physical care that is frequently part of the childhood experience of youth with spina bifida has created a situation where parents must be intimately involved in physical care at a time when children typically begin to do things for themselves. Parents must often provide total physical care during repeated hospitalizations and recuperation from surgical procedures, time-consuming bowel programs, and bladder catheterizations. In addition, the challenges of addressing medical and physical issues related to spina bifida are compounded when significant cognitive or learning issues are present. As a result, dependence on parents for care during childhood is a reality that has created a pattern of dependence that jeopardizes the development of skills necessary for independence. The tremendous degree of individual difference among individuals with spina bifida has complicated efforts to address independence issues systematically at all developmental levels. Acquiring age-appropriate skills related to independence has been and continues to be a priority, particularly during adolescence. Spina bifida continues to be recognized as a disability where those affected are likely to reach adulthood lacking the necessary life skills to live successfully (4). Research has yet to provide solid evidence to guide the development of independence skills in children or adolescents with spina bifida.

## THEORETICAL AND CONCEPTUAL PERSPECTIVES

A variety of theoretical perspectives can be used to explain the process through which adolescents with spina bifida achieve independence. Developmental theory, the theoretical framework most commonly used to understand the development of independence, identifies the emergence of autonomy as the developmental process particularly active during adolescence. The organization of this text illustrates the view that achieving independence is affected by human developmental stages regardless of the presence of a complicating condition such as spina bifida.

More recently, a holistic, interactional paradigm has been advocated as beneficial to understanding complex behaviors such as achieving independence. According to this perspective, individuals play an active, purposeful role, functioning within the context of their environment (5). This view is based on a strength perspective of human development and reflects the trend away from an emphasis on deficits and problems toward a developmental strengths-based and resilience-based approach (6). The construct of self-determination, with its basic characteristics of choice and control, has become widely accepted as crucial to achieving independence and therefore has significant implications for teens with spina bifida in their quest for independence (7).

## DEFINING INDEPENDENCE

Independence has been defined as "freedom from the control, influence, support, aid of others" (8) and as "not requiring or relying on others" (9). But, for individuals with spina bifida or those who live with or care for them, defining independence is far more complex. The term independence is generally used to refer to a constellation of factors that ultimately allow the individuals spina bifida to move beyond relying on others to meet their needs. The Disability Rights movement has influenced how independence is defined by shifting the focus toward individuals taking responsibility for their own behavior and making decisions regarding their own lives (10).

## FACTORS INFLUENCING INDEPENDENCE

From the moment of birth, a multitude of factors influence a young person's progress in developing the attitudes, skills, and assets that form building blocks for independence. Recognizing that an exhaustive account is virtually impossible, the following is an attempt to highlight some of the major factors thought to influence the success an adolescent with spina bifida will experience in achieving independence. To date, little research evidence exists to identify and explain the set of factors necessary to achieve independence during adolescence for individuals with spina bifida (11). Until evidence is available, research findings from related areas, clinical insight, and experience guide understanding for achieving independence. The adolescent's cognitive level, emotional status, self-care and self-management skills, social skills as well as the presence of key assets are critical factors. In addition, progress in assuming developmentally appropriate responsibility acquired through participation in activities in the home, school, or church provides an important base upon which to build during adolescence. The importance of entering adolescence with a set of attitudes and skills that form building blocks for achieving independence cannot be overstated.

Neurocognitive abilities affecting executive function, problem solving, and learning impact the process of achieving independence. Researchers examining the neuropsychological status of adolescents with spina bifida have documented the impact of hydrocephalus and shunting on spina bifida (12), although specific implications for independence have not been determined. Research has focused on higher-order cognitive abilities of conceptual reasoning, problem solving, and mental flexibility in adolescents with spina bifida and found that all subjects, regardless of IQ, had significant impairments of mental flexibility, efficiency of processing, conceptualization, or problem-solving ability (13).

Emotional or internal attributes play a tremendous role in achieving independence. This broad group of attributes includes initiative, self-concept, self-confidence, self-esteem, spirituality, locus of control, autonomy, self-determination, and resilience. Many of these have been identified as critical ingredients for psychosocial adjustment and achieving independence goals (14). Self-determination has been defined as the person's capacity to choose and have those choices as the determinants of one's own actions (15). The ability to make healthy, appropriate choices and act in self-determined way has been stressed as important for success in adult life (16). Resilience has been defined as the capability of individuals to cope successfully in the face of significant change, adversity, or risk (17). This ability to "bounce back" has been increasingly viewed as another critical ingredient for success in achieving independence.

Self-care has been a central issue for youth with spina bifida in their quest for independence. Children must have opportunities to learn and practice skills in self-care from as early an age as possible. By adolescence, readiness to assume responsibility for self-care, self-monitoring, and self-management is demonstrated by competence in specific aspects of care and the demonstration of established habits necessary for long-term successful independence (18). Children with spina bifida who enter adolescence having assumed responsibility for their own physical needs such as clean intermittent catheterization program, bowel program, and personal hygiene are in a better position to address other issues critical to achieving independence.

Social skills are critical to interacting with others, developing friendships, and building relationships. They are necessary if the adolescent is capable of the socialization and changing relationships that characterize adolescence. Developing and sustaining healthy relationship is critical to an adolescent's success in achieving independence. Of particular importance is the development of a network of relationships beyond the core family and healthy relationships with members of the opposite sex. Opportunities for developing positive relationships can occur through involvement in recreational activities, participation in a theatre group, in church activities, or as a team manager. Relationships that have the potential to grow and strengthen beyond a particular experience and beyond adolescence are of tremendous value.

Another aspect of developing healthy relationships and making healthy choices is sexuality. Sexuality can be addressed in a positive way as an example of making healthy choices. In a study that explored the sexual and reproductive health knowledge, attitudes, and behavior of 51 youths with spina bifida, 14 to 23 years old, researchers found that 95% of those interviewed reported inadequate knowledge about sexual and reproductive health relating to spina bifida, 60% reported an intimate relationship, and 25% reported sexual intercourse (19). Although early or precocious puberty has been considered common among youth with spina bifida, the influence of the timing of the onset of puberty on developing relationships during adolescence remains unclear (20).

The importance of becoming independent has been widely accepted but studies have also identified the need for interdependence between people and the importance of feeling accepted by others (21). Students who fail have been found to have few networks (15). Networking results in connections that build a support system, allowing an individual to function interdependently rather than in isolation. Networking skills are important in a variety of areas including job skills, recreation, and interacting with health professionals to meet health needs.

## ASSET DEVELOPMENT

The presence of basic assets that form the infrastructure for skills and abilities needed to develop independence is an important factor in increasing independence during adolescence. These assets function as tangible strengths that form the building blocks for achieving independence. Simple practices rooted in childhood lead to complicated behaviors in areas such as driving, money management, health promotion, job skills, and self-advocacy. Basic skills leading to self-advocacy, an integral part of self-determination, are tremendous assets as adolescents begin to make decisions. Asset development continues throughout adolescence providing additional strengths for achieving independence.

## ENVIRONMENTAL FACTORS

The adolescent's environment provides another significant factor that influences the development of independence. Sociocultural influences, including family variables, social environment, economics, and spiritual influence, have been found to impact the development of self-care practice in adolescents (22). An environment that provides experiences of success and focuses on an adolescent's strengths positively impacts the ability of a teen with spina bifida to achieve independence during adolescence.

## BARRIERS TO ACHIEVING INDEPENDENCE

Problems related to any of the factors influencing independence that have been discussed above can hinder the development of building block necessary for independence and become barriers for teens as they strive to achieve independence during adolescence. Learning problems related to nonverbal learning disabilities, memory, and math (23) create significant barriers to acquiring skills needed for independence. Researchers have identified specific tendencies associated with the neuropsychological issues and learning difficulties experienced by individuals with spina bifida, which may become barriers to achieving independence. They include an apparent disinterest in assuming responsibility for personal hygiene routines, failure to pursue hobbies or interests, and resistance to the motivational strategies that usually work for others (13). Poorly developed social skills represent a major barrier to building lasting positive relationships.

The development of physical problems, such as shunt infections necessitating revisions, pressure sores requiring long-term bed rest for healing, or surgical procedures, can become obstacles to the development of independence. Obesity can be a barrier to achieving independence by complicating mobility and participation in desired activities. Depression can complicate efforts to promote independence (24). In addition, physical issues that have not been resolved prior to adolescence can linger and become barriers to independence. For example, social incontinence places a tremendous barrier to normal adolescent experiences that promote independence. The situation becomes further complicated if the teen has developed an indifference to becoming continent. Reaching adolescence lacking necessary abilities in self-care adds additional barriers and makes it difficult for adolescents with spina bifida to experience success in achieving independence.

Overprotection by parents and/or other people with whom a teen with spina bifida interacts interferes with achieving independence. With the best of intentions, parents, family members, and caregivers often do things that the young people can and should do for themselves. Certain behavior patterns that promote dependence are simply a continuation of family habits that remain unrecognized. Overprotection may be the result of parental fear of perceived risk or parental perceptions of limitations in their child's abilities. As a result, young people growing up with disabilities often have decisions made for them and become conditioned to let others advocate for them creating a significant barrier to the development of skills in self-advocacy and self-determination.

Barriers to achieving independence undermine efforts to develop strengths that the teen began to develop during childhood. Identifying and altering behaviors or situations that have created barriers are crucial to further efforts to promote independence.

## ASSESSING PROGRESS OF DEVELOPING INDEPENDENCE

By the time a child with spina bifida reaches adolescence much has been gained (or lost) in the acquisition of attitudes, behaviors, and skills critical to achieving independence. Each young person enters adolescence at a unique point in this process. Multiple factors must be taken into consideration when assessing progress in achieving independence including the individual's personal traits, strengths and weaknesses, capacity for developing assets, experiences, and the environment.

Adolescence is framed by two critical transitions that provide key opportunities to assess progress in achieving independence. The first is the transition from childhood into adolescence and later, the transition from adolescence to adulthood. Although the transition from adolescence to adulthood has received greater attention, the transition to adolescence may offer an even greater potential benefit for assessing independence. An accurate assessment of the teen's "independence status" as the young person with spina bifida enters adolescence can maximize the opportunity to promote independence by building strengths and eliminating barriers throughout adolescence.

Few measurement tools have been developed specifically to assess independence. One early report from 1976, described a "functional activities scoring system" developed to quantitatively assess the status of daily living skills in individuals with spina bifida in an effort to provide a mechanism to set realistic goals (25). The Independent Behavior Inventory (26) was developed in 1989 to evaluate personal care skills, activities of daily living, communication, use of leisure, and general problem solving but reports of its use or effectiveness have not been published. More recent efforts to develop measures of independence have not been reported; a finding that supports the view that measuring independence is difficult and may explain why other tools and less formal methods have been more commonly used to gather information for assessing independence.

Neurocognitive testing can provide useful information regarding an adolescent's capacity for independence and may help identify potential barriers to achieving independence. Functional assessments, such as the functional independence measure for children (WeeFIM), the pediatric evaluation of disability inventory (PEDI), and the Vineland adaptive behavior scale have been used to assess selected domains related to independence. Assessments of adolescent decision making, self-management, and self-determination skills are becoming available (27). In addition, tools that identify potential problems, such as depression screening, may be useful.

Informal assessments can be used to evaluate the presence of behaviors necessary for independence. By adolescence, a young person with spina bifida has hopefully experienced success in achieving social continence, developed competencies in self-care, begun to develop abilities in self-management, and has interests outside the home. Learning about the teen's day-to-day activities, including how the teen functions in accomplishing daily routines, chores, or responsibilities at home, personal experiences with friends, at school, or camps is critical. In addition, answering questions such as: Do the adolescents with spina bifida answer questions directed to them? Do they demonstrate an understanding of their physical condition? Can they tell you about spina bifida, their level? Their shunt? What medications they take? How are their medications managed? Informal assessments allow questions to be tailored during an interview. Does the teen have personal goals? What are they? What is getting in the way of making them reality? How do they see themselves in 5 to 10 years? Does the teen spend the night away from parents or at a friend's house? It is particularly beneficial, when feasible, to observe actual behaviors as a component of assessing independence. It is difficult for parents and teens to recognize the extent to which parents or others actually provide assistance. They may inaccurately depict the teen as more independent than is actually true. In addition, observing the teen's behavior during interactions with others provides unique insight about social skills that are needed to develop and sustain meaningful friendships.

Individual progress in developing skills and assets related to independence is a process that can be assessed periodically throughout adolescence. The transition from adolescence to adulthood provides another key juncture to evaluate progress that has made in achieving independence during the teenage years and to identify strengths and weaknesses that exist as the young adult considers future goals.

## FOSTERING INDEPENDENCE

The stage for a teen's experience in achieving independence is set long before the onset of adolescence. The process of developing the building blocks necessary for achieving independence begins in infancy and continues through each stage of development (28). A major challenge for youth with spina bifida and those interacting with them is to recognize experiences that are critical to developing independence which may have been lost as a consequence of living with spina bifida and find ways to substitute other experiences that can provide missing building blocks.

Sparks of interest in increased independence and increased responsibility displayed by an adolescent with spina bifida should be encouraged. Adolescents must develop ownership of their own efforts toward independence. Looking ahead to anticipated roles and lifestyles can initiate a discussion with the teen about individual views of independence. Adolescents' perception about their control over life situations and the future influences their motivation and ability to develop independence skills. It is important to identify and alter perceptions that may undermine independence. These may include perceptions about lacking an understanding of the medical condition, having little control over medical treatment, being treated the same as other kids, ability to go out on dates, and future job opportunities (6). Involvement in experiences that enhance confidence and self-perception such as being a mentor for younger children can foster independence (29).

Adolescence is a time to review daily routines to consider their implications on future independence goals and make alterations to ensure that routines can be completely accomplished by the individual under anticipated conditions. Continence issues that have not been resolved prior to adolescence become a priority. Adolescents can use these years to become 'independent" in managing their own urological and bowel programs to achieve social continence. If independence does not seem feasible, adolescence is an appropriate time to begin a discussion about how to provide necessary assistance and how the adolescent can maintain control over the entire process even though unable to perform the actual task. Resolving the continence issue is a critical prerequisite to achieving future goals related to independent living and employment. An adolescent with spina bifida may also have to address any of a variety of other physical issues (including skin care, mobility, and medications) within the context of independence goals. Areas of self-management can be gradually expanded to include initiation of specific behaviors, minimizing the need for prompts and practicing when and how to contact help if a problem develops. In addition, health-promotion behaviors related to nutrition, exercise, and lifestyles should be reviewed and efforts made to establish them as part of the daily routine in an effort to facilitate developing the teen's self-concept as a healthy person who happens to have a disability.

Adolescents should be encouraged to speak for themselves and be given every opportunity to do so. Creating opportunities to actively teach social skills, including discussions of the subtleties and nuances of interpersonal interactions, can promote the development of successful relationships. Sexuality, including contraception must be addressed even when it is tempting to assume that young people are not sexually active. It is important to speak openly, encouraging frank discussion and questions.

Efforts directed toward realizing future independence goals, such as money management, driving, or employment, should continue throughout adolescence by identifying and providing stepping stones leading to these complicated tasks. The importance of developing an experiential base cannot be overstressed for most activities. Find easier, simpler ways, if necessary, to compensate for obstacles related to managing financial concerns. Beginning early allows time to establish realistic practices. Driving is a tremendous asset to achieving independence but requires consideration on an individualized basis. Formal driving evaluations are available. Practice through learning how to steer a riding lawn mower or other moving vehicle as a precursor to learning to drive a car is valuable. Job skills are built on other assets like social skills, organization skills, and reliability and fostered by elementary work experiences.

Self-determination has been considered critical to achieving independence and success in adulthood. Children growing up with disabilities frequently do not have typical opportunities to learn self-determination. Becoming self-determined may require systematic instruction in making choices (30) and participation in organized experiences that promote empowerment, perceived competence, and other self-determination skills (31), as well as experiencing personal achievement (32). It has also been suggested (33) that a shift in the attitudes and the perspectives of individuals with disabilities, their families, teachers, and human service providers must occur if self-determination is to be fostered. The adolescent's experience in achieving independence is affected by the people and institutions in their environment. The individuals and systems with which adolescents with spina bifida interact, day-to-day, play a critical role in fostering the development of independence.

## Family

An adolescent's family can foster independence in many ways. The importance of the family has been discussed in Chapter 12 but is stressed again to underscore the critical role the family plays in facilitating the adolescents experience in achieving independence. The major task of parenting during adolescence involves being responsive to the adolescents need for increased responsibility and behavioral autonomy while maintaining family cohesion (20). The increasing independence of teens can upset the dynamics of the family, particularly a family whose life has been centered on caring for a child with spina bifida.

By focusing on their adolescent's strengths, parents send positive messages fostering independence in the way they encourage, push, support, set expectations, provide opportunities, and accept mistakes (29). Families have the opportunity to instill confidence and set expectations for independence from early childhood. This includes minimizing the tendency to be overprotective by recognizing behavior patterns or habits that promote dependence. By treating their child with spina bifida no differently than other children in the family, providing opportunities to make choices and solve problems, giving them the freedom to fail, and helping them to become resilient, parents create an environment for achieving independence during adolescence. In addition, parents can provide opportunities for socialization and the development of a broad network of relationships.

Parents are, also, in a position to foster self-determination. It is important that an adolescent do the talking when interacting, in medical visits or meetings, with school staff. This requires that parents resist the temptation to speak and answer questions for their child. Children with disabilities who were raised in families that provided opportunities for self-determination have been shown to assume greater control over their lives (34).

## Friends

Friends play an important role in the quest of an adolescent with spina bifida to achieve independence. Friends, whether peers or adults, may be mentor, role model, sounding board, or one who gives a timely push. Successful young adults with spina bifida have described the important role their friends have played in encouraging and supporting them as they struggled to achieve independence (29). In another study (35), participants described wanting a personal relationship with an adult, whom they trusted and was available to "encourage their efforts, validate their fears, and celebrate their accomplishments" (p. 525).

Developing a broad group of friends and building relationships with other people create a social support network that can continue into adulthood when isolation poses a threat to success in living independently and quality of life. The need for interdependence and a supportive network of people has been emphasized (28). Too often, families have found themselves filling in for lack of friends and as a main resource for support and leisure time.

## School

During adolescence, school experiences have a tremendous influence on a teen's progress in achieving independence. The school provides a forum for social interaction with peers as well as adults. It provides varied opportunities for involvement in clubs, sports, and other activities. Independence, from the school's perspective, is typically considered within the context of the broad "transition" efforts that have emerged to prepare youth with disabilities for adulthood.

The active role schools have taken in assisting students to develop skills needed to achieve independence have been the result of a national effort that has focused on the transition from school to adult life for youth with disabilities. Transition efforts have been driven by federal legislation, particularly the passage of the 1990 amendments of the Individuals with Disabilities Education Act (P.L.101-476, IDEA) (36). Subsequently, the Individuals with Disabilities Education Act amendments of 1997 (P.L.105-17) (37) and its associated 1999 Regulations expanded transition concepts by initiating transition planning by age 14 and instituting a more holistic view of the transition process. Increasingly, the focus has been expanded to include elements directly related to achieving independence including "social" outcomes and developing the myriad of "life skills" requisite to achieve independence and success in adult life for individuals with disabilities. Student involvement in decision making has been emphasized as important to promote independence (38). Although the concept of student involvement in decision making preceded IDEA, and was mandated by IDEA (1990), implementation has been difficult. "Person-centered planning" has become popular as a mechanism for including the individual and parents as full participants in the transition planning process and building skills in self-determination and choice-making (39).

A number of best practices, identified through research, have implications for schools in their efforts to foster independence. They include parental involvement and student involvement (40), instruction in self-determination skills (41), acquisition of daily living skills, community instruction, social inclusion, functional vocational assessment, and vocation-related activities including work experiences (42). Although research has yet to be conducted specifically on youth with spina bifida, the findings of these studies of transition have implications for the process of achieving independence for teens with spina bifida.

## PROGRAMS/INTERVENTIONS

Programs designed to enhance levels of independence in adolescents with spina bifida have existed since the 1980s. Early reports suggested their effectiveness, particularly in providing support and socialization (43). Programs and interventions designed to promote independence have typically evolved as efforts of spina bifida clinics and local spina bifida associations. Many programs have been developed throughout the country as "camps" offering overnight experiences to develop skills related to independence (44). Camps, some of which have been hospital based, typically include developmentally appropriate efforts to encourage the development of skills in self-care, bowel and bladder management, social interaction, sports, and recreation.

A few adolescent or transition clinics have been created as a component of multidisciplinary spina bifida clinics to focus on adolescent and transition issues as a component of providing comprehensive health care. These programs are being developed to tackle issues related to independence, identify problem areas, address the prevention of secondary conditions, and include efforts to assist adolescents to begin assuming responsibility for health care and prepare for their transition into adult health-care settings. Occasionally, specific programs have been initiated to facilitate the development of specific skills related to independence. One, "GOAL independence, go out and learn independence," was created to promote the development of social skills and is available to teens with spina bifida in Wisconsin (45). Adolescents with spina bifida also have a continuously expanding set of resources available through Internet websites, particularly those offered by the Spina Bifida Association of America. These provide opportunities to interact with other adolescents and adults who live with spina bifida and personally address issues related to achieving independence.

## EVALUATING INDEPENDENCE OUTCOMES

Evidence related to desired outcomes for independence of teens with spina bifida has yet to be identified through research. Anticipated outcomes for adolescents with spina bifida that have been posed include appropriate growth and development, freedom from secondary disabilities, participation in self-care, and appropriate educational development (28). High-school graduation has been the key target for school efforts and selected outcomes after graduation have been of primary interest. Governmental agencies and legislative acts have identified employment as the accepted postschool outcome (46). Although employment remains a highly emphasized outcome, the language of IDEA acknowledged the relevance and importance of other desired postschool outcomes for individuals with disabilities. Additional outcomes that have been suggested include a sense of empowerment (38), self-determination (47), and independence/interdependence (33). The findings of one study support research documenting the benefit of student self-determination in terms of improved secondary and postsecondary outcomes. Researchers found that student identified transition goals, and personally meaningful activities including career-related work experiences were associated with improved graduation and employment outcomes (35).

Although not specific to individuals with spina bifida, numerous studies have raised concerns about postschool outcomes for students with disabilities in terms of employment, economic dependence, dependence on others, dissatisfaction with social lives, segregation, and quality of life (45,48). Youth with spina bifida have been reported to be lagging behind in social outcomes (49). Research specifically examining independence outcomes for individuals with spina bifida has yet to be reported. One study reviewed the outcomes of a 25-year cohort of individuals with spina bifida (50). This study, which focused primarily on physical and medical outcomes of patients ranging broadly in age included interesting educational, employment, and independence outcomes. Those surveyed reported educational outcomes in which greater than 50% had attended regular class and graduated from high school, employment outcomes in which approximately 50% were employed, and independent living outcomes in which far less than 50% were living independently. These findings suggest the need for an increased focus on achieving independence during adolescence in an effort to enhance postadolescent outcomes.

## RECOMMENDATIONS

1. Anticipate the long-term implications of achieving independence as early as possible—begin at birth.
2. Promote the development of independence skills as a normal part of every day life—never do for children or adolescents what they can do for themselves.
3. Facilitate broad life experiences allowing opportunities to fail.
4. Identify ways to compensate for lost opportunities related to independence—minimize barriers and remove obstacles to allow the development of autonomy and self-determination.
5. Assess individual strengths and barriers related to achieving independence as adolescence begins.
6. Capitalize on the transition into adolescence as a critical juncture to assess the development of independence skills.
7. Work collaboratively with the school system in transition efforts to empower adolescents with spina bifida to have full participation in making decisions that affect their life.
8. Utilize research findings related to promoting self-determination, resilience, and achieving desired independence outcomes as they become available.

The success young people with spina bifida experience in achieving independence during adolescence has a tremendous impact on their future transition to adulthood. Adolescents with spina bifida who have developed the skills and abilities they need to make healthy choices and decisions about how they want to live their lives, developed appropriated social skills and meaningful relationships, acquired necessary assets, built on personal strengths, and overcome obstacles can anticipate entering adult life successfully achieving personal goals and quality of life.

## REFERENCES


1. Lichtenstein S. Characteristics of youth and young adults. In: Rusch FR, Chadsey JG, eds. Beyond High School: Transition from School to Work. Belmont, CA: Wadsworth Publishing Co., 1998:3–35.
2. Edwards-Beckett J, Cedargren D. The sociocultural context of families with a child with myelomeningocele. Issues Compr Pediatr Nurs 1995; 18:27–42.
3. Holmbeck GN, Johnson SZ, Wills KE, McKernon W, Rose B, Erklin S, Kemper T. Observed and perceived parental overprotection in relation to psychosocial adjustment in pre-adolescents with a physical disability: the mediational role of behavioral autonomy. J Consult Clin Psychol 2002; 70(1):96–110.
4. Holmbeck GN, Faier-Routman J. Spinal lesion level, shunt status, family relationships, and psychosocial adjustment in children with spina bifida myelomeningocele. J Pediatr Psychol 1995; 20(6):817–832.
5. Bergman LR, Cairns RB, Nilsson LG, Nystedt L. Developmental Science and the Holistic Approach. New Jersey: Lawrence Erlbaum Associates, Publishers, 2000.
6. Sawin KJ, Brei TJ, Buran CF, Fastenau PS. Factors associated with quality of life in adolescents with spina bifida. J Holistic Nurs 2002; 20(3):279–304.
7. Wehmeyer ML. Self-determination and individuals with significant disabilities: Examining meanings and misinterpretations. JASH 1998; 23(1):5–16.
8. The Random House Dictionary of the English Language. 2nd ed. New York: Random House, 1987.
9. Merriam-Webster's Collegiate Dictionary. 10th ed. Springfield, Massachusetts: Merriam-Webster, Incorporated, 1997.
10. Ward MJ, Meyer RN. Self-determination for people with developmental disabilities and autism. Focus Autism Other Dev Disabil 1999; 14(3):133–139.
11. Liptak GS, ed. Evidence-Based Practice in Spina Bifida: Developing a Research Agenda. Wasington, D.C.: Spina Bifida Association of America, 2003.
12. Hommet C, Billiard C, Gillet P, et al. Neurologic and adaptive functioning in adolescents and young adults shunted for congenital hydrocephalus. J Child Neurol 1999; 14:144–150.
13. Dise JE, Lohr ME. Examination of deficits in conceptual reasoning abilities associated with spina bifida. Am J Phys Med Rehabil 1998; 77(3):247–251.
14. Holmbeck GN, Coakley RM, Hommeyer JS, Shapera WE, Westhoven VC. Observed and perceived dyadic and systemic functioning in families of preadolescents with spina bifida. J Pediatr Psychol 2002; 27(2):177–189.
15. Serna LA, Lau-Smith J. Learning with purpose: self-determination skills for students who are at risk for school and community failure. Interv Sch Clin 1995; 30:142–146.
16. Wehmeyer M, Sands DJ. Making It Happen. Baltimore: Paul H. Brookes Publishing Co., 1998.
17. Stewart M, Reid G, Mangham C. Fostering children's resilience. J Pediatr Nurs 1997; 12(1):21–31.
18. Williams J, Lyttle S. Mother and teacher reports of behaviour and perceived self-competence of children with hydrocephalus. Eur J Pediatr Surg 1998; 8(1):5–9.
19. Sawyer SM, Roberts KV. Sexual and reproductive health in young people with spina bifida. Dev Med Child Neurol 1999; 41(10):671–675.

20. Coakley RM, Holmbeck GN, Friedman D, Greenley RN, Thill AW. A longitudinal study of pubertal timing, parent–child conflict, and cohesion in families of young adolescents with spina bifida. J Pediatr Psychol 2002; 27(5):461–473.
21. King GA, Cathers T, Polgar JM, MacKinnon E, Havens L. Success in life for older adolescents with cerebral palsy. Qual Health Res 2000; 10(6):734–739.
22. McCaleb A, Cull VV. Sociocultural influences and self-care practices of middle adolescents. J Pediatr Nurs 2000; 15(1):30–35.
23. Dennis M, Barnes MA. Math and numeracy in young adults with spina bifida and hydrocephalus. Dev Neuropsychol 2002; 21:141–155.
24. Sandler A. Living with Spina Bifida. Chapel Hill: University of North Carolina Press, 1997:206–207.
25. Sousa JC, Gordon LH, Shurtleff DB. Assessing the development of daily living skills in patients with spina bifida. Dev Med Child Neurol Suppl 1976; 37:134–142.
26. Lollar DJ, Reinoehl JK, Leverette AT, Martin JC. Fascilitating and assessing progress toward independence: SPARX. Z Kinderchir 1989; 44:18–20.
27. Sawin KJ, Brei TJ, Adams RC. Issues related to independence in persons with spina bifida: an evidence based medicine review of the literature. Evidence-Based Practice in Spina Bifida: Developing a Research Agenda, Washington, 2003:1–9.
28. Peterson PM, Rauen K, Brown J, Cole J. Spina bifida: the transition into adulthood begins in infancy. Rehabil Nurs 1994; 19(4):229–238.
29. Zahra D. Living Successfully as Young Adults with Spina Bifida and Hydrocephalus. Ph.D. dissertation, University of Florida, Gainesville, Florida, 2002.
30. Hoffman A, Field S. Promoting self-determination through effective curriculum development. Interv Sch Clin 1995; 30(3):135–141.
31. Powers LE, Ellison R, Matuszewski J, Wilson R, Phillips A, Rein C. A multi-component intervention to promote adolescent self-determination. J Rehabil 2001; 67(4):13–19.
32. Owens TJ, Mortimer JT, Finch MD. Self-determination as a source of self-esteem in adolescence. Soc Forces 1996; 74(4):1377–1404.
33. Lehmann JP, Deniston TL, Tobin R, Howard D. Sharing the journey: an individual and integrated systems approach to self-determination. Career Dev Except Indiv 1996; 19:1–14.
34. Abery BH, Rudrud L, Arndt K, Schauben L, Eggebeen A. Evaluating a multi-component program for enhancing the self-determination of youth with disabilities. Interv Sch Clin 1995; 30:170–179.
35. Benz MR, Lindstrum L, Yovanoff P. Improving graduation and employment outcomes of students with disabilities: predictive factors and student perspectives. Except Child 2000; 66(4):502–529.
36. Individuals with Disabilities Education Act of 1990 (IDEA), PL. No. 101-476, 20 U.S.C. 1400 et seq.
37. Individuals with Disabilities Education Act Amendments of 1997, PL. 105-17, 20 U.S.C. 1400 et seq.
38. Wehmeyer M, Lawrence M. Whose future is it anyway? Promoting student involvement in transition planning. Career Dev Except Indiv 1995; 18:69–83.
39. Hanley-Maxwell C, Pogoloff S, Whitney-Thomas J. Families: the heart of transition. In: Rusch FR, Chadsey JG, eds. Beyond High School: Transition from School to Work. Belmont, CA:Wadsworth Publishing Co., 1998:234–264.

40. Martin JE, Marshall LH. Choicemaker: a comprehensive self-determination transition program. Interv Sch Clin 1995; 30:147–156.
41. Collet-Klingenberg LL. The reality of best practices in transition: a case study. Except Child 1998; 65(1):67–78.
42. Rusch FR, Chadsey JG. Beyond High School: The Transition from School to Work. New York: McGraw-Hill, 1998.
43. Sherman RG, Berling BS, Oppenheimer S. Increasing community independence for adolescents with spina bifida. Adolescence 1985; 20(77):1–13.
44. Telenko A. Penn State Hershey Medical Center Spina Bifida Camp. Presentation at the Nursing and Healthcare Professionals Council Education Program. SBAA National Conference, Orlando, Florida, 2002.
45. Rauen K. G.O.A.L. Independence: Go Out and Learn Independence. Presentation at the SBAA National Conference, Washington, DC, 2004.
46. Kohler PD. Implementing a transition perspective of education. In: Rusch FR, Chadsey JG, eds. Beyond High School: Transition from School to Work. Belmont, CA: Wadsworth Publishing Co., 1998:180.
47. Wehmeyer ML. A career education approach: self determination for youth with mild cognitive disabilities. Interv Sch Clin 1995; 30(3):157–163.
48. Thurlow M, Elliott J. Student assessment and evaluation. In: Rusch FR, Chadsey JG, eds. Beyond High School: Transition from School to Work. Belmont, CA: Wadsworth Publishing Co., 1998:234–264.
49. Loomis J, Javornisky JG, Monahan JJ, Burke G, Lindsay A. Relations between family environment and adjustment outcomes in young adults with spina bifida. Dev Med Child Neurol 1997; 39:620–627.
50. Bowman RM, McClone DG, Grant JA, Tomita T, Ito J. Spina bifida outcome: a 25 year prospective. J Pediatr Neurosurg 2001; 34(3):114–120.

# 7

# Adolescent Health-Care Transition

**Thomas S. Webb and Tena Benson**
*Division of Developmental and Behavioral Pediatrics, Cincinnati Children's Hospital Medical Center, Cincinnati, Ohio, U.S.A.*

## INTRODUCTION

Due to the success of medical technology, families, providers, advocacy groups, and public policies, up to 80% of children born with spina bifida are living well into adulthood (1). They represent some of the 500,000 to 750,000 children with special health-care needs who reach adult age each year in the United States (2). They also represent a new challenge for a health-care system that has only recently recognized this relatively new group of patients.

Historically, the adult and pediatric medical systems have operated mostly independent of each other. Pediatrics usually encompasses care from birth until an arbitrary age, usually 18 or 21, at which time patients would be released from the practice. Often, there is no formal transfer to adult-oriented health providers. With otherwise healthy adolescents and young adults, there usually is little interaction with the health-care system in mid-to-late adolescence and young adulthood. The healthy late adolescent rarely has a need for medical care, with the exception of required school, sports, or work physicals. During these years, the adolescent is leaving high school and entering college, vocational-technical school, or beginning work so that insurance for this age group is often transient (i.e., college health plans) or nonexistent (3). Therefore, the adolescent simply stops seeing the pediatric provider; receives occasional urgent medical care for illness and injury from nonspecific providers during post-high school training and initial employment; and eventually seeks out a long-term relationship with an adult provider only when new circumstances (i.e., a new chronic condition) develop (4). There may be many years and miles in between the end of the pediatric care and the beginning of routine, consistent adult care for most typically developing adolescents.

Conversely, adolescents with spina bifida have multiple chronic medical conditions requiring ongoing surveillance and treatment. As with other youth with special health-care needs (YSHCN), they usually have longstanding relationships with multiple pediatric providers and continue to have regularly scheduled medical visits to the pediatric system throughout their adolescent years. Like other YSHCN, adolescents with spina bifida reach a crossroads in care where their chronological age becomes an issue for the pediatric system. Because of historical hospital, insurance, and occasionally state regulations, as well as the comfort level of some pediatric providers, YSHCN are often requested or required to seek medical care from adult-oriented providers and locations that may or may not be prepared to assume care. Conversely, some patients with chronic childhood conditions continue to seek care at pediatric institutions through middle age or later (5).

Since the 1989 Surgeon General's conference "Growing Up and Getting Medical Care: Youth with Special Health Care Needs," there has been a growing awareness of this chasm in medical service (6). The importance of adolescent health-care transition for YSHCN has been recognized by the major organizations representing pediatrics, family medicine, adolescent medicine, and adult internal medicine (7). The need for adolescent health-care transition services to adult-oriented care has also been recognized in spina bifida care (8,9).

Despite this awareness by the health-care system, there remain inadequate services for health-care transition. There have been only a few specialty clinics in the United States that offer transition services (10). A national survey of children with special health-care needs (SHCN) revealed that only 50% parents of 14- to 17-year olds with SHCN had discussed transition issues with the adolescent's doctor and only 16% had discussed and developed a transition plan (11). Less is known about the services and plans offered to adolescents with spina bifida. Some have adapted general guidelines of health-care transition for adolescents with any developmental disability (9). Others have done descriptive studies on regional groups of adolescents with spina bifida (8). Most of the literature on adolescent health-care transition has not been evidence-based, but consists of consensus statements, expert opinion, and regional experiences incorporating a broad variety of chronic childhood conditions.

## PRINCIPLES OF ADOLESCENT HEALTH-CARE TRANSITION

Adolescent health-care transition is defined as "the purposeful, planned movement of adolescents and young adults with chronic physical and medical conditions from child-centered to adult-centered systems" (12). Health-care transition is one of several concurrent developmental changes that also include the adolescent learning to move (*i*) from parental home life to living in the community, (*ii*) from high school to postsecondary education, training, or work, (*iii*) to independent participation in leisure activities, and (*iv*) toward the formation and maintenance of adult relationships (13). Health plays an important role in each of these transitions, and the complex medical and developmental issues in spina bifida impact each adolescent's rate and route through these changes. While this chapter will focus on adolescent health-care transition, the reader should be aware of the reciprocal relationships among all the facets of adolescent transition. Information on the educational, vocational, and community living aspects of transition are reviewed elsewhere (13) and will be highlighted here with respect to their impact on health-care transition.

The general principles of adolescent health-care transition include the following:

1. Health-care transition is a process and not an event (14). It involves more than just the transfer of care from pediatricians to adult providers. As a process, transition includes three stages: early, future orientation; middle, skills development; and late, actual transitions (15).
2. The process of transition should begin long before the anticipated transfer of care. Many believe transition should begin at the time of diagnosis; for spina bifida, this would be following the prenatal diagnosis or the delivery of the infant (16). While there will be numerous more immediate concerns for the health team, family, and infant, maintaining the expectation that the child will eventually be an adult helps the family develop a future orientation. Parents have identified this advice as important to their overall focus for the child and helped the parents to foster independence in the child (17).
3. A formalized transition plan should begin by age 14. This correlates with the timeline for transition plan development in the public school system (18). The health-care team, in concert with the adolescent and family, should develop a health-care transition plan outlining the skills, services, providers, finances, and agencies needed to maximize the autonomy of the future adult patient. The written plan should be reviewed and updated annually and include specifically identified adult-oriented health-care providers, community-based adult services, and financial assistance (7,14).
4. At each phase of the transition process, there should be a specifically identified health-care professional who understands the unique issues of transition and assumes responsibility for current health-care, care coordination, and future planning (7). The actual individual responsible for coordination of care can change as the needs and services move from pediatrics to adult-oriented care. Ideally, this transition coordinator would use the medical home concept of "accessible, continuous, comprehensive, family centered, coordinated, compassionate, and culturally effective" care (19).

5. The course of transition should be flexible and developmentally appropriate to meet the individual needs of the adolescent; therefore, the actual timeline can be variable and should not be determined or completed based only on age (14).
6. Transition should encourage and promote increasing autonomy, personal responsibility, and self-reliance by the adolescent. Families should be continuously encouraged to change their focus from providers of care to advocates for the adolescent. The adolescent should be allowed to attempt self-care and occasionally fail rather than wait until the caregivers are assured of success (14).
7. A comprehensive but concise medical summary should be prepared for transfer of important medical history to the receiving providers (7,8,20). Inadequate medical history has been identified by adult providers as a significant barrier to successful transition of care (21). Ideally, the adolescent would play a significant role in the development of the medical history summary, which could facilitate improved self-care knowledge and skills (9).
8. Transition should include typical adolescent preventive care, services, and education, including access to information on typical adolescent issues, such as growth and development, sexuality, mood and other mental health disorders, substance abuse, and health promotion and disease prevention (7,14). These topics should be modified to incorporate the impact of spina bifida, hydrocephalus, neurogenic bowel and bladder, mobility, and learning differences for the individual adolescent (22,23).
9. Transfer should occur at a time of medical stability (24).
10. Adolescents and families should be prepared for the differences in culture and style that exists between pediatric and adult-oriented providers and systems (4).

## POTENTIAL BARRIERS TO SUCCESSFUL HEALTH-CARE TRANSITION

Each of these 10 principles attempts to alleviate the problems that have been previously identified as potential barriers to successful health-care transition. These barriers can come from the pediatric or adult systems, the family, or the adolescent (24). The adolescent may have concerns about working with the new health-care team due to a lack of familiarity and trust, the noticeable difference in age between themselves and the other adult patients in the adult providers' practices, the level of autonomy expected of the adolescent by the adult providers, and the lack of input from the adolescent's family allowed by the adult providers.

The family may also feel left out of the decisions and discussions between the adult providers and the young adult patient. While the parents and caregivers were previously integral to the pediatric care plans, the adult system is much less familiar with this type of family-centered care. The pediatric providers admit concerns with the practice style and knowledge base of the adult providers and systems with respect to the issues and needs of YSHCN, and often hold on to patients longer than the typical 18- to 21-year cut-off. The adult providers may be uncertain how to handle the inconsistent knowledge base, potentially delayed self-care and self-advocacy skills, and different expectations of the young adults. The adult providers may feel uncomfortable receiving input and sharing clinical decision making with parents and guardians in addition to the patient. Finally, the adult providers may have additional concerns regarding their own knowledge and abilities caring for patients with previously uncommon diagnoses in the adult population.

## Transition Begins at Diagnosis

Transition is a process not an event. The ideal beginning of transition is at the time of diagnosis so that the parents, caregivers, health-care team, and child continually focus on the need to develop personal skills, family expectations, financial resources, school and vocational supports, and community services that will eventually lead to a maximally autonomous adult life (16). Those without this future orientation often find themselves surprised and unprepared for the simultaneous graduations from public education, pediatric healthcare, and child-oriented community services. Reiss calls this stage "envisioning the future" (15). Detailed plans are not necessary and revisions are expected to occur as the chronic condition changes over time. By considering a 20- to 30-year vision, families can more effectively research school districts, community services, insurance plans, retirement and personal financial plans, home designs, and other issues that will eventually be impacted by this special needs child. Invaluable resources in this future planning are national organizations such as the Spina Bifida Association of America (SBAA) and other families who have already traveled these paths (25).

## Individualized Transition Plans

The concept of adolescent health-care transition derives from the education system, which developed transition planning in response to several important federal legislative polices. As a result of the Individuals with Disabilities Education Act (IDEA) of 1997 (Public Law 105-17), individualized transition plans (ITP) must be incorporated into the individualized education program (IEP) by age 14–16. Transition services are defined as a "coordinated set of activities" that include "instruction, related services, community experiences, the development of employment and other postschool adult living objectives and, when appropriate, acquisition of daily living skills and functional vocational evaluation" [§602(30)]. Therefore, the adolescent's school can become an active partner in teaching self-advocacy and self-care skills, including functional health skills, such as learning how to fill prescriptions, understanding the importance of medical procedures, learning the signs and symptoms of acute illness or exacerbations of chronic illness, learning how to make appointments, developing interview skills, and making lists of questions for doctor visits. The health-care provider can participate in the IEP as team member and/or consultant (26).

While incorporating functional health skills into the school ITP will exponentially increase the adolescent's exposure to these important self-care skills, the full health-care transition plan should be designed by the adolescent, family, and medical team independent of the IEP. The plan should address each medical issue affecting the adolescent, what is needed to facilitate transition, who will be responsible for monitoring progress for that issue, what will constitute readiness for transfer of care, and what financial issues will need to be addressed. For the typical adolescent with spina bifida, the usual medical issues to include are:

1. Medication management
2. Neurological/neurosurgical needs
3. Ophthalmologic needs
4. Orthopedic needs
5. Bowel/continence issues
6. Urologic needs
7. Skin issues
8. Mental health issues
9. Primary and preventive care needs
10. Equipment needs
11. Activities of daily living skills
12. Functional health skills needs
13. Transportation issues

The transition plan would include the current and future provider for each service, when transition is likely, and the information needed by the receiving team.

## Self-Care Skills

An integral part of successful transition planning is the adolescent's development of independent self-care skills. Due to cognitive, motor, and specific learning disabilities, not all adolescents with spina bifida will become completely independent in functional health and self-care skills; however, all can and should be encouraged to reach their maximum autonomy (16). Often, the inability to perform a self-care skill is attributed to a mood or motivational issue when, in fact, the problem is an unrecognized learning, motor, or coordination (visual-motor or visual-perceptual) impairment (27). Screening for executive function, attention, and working memory problems, such as with attention deficit hyperactivity disorder screening tools, can identify learning disabilities that can respond to pharmacologic and cognitive-behavioral interventions. Simple adaptations such as reminder signs in the bedroom or bathroom, laying out pills in a conspicuous area, or setting alarms on watches, beepers, and cell phones can markedly increase a young person's adherence to medication, bladder, and bowel regimens. Similarly, an occupational therapy evaluation can identify motor and coordination difficulties and either provide therapeutic interventions or adaptive equipment to facilitate greater autonomy. An example is an evaluation that identifies adaptations to help an adolescent with fine motor difficulties to independently unbutton and unzip his pants, cleanly self-catheterize, and clean-up his materials in a public restroom.

One approach to determining the current health-related knowledge base and educational needs of an adolescent is through an interpretive interview and teaching physical exam (28). Although this evaluation requires significantly greater time than a typical medical encounter, it serves multiple important roles in the transition process. In preparation for the interview, the provider reviews and summarizes the adolescent's pertinent medical and developmental history that can serve as the medical summary delivered to the adult team. Through the chart review and interview, the provider better understands the adolescent's cognitive, academic, language, and self-advocacy skills and can make recommendations for further evaluation or therapy. In addition to identifying learning issues, the adolescent's mental health, motivation, and autonomy can be assessed. The comprehensive interview covers the etiology and impact of spina bifida on each body system, the possible treatments and procedures to maximize function, and the preventive health recommended to minimize the development of secondary conditions. The adolescent's current knowledge is assessed and recommendations for ongoing education can be made. In addition, the adolescent can discuss his own values and desires regarding the management of these medical issues.

The teaching physical examination is a companion educational and evaluative opportunity where the adolescent can utilize visual learning. With the assistance of adaptive equipment such as long handle mirrors, the clinician can show the adolescent their myelomeningocele scars, subcutaneous shunt tubing, pressure areas susceptible to skin breakdown, problem areas developing under orthotics or on the feet, ostomies, and the perineal and genitourinary areas. Because of physical limitations and altered sensation, many adolescents with spina bifida will not have explored their own bodies like their typically developing peers and may never have seen or felt these parts of their body. Similarly, neither the adolescent nor the parents may have felt comfortable examining these areas together at home.

The optimal timing for the interpretive interview and teaching physical exam is not chronologically based, but could be started when developmentally appropriate. It can be performed intermittently throughout adolescence to both reinforce knowledge and assess progress. Due to the extended time needed to cover all the material, as well as the privacy required to make the adolescent feel comfortable, this evaluation should not occur during a busy, crowded multidisciplinary clinic visit. As much as possible, visual materials should be used as part of the interpretive interview. There are many handouts and pamphlets available from the SBAA (29) as well as other spina bifida websites (30,31). These handouts are helpful by utilizing common, nontechnical language. The goal of the interpretive interview is ultimately for the adolescent to understand the effects of spina bifida on their health and to be able to summarize the important clinical information. Encouraging the adolescent to develop his own portable medical record in preparation for these teaching clinical encounters may facilitate learning the specific medical issues while also developing general health literacy.

### Fostering Autonomy

The transition process necessitates significant changes for the parents and caregivers separate from the adolescent. Until this phase of the adolescent's life, the parents and caregivers have directed, decided, and advocated for most of the child's complicated medical care. Now these caregivers need to be encouraged to gradually, but continually, transfer control of these decisions to the adolescent. Because of previous experience with a complex, and often difficult, health-care system, parents can be wary of releasing too much control to the adolescent (8,15). Failure of the adolescent may be viewed as failure by the parent. There may be excessive parental concern that failure by the adolescent may result in severe illness or incapacity. Thus, parents should be counseled about the realistic potential outcomes from transferring some control to the adolescent. Also, the health-care team can help the parent determine whether the adolescent is ready to attempt independence in a given area. There are tools available to monitor progress toward autonomy. An example of a checklist for health-care autonomy is in Figure 1 (32).

Parents often ask what they can do to help foster autonomy and self-care. Children with special needs who have been given chores similar to other children of the same developmental age attain higher self-esteem and self-care skills than children who are protected from responsibilities because of their disability (33,34). Similarly, adolescents who report spending time with friends other than a single best friend and those who believe they are not viewed by others as being disabled have greater individual competence and self-concept (33).

## PSYCHOSOCIAL ASPECTS OF TRANSITION

Adolescence, combined with a chronic multisystem developmental disability, can greatly impact the psychosocial health of a teenager or young adult with spina bifida. The middle to late teen with spina bifida may already be struggling with body-image issues, ineffective social skills, increased awareness of learning difficulties, and the negative impact of limited mobility (35). Concurrently the teen may be frustrated by missed school and social opportunities due to multiple medical appointments, complex routine care, and social (bowel/bladder) continence issues.

Classically, health-care transition/transfer occurs at a time of considerable anxiety for the adolescent, who is simultaneously experiencing significant

| Health Care Skills | Can Do Already | Needs Practice | Plan to Start | Accomplished |
|---|---|---|---|---|
| Understand health condition | | | | |
| Perform self-care skills, i.e., bowel and bladder care | | | | |
| Prepare questions for doctors, nurses, therapists | | | | |
| Respond to questions from doctors, nurses, therapists | | | | |
| Know medications and what they're for | | | | |
| Get a prescription refilled | | | | |
| Keep a calendar of doctor, dentist appointments | | | | |
| Know height, weight, birth date | | | | |
| Learn how to read a thermometer | | | | |
| Know health emergency telephone numbers | | | | |
| Know medical coverage numbers | | | | |
| Obtain sex education materials/birth control if indicated | | | | |
| Discuss role in health maintenance | | | | |
| Have genetic counseling if appropriate | | | | |
| Discuss drugs and alcohol with family | | | | |
| Make contact with appropriate community advocacy organization | | | | |
| Take care of own menstrual needs and keep a record of monthly periods | | | | |

Developed by the Youth in Transition Project (1984-1987) University of Washington Division of Adolescent Medicine and based on a model developed by the Children's Rehabilitation Center at the University of Virginia.

**Figure 1** This is an example of a worksheet used to assess adolescents' readiness to independently manage their own health-care needs.

changes at school, either by graduating or remaining in school due to deferred graduation. In either case, the adolescent may have mixed emotions about leaving school or remaining behind, which may adversely affect previous progress in self-care and transition skills. When asked, YSHCN acknowledge that the concurrent educational transitions (high school graduation, starting college, or vocational-technical school) and life changes (moving away from home, beginning work, marriage) are more important than addressing health-care transition (36). Some young adults admit to health-care "burnout" and exercise their new adult rights to avoid any health services.

Since the timeline for health-care transition can be more fluid than the educational system, which is designated by state and federal laws, delaying the transfer of care until the educational and life changes have occurred may alleviate some unnecessary stress on the adolescent (14). Having available counseling during the transition process was considered very important by clinicians providing transition services to YSHCN (11). The consensus statement by the three leading primary care professional organizations listed counseling and mental health services as one of the six first steps to developing good transition care (7). It is also important to recognize that adolescents with cognitive disabilities can have a delayed response to these life changes and may not manifest behaviors until several months later.

Preventive measures include facilitating the development of self-esteem and independence skills, maximizing social opportunities and connectedness, and providing mentorship by other self-advocates (1,36). Adolescents listed the ability to feel involved and to be given choices in the management of their disability as extremely important to their self-esteem and willingness to participate in their health-care (36).

### Sexuality

The topic of sexuality for adolescents with developmental disabilities is often ignored by parents and professionals. Persons with disabilities, both physical and intellectual, are frequently viewed as nonsexual persons. However, sexuality is integral to physical and psychological health with reciprocal influence on self-esteem, self-identity, personal and family values, social aptitude, and adult relationships. In a state survey of children receiving Title V services, parents of adolescents with developmental disabilities were less likely than parents of children with other chronic medical conditions to view sexuality counseling as an important health-care service (37). A recent study found that while most patients seen in a Dutch multidisciplinary spina bifida clinic received sexuality information, less than 25% of those patients received information specific to spina bifida (23). A 1990 study found only 16% of sexually active adolescents with spina bifida used contraception compared to 60% of similarly-aged adolescents with cystic fibrosis and 60% of age-matched typically developing controls (38). Hopefully, the public education efforts resulting from the HIV/AIDS epidemic have impacted these percentages; however, there is no current information available in the literature.

While they can be embarrassed to talk about sex, most adolescents share common sexuality questions and concerns. Adolescents and young adults with spina bifida may have additional sexuality questions related specifically to their disability including the impact of neurogenic bowel and bladder, contractures, scoliosis, latex allergy, genital insensitivity, erectile function, and medication side effects.

Specific information on sexuality in spina bifida is in the adult chapter of this textbook. The important transition issues are to ensure that (*i*) sexuality information is integrated into the health-care visit, (*ii*) the adolescent is routinely afforded private visit time to discuss sexuality with the health provider (i.e., during the teaching physical exam), and (*iii*) the information provided takes into account the cognitive ability, developmental level, communication skills, and specific learning disabilities of the adolescent (14).

## PREPARING FOR THE ADULT HEALTH SYSTEM

The differences between the adult and pediatric health systems are frequently listed as a barrier by all involved in the health-care transition process (15,39).

The adult system and its providers predominantly interact with previously able-bodied, developmentally typical adults who are now facing acute or chronic medical problems. With the exception of geriatrics and oncology (not typically utilized by young adults with spina bifida), most of these adult-oriented health-care providers are not familiar with the concept of graduated responsibility nor understand how to work with patients who utilize supports for self-care, medical decision making, and community living.

Because most of the adult-aged patients seen by adult providers are cognitively and developmentally mature, they are expected to know most of their health history and to have the necessary skills to manage their own care (4). When these adult-aged patients fail to participate in their care it is usually for reasons deemed under their control. Therefore, adult providers may be less likely to legitimize perceived noncompliance and may not provide as much support or assistance when patients struggle to adhere to treatment plans. Completing a skillset worksheet (Fig. 1) may help the adult provider to better understand the transitioning young adult's current abilities, as well as identify skills not yet developed. Training the adolescent to prepare for the adult visit can facilitate efficient communication between the patient and adult provider. Adolescents can prepare a list of complaints and questions prior to the visit. They can also keep a list of medications and allergies readily available. Keeping a portable medical record or written summary, which can be copied and given to each new provider, will help to maximize the exchange of information during the time-limited office visit and will likely endear the patient to the adult provider.

The transfer of medical history is an essential, yet complicated component of the health-care transition process. Young adults with spina bifida often have volumes of records due to multiple office visits, procedures, and hospitalizations. Medical record departments are unlikely to copy multiple volumes of charts for multiple new providers. The costs to families may be prohibitive. Regardless, the new providers are unlikely to wade through volumes of old records to summarize previous care. Therefore, a medical summary is a useful tool to begin developing early in the transition process. The summary should at least include:

1. Information from the birth history, including lesion level, date of primary closure and/or shunting, and orthopedic procedures, with the names and contact information of the surgeons who performed them
2. Major previous hospitalizations and procedures, including surgeons' names, and contact information
3. Previous medications, indications, and reasons for discontinuing
4. Current medications and allergies
5. Most recent tests results including radiological (CT head, shunt series, renal ultrasound, voiding cystourethrogram, scoliosis, and hip films), urodynamic, and laboratory procedures
6. Orthotic and adaptive equipment needs with the names and contact information for the durable medical equipment providers

In a pilot study on spina bifida health-care transition, it took the team an average of four hours per adolescent to compile a medical summary (8). Since it is unlikely a multidisciplinary team could provide this amount of time for each patient at the time of transfer, it would be better to continuously develop a working document throughout the transition process. With many hospital systems developing electronic medical records and pilot projects examining the role of internet portals and Web-based portable medical records, the need for paper records may diminish in the future. For now, any system to transfer the medical history involving multiple organ systems to multiple health-care providers is a critical aspect of successful health-care transition. Examples of paper-based medical summaries and portable medical records are available at several adolescent transition websites, including the American Academy of Pediatrics' National Center of Medical Home Initiatives for Children with Special Health Care Needs (40). There is an annotated list of these adolescent health-care transition websites at the end of this chapter.

Another frequent concern of adolescents, families, and pediatric providers is that adult systems are not familiar with family-centered care (4). They emphasize patient confidentiality, which can inadvertently alienate family caregivers and guardians. Care can be improved by proactively establishing that the patient would like the family to remain involved in health-care decisions and completing the necessary legal forms (see Future Planning, this chapter).

Adult health care has only recently begun recognizing the systems needed to provide comprehensive chronic care. Interdisciplinary care coordination is uncommon for any condition and multidisciplinary adult spina bifida clinics are rare. While pediatric specialists are often localized within pediatric hospitals, recommended adult specialists with expertise in spina bifida may not all be in one outpatient or hospital setting so that coordinated appointments may not be possible. There may need to be separate appointments with orthopedics, neurosurgery, urology, pulmonology, gastroenterology, rehabilitation/physiatry, physical therapy, and other needed providers. The patients should be advised against attempting to maximize the number of visits per day. Due to the uncertainty of competing hospital and surgical emergencies and schedules, these providers may not be able to keep to planned appointment schedules. Both providers and patients are advised to select first and last appointments of the day to assist patients in seeing at least two providers in one day, if possible.

Some adult providers have been described as cognitive specialists who pursue extensive testing in order to achieve diagnostic certainty (4). Whether the typical adult surgical specialists in spina bifida care would require extensive new testing upon receiving a new patient from pediatrics is uncertain. While these new providers may wish to repeat tests or "obtain a new baseline," it is important to consider the time, expense, and discomfort this may cause the new patient, who may have just undergone testing prior to the transfer. Having previous relevant test reports in the medical summary or portable medical record may be sufficient. However, it is important for the new patient to realize that this is also a new relationship for the provider, and information or tests from familiar sources may help to increase the comfort level of the new provider, particularly if they are less familiar with the diagnosis.

Insurance requirements may mandate care by providers other than those recommended by the transferring pediatric specialist. A letter to the insurance company explaining the need for a particular out-of-network provider may suffice. Alternatively, paying out-of-network fees in order to receive more expertise may be worth the added expense.

Ideally, transition teams should include the pediatric team and the receiving adult health-care team (7,14). Given the time constraints and financial limitations of the current health system, this may not be possible. Adult health systems are less likely to be familiar with or open to coordinated visits or multidisciplinary teams. Hopefully, as the adult health system increases its awareness of this new patient population of adults with chronic, complex, multisystem medical conditions, adult providers will recognize the benefits of coordinated care clinics. Advocacy groups are needed to increase the awareness by hospitals, public and private health insurers, state Title V programs, and professional health organizations of the need for this type of adult care. There are few outcome studies of multidisciplinary clinics for any age group, which limits the arguments for developing the same type of system for adults.

## INSURANCE

As adolescents reach between 18 and 21 years of age, they begin to "age out" of their parents' insurance plans. Approximately 22% of young adults (19–29 years old) with a disability in the United States are without health insurance (3). Some insurance plans allow for the dependent adolescent to remain on the parents' insurance while they continue to live at home and/or remain a student. Usually the adolescent is required to attend school full-time, which may be difficult for the college student with learning difficulties. Other insurance companies extend benefits to age 23 to 25, and some offer continued benefits, at sometimes higher rates, provided the adolescent is deemed disabled and dependent on the covered family member.

Some adolescents with spina bifida qualify for Title V financial assistance to cover equipment, supplies, and services not provided under their insurance plans. Most states end Title V services at 18 to 21 years old, and only Pennsylvania provides for adult coverage in spina bifida (41). Therefore, the adolescent, family, and health providers need to discuss how these previously covered services will be handled during the adult years. Fortunately, most adolescents with spina bifida over 18 will qualify for Medicaid services regardless of whether they continue to live with their family or not. Therefore, adolescents and their families should be encouraged to apply for Medicaid as soon as possible after the 18th birthday.

Some adolescents and their families receive supplemental security income (SSI) during childhood based on their disability, family resources, and medical needs from spina bifida. Following their 18th birthday, all children receiving SSI must reapply under the adult criteria (41). Many adolescents with spina bifida continue to qualify for SSI under the adult criteria. Those who did not qualify for SSI as a child due to the family's income should be encouraged to apply as an adult because their need is determined based only on their own income, not that of the family, even if the adolescent continues to live at home (42). Having qualified for SSI, most recipients can also apply for and receive Medicaid. The combination of SSI income and Medicaid insurance can offset some of the expenses incurred from the loss of Title V benefits. It is important for families to understand that these benefits can be sought in addition to parental insurance coverage. Even if the adolescent remains on the parents' insurance, Medicaid can become a secondary payer, covering copayments and items not covered by the primary insurance.

Some adolescents who apply for SSI may instead receive social security disability benefits (SSDI) under Title II of the social security program. These benefits are not needs based and do not take into account income or assets. The adolescent qualifies if the disability occurred before 21 years old (as in spina bifida) and the parent has worked a sufficient number of years and is currently disabled, retired, or deceased. With SSDI the adolescent receives Medicare insurance benefits after a two-year waiting period. Unfortunately, these benefits often disqualify the adolescent from receiving SSI and Medicaid (3).

Some adolescents and families are surprised and discouraged when they are denied SSI benefits. This is a common occurrence following the initial application. Families should be encouraged to appeal the denial and seek representation from a lawyer with experience in disability applications. A significant proportion of those who were initially denied benefits are eventually accepted. The lawyer fees are generally covered by a portion of the benefits retroactively due to the recipient from the time of the original application. Thus, there are no out-of-pocket fees required of the adolescent to appeal a denial.

Adolescents and families are also often concerned about attempting any work opportunities once they have qualified for SSI benefits. The federal government has approved Ticket to Work legislation, which addresses these concerns (41,43). This legislation allows individuals with disabilities to seek employment without losing all of their benefits, realizing that most employment opportunities will not provide enough income and benefits to offset the costs of care for the disability. Unfortunately, this legislation is complicated with complex rules for adjusting benefits based on the employment income. Additionally, not all states have fully enacted this program. While it is important not to let the potential loss of benefits hinder an adolescent from seeking job training and eventual employment, the family should be counseled to discuss these issues with an experienced lawyer who understands the local state regulations.

## FUTURE PLANNING

It is important that parents as well as providers understand the importance of future planning. Future planning is more than financial and legal planning. It addresses all significant areas of the individual's life including living arrangements, financial arrangements, educational programs, employment, health care, recreation, and personal needs (44). Careful future planning allows parents to provide for their children even after their death. There are many components to future planning, which could be as a simple as a will or as complex as guardianship and special needs trust.

Once an individual reaches the age of majority (in most states at age 18), he legally becomes an adult. This is true regardless of disability status and includes those individuals with developmental, cognitive, and/or physical disabilities. Parents no longer have the legal right to make decisions or consent to treatment on behalf of the adult child. This transfer of rights does not occur if the court has appointed a guardian. To establish guardianship, the courts must determine the individual to be "incompetent." Alternatively, some adults with developmental disabilities do not relinquish their decision-making rights, but allow family members to have health care power of attorney. Another option is to have the competent adult sign release forms to enable health-care providers to discuss medical management with designated family. The decision to choose among these legal pathways should be individualized based on the capacity of the individual. The overall goal should be to maximize autonomy and self-determination while ensuring safety and minimizing legal risks to the individual.

These issues of competency, health-care decision making, and confidentiality have received more consideration since The Administrative Simplification section of the Health Insurance Portability and Accountability Act of 1996 (HIPAA) on healthcare (45). Prior to the age of majority, parents or guardians have the authority to act on behalf of the minor to make health-care decisions, sign consents, and review or discuss care with health providers. Once an individual reaches the age of majority, he is deemed able to make all his own health-care decisions and can control access to personal health-care information. Therefore, under these regulations, health providers can only share information with family if that family member has guardianship, power of attorney for health-care decisions, or there is a signed release from the competent adult patient. For these reasons, it is no longer advisable for families to approach these legal issues with benign neglect. While previously families were often counseled to remain outside the legal system and preserve the rights of adults with developmental disabilities through inaction, a plan must be enacted to ensure that families can remain involved in the health care of their adult children, if desired. Additional information on how to approach guardianship and HIPAA issues but preserve autonomy and individual rights can be obtained from the Center for Self-Determination (46).

## SUMMARY

Most adolescents with spina bifida are surviving to adulthood and will need to address the issues of transitioning to adult health care. Preparation for transition by the adolescent, family, and pediatric providers should start in infancy. Adolescents should continuously be encouraged to develop self-care skills to maximize autonomy. During mid-adolescence a formalized, comprehensive, patient-centered transition plan should be developed and updated annually. All adolescents should eventually transition to a well-informed, adult-oriented care team when developmentally appropriate.

## TRANSITION AND INTERNET RESOURCES

### Adolescent Health Transition Project

http://depts.washington.edu/healthtr/

This project is housed at the University of Washington, Seattle, Washington, U.S.A., and sponsored by the Children with Special Health Care Needs Program, Washington State Department of Health.

This site includes Transition Timeline, Adolescent Autonomy Checklist, Health History Summary for Teens, and Working Together for Successful Transition: Washington State Adolescent Transition Resource Notebook. Information for health-care providers and educators, parents and families, and teens and young adults.

### American Academy of Pediatrics

http://www.medicalhomeinfo.org/tools/youthstart.html

Topics include information on roles in transition for youth and families and physicians, as well as a transition guide, information and links regarding transitions from pediatric to adult health, school to work and home to the community, and sexuality.

### ARC of the United States

http://www.thearc.org/

National organization of and for people with mental retardation and related developmental disabilities and their families. Publications available for free download include information regarding Americans with Disabilities Act, Money Management for Consumers, Futures Planning/Trusts/Guardianship, and mental retardation. Links to resources including tri-State area ARC chapters.

### Center for Self-Determination

http://www.self-determination.com/

This site reviews the principles of self-determination, provides state listings of advocacy providers and events, and includes resources and position papers.

### Family Village

http://www.familyvillage.wisc.edu

Family Village is sponsored by the Waisman Center, University of Wisconsin, Madison, Wisconsin, U.S.A.

Has extensive listing of transition and internet resources as well as resources for people with cognitive and other disabilities, their families and those that provide them with services and support. It includes resources about specific diagnoses and general disability-related topics, such as adaptive products and technology, advocacy, childcare, education, respite care, and worship. The site links to disability research programs and projects, statistics, and surveys.

### Heath Resource Center, The George Washington University

http://www.heath.gwu.edu/

The Web site is sponsored through cooperative agreement between The George Washington University and the Office of Special Education Programs of the U.S. Department of Education.

This is a national clearinghouse on postsecondary education for individual with disabilities. Have a variety of topics such as Summer PreCollege for Students with Disabilities, publications, links, and a Quarterly Newsletter.

### Health-Care Transitions

http://hctransitions.ichp.edu/

This site is supported by the promising practices in health-care transition research project based at the Institute for Child Health Policy ate the University of Florida.

The focus of this site is health-care transition for youth with disabilities and SHCN. Has annotated bibliography, health-care transitions, and excellent transition digest list serve for youth/young adults with disabilities, family members and health-care providers, policy makers, insurers, and others with knowledge and experience in the transition from child-centered (pediatric) to adult-oriented health care.

### Health and Ready to Work National Center

http://www.hrtw.org/index.html

Health and Ready to Work National Center (HRTW) funded through Federal Maternal and Child Health Bureau, Health Resources and Service Administration, and Department of Health and Human Services.

Excellent Web site includes a description of a wide range of topics such as transition checklists, transition planning manuals guidelines, screening and assessment tools, and where to obtain them. Resources can be used by adolescents, families, and health-care providers.

### National Information Center for Children and Youth with Disabilities

http://www.nichcy.org

National Information Center for Children and Youth with Disabilities (NICHY) is funded by the U.S. Department of Education, Office of Special Education.

NICHY provides information, publications, and assistance to families, educators, and other professionals on disabilities and disability-related services, individualized education programs (IEP), family issues, disability organizations, education rights, and transition to adult life. Have state-by-state resources lists, disability specific organizations, parent groups and parent training and information centers, and other organizations within each state that address disability-related issues.

### North Carolina Office of Disability and Health

http://www.fpg.unc.edu/~ncodh/

Receives primary funding from the Centers for Disease Control and Prevention as a collaborative endeavor between the Division of Public Health of the Department of Health and Human Services and the Frank Porter Graham Center, University of North Carolina, Chapel Hill, North Carolina, U.S.A.

Online articles, links, and publications regarding: Adolescents and Young Adults, Recreation, Accommodations for College, Women's Health, Recreation.

### Parent Advocacy Coalition for Educational Rights

http://www.pacer.org

This is a national center based in Minnesota.

Has transition to work and health information along with many other resources, links. Excellent publications, videos regarding transition, health, vocational-educational planning.

### Spina Bifida Association of America

http://www.sbaa.org

Click on "About Spina Bifida" then click on "Fact Sheets" for Transitions into Adolescence regarding teens with spina bifida and for Health Issues for Adults with Spina Bifida click on "Insights" then "Adults."

## REFERENCES

1. Blum RW. Transition to adult health care: setting the stage. J Adolesc Health 1995; 17:3–5.
2. Newacheck PW, Taylor WR. Childhood chronic illness: prevalence, severity, and impact. Am J Public Health 1994; 82:364–371.
3. White PH. Access to health care: health insurance considerations for young adults with special health care needs/disabilities. Pediatrics 2002; 110:1328–1335.
4. Rosen D. Between two worlds: bridging the cultures of child health and adult medicine. J Adolesc Health 1995; 17:10–16.

5. Goodman DM, Mendez E, Throop C, Ogata ES. Adult survivors of pediatric illness: the impact on pediatric hospitals. Pediatrics 2002; 110(3):583–589.
6. Magrab PR, Millar HEC. Growing up and getting medical care: youth with special health care needs. Surgeon General's Conference, Jekyll Island, 1989.
7. American Academy of Pediatrics, American Academy of Family Medicine, American College of Medicine–American Society of Internal Medicine. A consensus statement on health care transitions for young adults with special health care needs. Pediatrics 2002; 110(6 Pt 2):1304–1306.
8. Sawyer SM, Collins N, Bryan D, Brown D, Hope MA, Bowes G. Young people with spina bifida: transfer from paediatric to adult health care. J Paediatr Child Health 1998; 34:414–417.
9. Johnson CP, Dorval J. Transitions into Adolescence Fact Sheet. Spina Bifida Association of America, April 2001.
10. Scal P, Evans T, Blozis S, Okinow N, Blum R. Trends in transition from pediatric to adult health care services for young adults with chronic conditions. J Adolesc Health 1999; 24(4):259–264.
11. Scal P, Ireland M. Addressing transition to adult health care for adolescents with special health care needs. Pediatrics 2005; 115(6):1607–1612.
12. Blum RW, Garell D, Hodgman CH, et al. Transition from child-centered to adult health care systems for adolescents with chronic conditions. A position paper of the society for adolescent medicine. J Adolesc Med 1993; 14:570–576.
13. White PH, Schuyler V, Edelman A, Hayes A, Batshaw ML. Future expectations: transition from adolescence to adulthood. In: ML Batshaw, ed. Children with Disabilities. Baltimore: Brookes, 2002:693–705.
14. Society for Adolescent Medicine. Moving on: transition from pediatric to adult health care. J Adolesc Health 1995; 17:6–9.
15. Reiss JG, Gibson RW, Walker LR. Health care transition: youth, family, and provider perspectives. Pediatrics 2005; 115:112–120.
16. Peterson PM, Rauen KK, Brown J, Cole J. Spina bifida: the transition into adulthood begins in infancy. Rehabil Nurs 1994; 19(4):229–238.
17. Olsen DG, Swigonski NL. Transition to adulthood: the important role of the pediatrician. Pediatrics 2004; 113(3 Pt 1):e159–e162.
18. Individuals with Disabilities Education Act. Public Law No. 105-17, 1997.
19. Kelly AM, Kratz B, Bielski M, Rinehart PM. Implementing transitions for youth with complex chronic conditions using the medical home model. Pediatrics 2002; 11:1322–1327.
20. Blum RW. Overview of transition services for youth with disabilities. Paediatrician 1991; 18:101–104.
21. Charvat KA, Nebrig DM. Adolescents with Developmental Disorders: Smoothing Bumps in the Road to Adulthood. Grand Rounds Presentation. Cincinnati Children's Hospital, 1997.
22. Sloan L, Leibold SR, Henry-Atkinson J. Sexuality and the Person with Spina Bifida. Spina Bifida Association of America, 1993.
23. Verhoef M, Barf HA, Vroege JA, et al. Sex education, relationships, and sexuality in young adults with spina bifida. Arch Phys Med Rehabil 2005; 86:979–987.
24. Sawyer SM, Blair S, Bowes G. Chronic illness in adolescents: transfer or transition to adult services. J Paediatr Child Health 1997; 33:88–90.

25. Rauen K. Guidelines for Spina Bifida Health Care Services Throughout Life. Spina Bifida Association of America, 1995.
26. Committee on Children With Disabilities. The pediatrician's role in the development and implementation of an individual education plan (IEP) and/or an individual family service plan (IFSP). Pediatrics 1999; 104(1):124–127.
27. Hommet C, Billard C, Gillet P, et al. Neuropsychologic and adaptive functioning in adolescents and young adults shunted for congenital hydrocephalus. J Child Neurol 1999; 14(3):144–150.
28. Johnson CP. Transition in adolescents with disabilities. In: Capute AJ, Accardo PJ, eds. Developmental Disabilities in Infancy and Childhood. 2nd ed. Baltimore: Brookes Publishing Company, 1996:549–570.
29. Fact Sheets. Spina Bifida Association of America. Retrieved September 1, 2005, from http://www.sbaa.org/site/PageServer?pagename=asb_facts
30. Body Owner's Manual. Adolescent Services, Glenrose Rehabilitation Hospital. Retrieved September 1, 2005 from http://www.adolescentservices.net/bodyowners manual.htm
31. Fact Sheets. Australian Spina Bifida and Hydrocephalus Association. Retrieved September 1, 2005 from http://www.asbha.org.au/FactSheets.htm
32. Adolescent Autonomy Checklist. Youth in Transition Project. University of Washington. Retrieved September 1, 2005 from http://depts.washington.edu/healthtr/checklist_print.doc
33. Resnick MD, Hutton L. Resilience among physically disabled adolescents. Psychiatric Annals 1987; 17:796–800.
34. Wolman C, Basco DE. Factors influencing self-esteem and self-consciousness in adolescents with spina bifida. J Adolesc Health 1994; 15:543–548.
35. Appleton PL, Minchom PE, Ellis NC, Elliott CE, Boll V, Jones P. The self-concept of young people with spina bifida: a population-based study. Dev Med Child Neurol 1994; 36:198–215.
36. Patterson DL, Lanier C. Adolescent health transitions: focus group study of teens and young adults with special health care needs. Fam Community Health 1999; 22(2):43–58.
37. Geenen SJ, Powers LE, Sells W. Understanding the role of health care providers during the transition of adolescents with disabilities and special health care needs. J Adolesc Health 2003; 32:225–233.
38. Cromer BA, Enrile B, McCoy K, Gerhardstein MJ, Fitzpatrick M, Judis J. Knowledge, attitudes, and behavior related to sexuality in adolescents with chronic disability. Dev Med Child Neurol 1990; 41:671–675.
39. Scal P. Transition for youth with chronic conditions: primary care physicians' approaches. Pediatrics 2002; 110(6):1315–1321.
40. AAP. Build Your Own Care Notebook. National Center of Medical Home Initiatives for Children with Special health Care Needs. Retrieved on September 1, 2005 from http://www.medicalhomeinfo.org/tools/care_notebook.html
41. Fishman E. Aging out of coverage: young adults with special health needs. Health Affairs 2001; 20(6):254–266.
42. Understanding Supplemental Security Income SSI Income Social Security Administration. Retrieved September 1, 2005 from http://www.ssa.gov/notices/Supplemental_security Income/income_htm

43. Ticket to Work. Social Security Administration. Retrieved September 1, 2005 from http://www.yourtickettowork.com
44. The ARC. A Family Handbook on Future Planning. Retrieved on September 1, 2005 from http://www.thearc.org/afcsp/futureplanning.htm
45. Standards for the Privacy of Individually Identified health Information; Final Rule. Federal Registry. Retrieved on September 1, 2005 from http://www.cms.hhs.gov/hipaa/hipaa2/regulations/privacy/default.asp
46. Herr SS. Self-determination, autonomy, and alternatives for guardianship. Retrieved on September 1, 2005 from http://www.self-determination.com/publications/position_papers_index.html

# 8

# Adults Who Have Spina Bifida: Work and Mental Health

**Gregory S. Liptak**
*Department of Pediatrics, Upstate Medical University, Syracuse, New York, U.S.A.*

*The past is never dead; it's not even past.*
—William Faulkner, *Requiem for a Nun*, Act I, Scene iii

## INTRODUCTION

Adults who have spina bifida carry the past with them, both personally and culturally. Their personal past includes their abilities, physical impairments, coping strategies, and social skills. These affect their well-being and functioning as adults. As reviewed in earlier chapters of this book, impairments and disabilities that occur with spina bifida include nonverbal and verbal learning disabilities as well as problems with attention; and executive function these can affect performance in postsecondary education, employment, communication, and socialization. Adults with spina bifida typically have limited mobility with paraplegia and may have impaired fine motor skills. They may have problems accessing transportation. They may have recurrent medical problems such as urinary tract infection, skin breakdown, and ventricular shunt malfunction that can limit them from participating in school or work for an extended time. They may have urinary or fecal incontinence, which can affect social interactions and self-esteem. For each of these challenges, they possess coping skills, with some individuals being more resilient than others.

In addition, they carry their cultural heritage, which, in many places, includes diminished opportunities for work or education for individuals who have disabilities. It may mean limited access to knowledgeable mental health professionals (1) as well as the inability of part-time employees to obtain adequate health insurance. If a job that they can manage physically (e.g., a part-time job) does not offer them adequate insurance coverage, they may be better off financially remaining unemployed and relying on governmental assistance like Medicaid. The physical and cultural factors that they bring with them to adulthood affect their mental health and well-being as well as their ability to participate in society.

## THEORETICAL BASES

The World Health Organization (WHO) has developed a model for evaluating the impact of health status on the functioning of individuals (2). This conceptual framework describes and classifies components of health. Functioning is described as the interaction among three dimensions: body functions/structures, activity/participation, and environmental/personal factors. Every component is subdivided into domains that encompass anatomical or physiological systems (body functions and structures), life areas (activity and participation), and physical, social, and attitudinal environment (environmental and personal factors). Figure 1 illustrates the ICF model as applied to some issues faced by an adult with spina bifida. For example, if a child with spina bifida has hydrocephalus and a small corpus callosum (body function and structure), they will have difficulty understanding mathematics and certain aspects of language, for example,

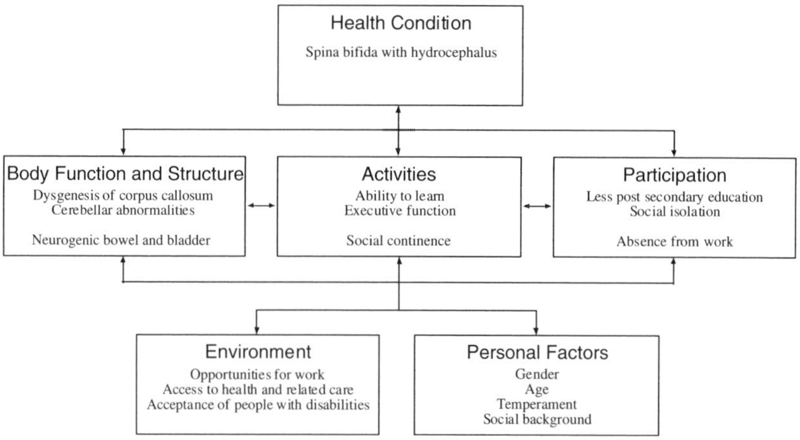


**Figure 1** World Health Organization International Classification of Functioning, Disability, and Health applied to some issues of adults with spina bifida and hydrocephalus. *Source*: From Ref. 2.

idioms (activities). They likely will not do as well in school, and will not be able to obtain a rewarding job when they are adults (participation). (This has been called a chain of adversity.) However, (*i*) providing remediation (additional instructional time or different instructional approaches to "fix" a certain area of weakness and build strength in a particular area to facilitate potential learning) and compensation [alternative approaches (e.g., assistive technology) to offset, or counter balance, a learning disability and produce the desired level of performance] in the school, (*ii*) having parents who help the child with homework (environment), and (*iii*) having a child who has a persistent temperament (personal factor) can ameliorate the adverse effects of the impairments and lead to better outcomes.

Erikson (3) has argued that an individual has to master certain stages in order to develop a healthy personality. During elementary school, children need to develop a sense of industry. During adolescence, the teen develops a sense of identity (the identity crisis). During adulthood, the individual must develop a sense of intimacy (vs. isolation) and a sense of generativity (typically manifest by having children). Factors that interfere with the successful resolution of these crises adversely affect mental health. These issues (crises) do not completely disappear as the person ages but continue in different manifestations throughout development.

Bandura (4) hypothesized as part of his Social Learning Theory that individuals develop a sense of self-efficacy, which is related to self-concept and self-esteem. This is defined as people's belief in their ability to successfully perform specified tasks, expend greater effort, and persevere in the face of adversity. If people are subjected to repeated failures, for example, people with learning disabilities in a classroom, they may develop the opposite of self-efficacy, which is learned helplessness. Learned helplessness occurs when individuals believe that they have no control over a situation. This feeling of helplessness occurs because of repeated failures in similar situations. It causes individuals to think that they should not even try, because they believe they will not be successful. Learned helplessness has been linked to depression (5).

Finally, Evans and Stoddard developed a model to explain the determinants of individual health. Figure 2 illustrates this model in terms of depression in an individual with spina bifida (6). The physical and social environments, genetic endowment, and prosperity affect health and well-being in addition to the presence of disease and the availability and quality of health care.

## BACKGROUND

Very few scientific studies of adults with spina bifida have been conducted. The ones that have been published often are descriptive and limited by small or non-representative samples. However, the picture they paint of the life of an adult with spina bifida is not bright. For example, in a study of 53 adults who had spina bifida, lived in Kentucky, and had a mean age of 27.8 years at interview, 86% completed at least 12 years of school, but 80% earned less than $10,000 per

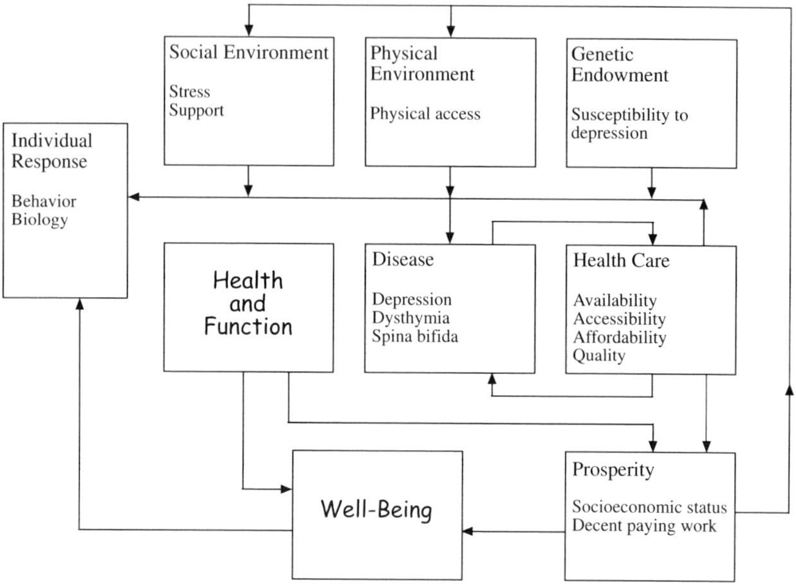


**Figure 2** Evans and Stoddard model applied to depression in persons with spina bifida. *Source*: From Ref. 6.

year, and 82% had been on Supplemental Security Income for an average of nine years. Ninety-three percent had never been married, 24% were currently sexually active, only 30% were employed, and 23% were driving. They spent an average of 29 hours per week watching television (their prime activity) and six hours talking on the telephone. Only 16% made all their monetary decisions on their own, 66% were using intermittent catheterization for bladder continence, only 51% were using a bowel program, and only 41% were continent of stool (7). In a study from Ireland, McDonnell and McCann found that only 36% of adults with spina bifida were employed, 33% were regular drivers, 17% were married or engaged, and 8% were parents (8). Secondary medical conditions that interfere with functioning occur commonly. For example, a group of 98 adults with spina bifida accounted for 353 admissions to Johns Hopkins Medical Center during the study period; 166 (47.0%) of the admissions were due to potentially preventable secondary conditions such as serious urological infections, renal calculi, pressure ulcers, and osteomyelitis (9).

## WORK

### Current Status

Work is a major way in which adults participate in society. As shown in Figure 1, impairments that affect body functions and structures, as well as activities, impact the ability to work (i.e., participation in society). On the basis of Figure 2, work is critical for prosperity, which in turn affects the physical and social environment, and has direct effects on health and well-being. Work too helps give individuals a sense of identity (as discussed by Erikson earlier), which is an ongoing process. It may also provide opportunities for intimacy (as opposed to staying home alone) and can help contribute to a sense of industry (another earlier but ongoing process).

Very few studies relating to work in individuals who have spina bifida have been published. The few studies of adults with physical disabilities in general that have been done confirm the importance of work. The life goals of adults who have disabilities include the same ideals as those of adults without disabilities. In general terms, they include being independent, living on one's own terms, and feeling that life is meaningful (10). In more specific terms, they include having adequate financial status, leisure activities (which often require adequate finances), and work (11). Poverty continues to be one of the most important determinants of health and well-being (12) and clearly is based in large part on the ability to hold a meaningful job.

A number of descriptive studies have evaluated employment in adults with spina bifida. The rates for employment reported in these studies ranged from 4% to 88%, whereas unemployment rates ranged from 25% to 72%. The employment rate of 88% was found in a study of individuals with spina bifida without shunted hydrocephalus. For persons with shunts, the employment rate in that study was 42% (13). The outcome was worse in those who had revisions of their ventricular shunts, especially if the revisions had occurred after the age of two years. Significantly fewer of those who had had a shunt revision lived independently or drove a car. In more recent studies by the same group, adults with an age range of 26 to 33 years were evaluated; 37% lived independently in the community, 39% drove a car, 30% could walk more than 50 m, and 26% were in open (not sheltered) employment (a worse outcome than before). Attainment and independence were reduced in those who had needed revision of their ventricular shunts (14). In another study by the same group, out of 54 adults with a mean age of 35 years (range 32–38 years), 22 lived independently in the community and managed their own lives including transportation, continence care, pressure areas, and all medical needs. Thirteen worked in open employment (15).

Tew (16) found that employment of adolescents with spina bifida was 11%, whereas that for matched peers without disabilities was 37%. In a study from Ireland, McDonnell and McCann (8) found that 36% of adults with spina bifida were employed, 33% were regular drivers, 17% were married or engaged, and only 8% were parents.

## Factors Affecting Employment

Cognitive abilities have been found to affect employment. In a study of 98 young adults, Tew et al. (17) found that 33% were employed and 32% were unemployed. The other individuals followed in the study were either in sheltered work programs or in educational settings. The most important factor differentiating those employed in nonsheltered settings from those employed in sheltered settings or unemployed was intellectual level. Hurley and Bell (18) in a study of 36 adults also found that level of cognitive abilities and academic achievement discriminated the 14 persons who were employed from the 22 who were unemployed. Statistically significant differences were found for IQ scores, achievement scores, language ability, and visual-spatial skills.

Castree and Walker (19) compared the employment experiences of 45 young adults with spina bifida with those of 31 persons with cerebral palsy. At the time of follow-up, 90% of the young adults with cerebral palsy were employed, whereas only 69% of young adults with spina bifida were employed. Young adults with both spina bifida (76%) and cerebral palsy (93%) had obtained career advice and had visited work places (44% and 60%, respectively) prior to leaving school; however, 44% of the persons with spina bifida experienced several months of delay in job placement compared to 26% for those with cerebral palsy. One factor accounting for differences in employment between the two groups in this study was access to travel, with individuals with cerebral palsy being characterized by greater mobility.

Bomalski et al. (20) compared the employment status of 38 adults with spina bifida with a reference population based on U.S. census data. In comparison with the employment rate of 69% for the general population, the rate for adults with spina bifida was 33%, the same as that of individuals with a work-related disability. Females were more likely to be employed, but no relationships were found between employment and urological management or continence level.

In a study of 32 adults with spina bifida, ranging between 18 and 48 years of age (21), 17 were employed. Regression models indicated that family encouragement of achievement was positively predictive of employment, independent of the contribution of IQ, lesion level, and gender.

## Findings from Spinal Cord Injury Occurring During Childhood

A few studies of individuals examined adults who had acquired spinal cord injury in childhood have been performed. Since in-depth studies of adults with spina bifida are lacking, these may provide insight into the issues that relate to adults with spina bifida. Adults with spinal cord injury share the motor and sensory neurological losses seen in spina bifida as well as in the neurogenic bowel and bladder. However, unless they also have had a brain injury, they do not share the learning disabilities and other cognitive problems seen in spina bifida. In one study (22), 54% of those adults were employed, 48% lived independently, and 15% were married. These numbers are higher than the average for individuals with spina bifida.

Life satisfaction in adults with spinal cord injury has been found to be associated with education, income, satisfaction with employment, and social/

recreation opportunities and was inversely associated with medical complications. Life satisfaction was not significantly associated with level of injury, age at injury, or duration of injury (23). Dating opportunities, job opportunities, and income have been identified as the three areas in which adults with pediatric-onset spinal cord injury are least satisfied and those domains have a significant impact on overall satisfaction (24). A predictive model of employment identified four factors associated with employment: education, community mobility, functional independence, and decreased medical complications. Other variables significantly associated with employment included community integration, independent driving, independent living, higher income, and life satisfaction (22). As found in individuals with spina bifida, higher levels of education and being employed were both associated with greater community integration (25).

## Postsecondary Education and Training

Children with meningomyelocele are less likely to advance to postsecondary education and training than children without meningomyelocele. Learning disabilities that occur in childhood, for example, problems with mathematics, evolve into learning problems in adulthood, such as an inability to use numbers in everyday life. These significantly limit functional independence, affect the quality of adult life, and decrease the ability to get into higher educational institutions. In one study, 34% of children were involved in postsecondary education compared to 47% of the general population. Young adults with meningomyelocele were one to two years delayed in educational attainment compared to age-matched peers (20). In a study published in 1983 (26), 52% of individuals with spina bifida had attended college, whereas in a study of 48 adults published in 1994, only seven (15%) had attended college. Achievement and IQ scores as well as measures of language and visual-spatial ability differentiated those who attended college from those who did not (18). Attending college is no guarantee of finding employment. Individuals with spina bifida who attend a very supportive college or university may still be unable to find meaningful (unsupported) work after graduation.

## Potential Interventions

Very little is known about successful ways to increase employment for adults who have spina bifida. Interventions to prepare individuals with spina bifida to enter the world of work may need to begin well before the end of secondary education. An emphasis on prevocational and vocational skills would be appropriate to begin in middle adolescence (27). Such skills include using transportation and following schedules. Because individuals with spina bifida have disabilities with nonverbal learning and executive function, providing strategies to help them to organize and plan and teaching them social skills could be helpful. Adults with spina bifida have identified self-confidence and work benefits among positive factors related to employment; thus, efforts to promote personal and social skills could address those needs. Inadequate health insurance and discrimination in hiring have been identified as significant problems for individuals with spina bifida (28). Therefore, changes in the employment system may be required as well.

Although some information is available about the employment status of adults, little is known about specific self-care skills, including their acquisition and retention. Assistive technologies can help the self-care of individuals with spina bifida and be invaluable for employment; yet, information about their actual use is rare. For instance, the prevalence of use of different types of assistive devices for academic remediation or accommodation by people with spina bifida is unknown. Nor are the benefits achieved by the use of these devices known.

Supported employment programs appear to work by helping individuals compensate for problematic symptoms and cognitive impairments and, to a lesser extent, by finding or developing environmental niches in which these impairments do not impede their ability to perform the necessary job-related tasks. Supported employment includes (*i*) training and support to learn the job, (*ii*) helpful interpersonal relationships at work, (*iii*) an accepting workplace culture, and (*iv*) approaches to self-management. Although no form of job accommodation has been reported with great frequency, in a study of adults with arthritis, the most commonly used ones included getting someone to help do one's job (12.1%), scheduling more breaks during the work day (9.5%), changing the time that the work day started and stopped (6.3%), having a shorter work day (5.6%), getting special equipment (5.3%), and changing the work tasks (5.3%) (29). These programs may benefit adults with spina bifida as well.

In summary, although increasing numbers of individuals with spina bifida are surviving into adulthood, the rate of employment remains low and unchanging. The percent of individuals with spina bifida who attend postsecondary education also is low. No studies have been published that evaluate interventions to increase the rate of employment. On the basis of the findings of studies conducted on adults who acquired spinal cord injuries during childhood, focusing resources and rehabilitation strategies on improving education level, employment potential, independence, income, and health of individuals with spina bifida might improve both their community integration and their life satisfaction. Issues of personal choice, environmental barriers, motivation, interests, and skills need to be addressed. Strategies for intervening could include improving job training in school and immediately after graduation from high school, providing better assistive technology and supported employment programs.

## MENTAL HEALTH

Mental health can be defined in a number of ways and includes the subjective sense of emotional well-being in which individuals feel that they are coping, relatively in control of their lives, able to face challenges, and take on responsibilities. The definition also includes the absence of mental disorders, for example, those conditions listed in the Diagnostic and Statistical Manual of Mental Disorders (30). Good mental health is strongly tied to quality of life, as well as to healthy, happy personal relationships. It can be influenced by genes, physical health, individual behavior, and external environments (Fig. 2).

Children with spina bifida and hydrocephalus have a high frequency of learning disabilities, both verbal and nonverbal. Individuals with nonverbal learning disabilities have difficulty with visual attention and visual-spatial perception, flexibility, abstract thinking, executive function and organizational skills, the pragmatics of language (31), generalizing information, and motor coordination. They have significant problems with social skills because of difficulties understanding the nonverbal aspects of communication. Young adults with spina bifida have been found to have the same pattern of higher verbal to performance (nonverbal) scores on intelligence tests (32,33). This difficulty in understanding communication adds to the physical disabilities of the condition, including impaired mobility and social incontinence. Coupled with the failure of most communities willingly to accept people with disabilities, individuals with spina bifida must face formidable odds to achieve normal social interactions and a sense of mental health.

In a population-based study in Canada, children with both chronic illness and associated disability were at greater than three-fold risk for psychiatric disorders and considerable risk for social adjustment problems (34). Empirically, studies of children with spina bifida have found that they tend to be socially immature and passive. They are less likely to have social contacts outside school, more dependent on adults for guidance, less competent scholastically, less physically active, less likely to make independent decisions, and more likely to exhibit impairments with attention and concentration (35). Teens with spina bifida have been found to have low levels of responsibility at home, extremely limited out-of-school contacts, negligible participation with organized social activities, and a primary orientation toward sedentary activities (36). As the descriptive studies of adults with spina bifida cited in the Background section would indicate, social isolation, decreased responsibilities, and the orientation toward sedentary activities continue into adulthood.

## Sexuality

Sexuality is an important part of mental health and includes an individual's concept of himself or herself in a social context as well as biological capabilities. Sexuality is affected by biological maturation, progression through the socially defined stages of childhood, adolescence, and adulthood, and by the person's relationships with others, including family members, intimate partners, and friends. These forces shape the person's gender and sexual identities, sexual attitudes, and sexual behavior (37). Sexuality includes puberty, sexual functioning (including fertility), and psychosexual development. Between 10% and 30% of girls with meningomyelocele and hydrocephalus experience precocious puberty (38). The average age of menarche in girls with spina bifida has been reported from 10.9 (39) to 11.4 years (40), compared with a mean of 12.7 years for girls without spina bifida (40). In one study, early pubertal timing in girls with spina bifida was associated with lower levels of self-concept and higher levels of depression (41).

Both males and females with spina bifida typically have decreased sensation in the perineum, which can impair the ability to experience orgasm. Erectile dysfunction and retrograde ejaculation, which are common in adult men with spina bifida, and urinary and fecal incontinence, which are common in all adults with spina bifida, directly affect sexual function. Around 70% men with spina bifida report having erections (42,43). Yet, in another study, only 27% were satisfied with the quality of their tumescence (44). The ability to have erections has been found to be related to the person's sensory level (45); erections are mainly achieved reflexively by stimulation rather than occurring by psychogenic means (46). Ejaculation and orgasm are reported in around two-thirds of men (42); however, many men experience retrograde ejaculation, and thus are infertile through the usual route of intercourse.

Very few studies have been published relating to female sexual function in spina bifida. Women with spina bifida are reported to have fewer orgasms and less sexually related lubrication. Two studies (47,48) have documented that 37% to 39% of women reported the ability to perceive orgasm, and in one of these studies (48), 77% reported the ability to achieve lubrication. Studies of women with spinal cord injury may provide some physiological insights on this topic. In a study of women with spinal cord injury (49), the maintenance of psychogenic lubrication was related to the degree of preservation of touch and pinprick sensation in the T11-L2 dermatomes. Moreover, the ability to achieve orgasm was decreased in women who had complete lower motor neuron dysfunction affecting their sacral spinal segments when compared with women with all other degrees of spinal cord injury.

Adults with spina bifida are described as being more socially isolated than those without disabilities. This may decrease opportunities for sexual intimacy. Problems with understanding social cues related to nonverbal learning disabilities may make intimacy more difficult as well. Although sexual abuse of individuals (especially females) with spina bifida has been reported, the frequency is unknown (50).

## Self-Concept

Self-concept and self-esteem are important components of mental health. Studies of self-concept in children with meningomyelocele are equivocal. Some (51,52) have not shown a difference between children with meningomyelocele and controls without disabilities. Others, however, have found significant differences in self-concept between children with meningomyelocele and matched controls

(53–56). In a recent study, children with spina bifida in general were found to have lower self-concept than controls. This was particularly true for girls. However, urinary continence (as opposed to incontinence) was associated with normal self-concept (57). In a related study, children who had a Malone antegrade colonic enema implanted surgically reported increased self-reliance, independence, and a feeling of security, which led to significant improvement in self-esteem (58). These results suggest that better urinary and fecal continence are associated with better self-concept. In a study of adolescents who had a physical disability, increased exposure to normal daily activities and social interactions was found to be related to a healthy self-concept (59).

## Depression, Anxiety, and Internalizing Symptoms

Because of severe learning disabilities as well as the impairments that affect physical functioning, some children with spina bifida may develop learned helplessness. They believe that unpleasant or aversive stimuli cannot be controlled and, therefore, cease trying to fix an aversive circumstance, even if they can exert some influence. Learned helplessness has been linked to depression and other internalizing symptoms (such as anxiety, somatic problems, and social withdrawal) (5). Loss and humiliating events that directly devalue an individual (such as teasing or bullying at school) also are linked with major depression (60). A few published studies have shown that persons with disabilities are at greater risk of having behavioral issues. Internalizing behavior problems are more likely than externalizing behavior problems. Using specific measures of depression, Appleton et al. (55) found a higher incidence of depression in a group of youth with spina bifida (nine years or older). Other studies in children of other age groups that used different assessments also have identified higher mean scores on measures of depression (61,62). Children with spina bifida have been found to exhibit more internalizing symptoms than able-bodied children (63).

Classic symptoms of major depression include depressed mood, irritability, reduced concentration, loss of interest/motivation, inability to enjoy things (anhedonia), feelings of hopelessness or helplessness, and preoccupation with one's self. Many of these also characterize normal adolescence. Other symptoms include insomnia, altered appetite (usually decreased), and psychomotor agitation or retardation. Whether individuals with spina bifida experience these same signs and symptoms of depression is not clear.

Depression is closely linked with anxiety, with both cooccurring in many individuals. Depression also commonly presents with somatic symptoms, such as headache (64). This may make diagnosis difficult, especially in an individual who has shunted hydrocephalus. In addition, infections, metabolic disturbances, endocrinopathies (e.g., hypothyroidism), other serious illness, medications (e.g., anticonvulsants), and even shunt failure may present with signs and symptoms similar to those found in depression. Screening questions are used in individuals without spina bifida, such as (*i*) during the past month, have you been bothered by feeling down, depressed, or hopeless? and (*ii*) during the past month, have you often been bothered by little interest or pleasure in things? (65). These have not been tested in individuals with spina bifida.

## Behavioral Outcomes

Behavioral factors strongly contribute to physical health outcomes and have been implicated in the etiology and management of most acute and chronic illnesses. For example, obesity is directly affected by eating patterns and physical activity. The factors associated with behavioral outcomes in individuals who have spina bifida have not been well characterized. Most evidence suggests that the severity of spina bifida plays relatively little role. This is similar to the finding noted above in individuals with spinal cord injury that level of injury was not significantly associated with life satisfaction. In fact, in one study, the mental aspects of quality of life of individuals with spina bifida were inversely associated with disability, that is, less disability was associated ($r = -0.70$, $P < 0.05$) with higher psychological distress and severe role disability because of emotional problems (66). This finding has been documented in the past in individuals with other chronic conditions (67,68). Children with less physical involvement may not be able to be part of the disability culture (e.g., they cannot participate in wheelchair sports); yet, they do not fit in the world of able-bodied individuals, though their near-normal appearance may give the perception that they should be functioning in the able-bodied world.

Issues related to self-concept, family cohesion, and maternal adjustment have been correlated to the presence of behavior or mental health problems. For example, children with spina bifida who had significant symptoms of depression and sadness had increased family conflict, lower socio-economic status and were more likely to be female; high levels of parental control predicted better adjustment (69). In a separate study, positive relations between perceived family encouragement of independence and achievement and young adult outcomes were found (21). Social support from both family and peers has been shown to decrease behavioral problems (70). The nature of these relationships remains unclear. Published studies evaluating factors that affect mental health have been cross-sectional. Thus, cause and effect are impossible to elucidate. Nor have the effects of interventions been evaluated.

## Potential Interventions

Mental health promotion is the attempt to enhance mental health and quality of life by improving the social, physical, and economic environments that determine mental health (Fig. 2), the social connectedness (sense of belonging), coping skills (71), and resilience (72) of individuals. One approach used in adolescence has been to focus on positive aspects in the internal and external environments that increase resilience and coping, for example, the "developmental assets of youth" (73). Study of a large sample of youth has shown a cumulative effect of assets linked to reduced likelihood of engagement in high-risk behaviors and increased likelihood of participation in positive behaviors (74,75). Whether such assets are relevant to adults in general or to adults who have spina bifida is uncertain, because virtually no scientific evidence has been published on any interventions to improve mental health in adults who have spina bifida.

Interventions that address sexuality include the use of medications such as sildenafil (Viagra®) (76) or vacuum pumps to enhance male sexual function. The use of assisted reproductive technology such as artificial insemination can increase the ability to produce children (generativity) in couples who are ready for that step. The effective medical treatment of continence could enhance self-esteem as well as sexual functioning. Programs that address teasing and bullying in school (77) may be able to decrease the occurrence of depression while enhancing self-esteem.

Studies in children and adolescents with spina bifida have shown that community-based support programs, such as summer camps, are able to enhance self-help skills, independence, and socialization at least for the short term (78,79). Again, whether similar recreational programs would be helpful for adults with spina bifida is uncertain.

Interventions that address specific components of mental health in younger individuals who have spina bifida have been published. For example, King et al. (80) ran a program to improve social skills. It included two 90 minutes group sessions for 10 weeks. They targeted problem solving, verbal and nonverbal communication, initiating interactions, and coping with difficult peers. They used video modeling, instruction, role play, and homework. Individuals in the program experienced an improvement in self-perceived social acceptance at the end of treatment and a decrease in self-reported loneliness at the six-month follow-up. Whether a similar program that addresses specific social skills (81,82) in an adult population would be as successful is unknown.

Mental health promotion also includes prevention, early diagnosis, and effective treatment of conditions like depression and anxiety. The issue of depression has been addressed in adults without disabilities. Cross-sectional studies have shown that factors that protect against the development of depression include well-developed intrapersonal skills and social connectedness (83). In a different study, characteristics found in mid-adolescence that predicted subsequent depression included low self-esteem, dissatisfaction with academic achievement, poor atmosphere at home, and having no close friends—features found to be increased in individuals who have spina bifida (84). However, whether enhancing social connectedness can prevent depression in adults with spina bifida is unknown. Early recognition and effective treatment of depression has been shown to be feasible and beneficial in the treatment of adults without disabilities (85) and is a useful concept for adults with spina bifida as well.

## FUTURE DIRECTIONS

Adults comprise an ever increasing proportion of the population of people with spina bifida. Maximizing their health and well-being includes effective screening, early intervention, and prevention. These require knowledge of the issues that adults with spina bifida currently face, including their magnitude and mediating factors: the etiology of conditions, risk and protective factors, and mechanisms of occurrence. It also includes ascertaining what individuals with spina bifida want for themselves. Such knowledge can help in the development of effective intervention strategies. These strategies include changes in systems and in policies (e.g., supportive employment) that will assist the development of a society in which all people are fully valued. The promotion of health and well-being should be emphasized along with the prevention of secondary conditions. The development of effective strategies for preventive intervention requires scientifically based trials, tailoring, implementing and sustaining prevention practice through a clear understanding of the community context, and partnerships with the community.

A cross-sectional population-based study of adults with spina bifida should be undertaken emphasizing long-term follow-up, complications, challenges, and outcomes for this group. Outcome measures should use the WHO model of disability and examine participation in society [e.g., employment (86)], survival, cognitive and functional outcomes, quality of life issues, costs and benefits of interventions, and ready access to services in a coordinated fashion. Studies of various models of transition to adult healthcare services should be undertaken to find the best practice in caring for these individuals (87,88). Finally, training grants should be offered to help health-care and other providers whose practice involves adults to better understand the issues facing this population and to learn the best interventions for them.

A civil rights song says that we should "keep our eyes on the prize." The "prize" for people who have spina bifida is having the same opportunities during adulthood for health and well-being as experienced by people without spina bifida. This should be the goal of all that is done in health and related areas during childhood and adolescence as well as during the transition from adolescence to adulthood. Helping individuals who have spina bifida develop a better past that they can bring with them to adult life should ensure that they have a brighter future than they do now.

## REFERENCES

1. Mental Health: A Report of the Surgeon General. http://www.surgeongeneral.gov/library/mentalhealth/home.html; accessed April 27, 2004.
2. World Health Organization. International Classification of Functioning, Disability and Health. Geneva: World Health Organization, 2001.
3. Erikson E. Identity and the life cycle. Psychol Issues 1959; 1(1):1–171.

4. Bandura A. Self-efficacy mechanism in human agency. Am Psychol 1982; 37: 122–147.
5. Shumake J, Gonzalez-Lima F. Brain systems underlying susceptibility to helplessness and depression. Behav Cogn Neurosci Rev 2003; 2(3):198–221.
6. Evans RG, Barer ML, Marmor TR, eds. Why are some people healthy and others not?: the determinants of health of populations. New York: A. de Gruyter, 1994:53.
7. Mier R, Holcomb LA, Minter C. Community functioning among adult spina bifida patients [abstr]. Dev Med Child Neurol 2003; 45(9):29.
8. McDonnell GV, McCann JP. Link between the CSF shunt and achievement in adults with spina bifida. J Neurol Neurosurg Psychiatry 2000; 68(6):800.
9. Kinsman SL, Doehring MC. The cost of preventable conditions in adults with spina bifida. Eur J Pediatr Surg 1996; 6(suppl 1):17–20.
10. Engstrom B, Nordeson A. What neurological patients regard as quality of life. J Clin Nurs 1995; 4(3):177–183.
11. Sivaraman Nair KP, Wade DT. Life goals of people with disabilities due to neurological disorders. Clin Rehabil 2003; 17(5):521–527.
12. Bronfenbrenner U, Hembrooke H, Morris PA. Poverty and the next generation. In: Bronfenbrenner U, McClelland P, Wethington E, Moen P, Ceci SJ, eds. The State of Americans: This Generation and the Next. NY: The Free Press, 1996:150–188.
13. Hunt GM, Oakeshott P, Kerry S. Link between CSF shunt and achievement in adults with spina bifida. J Neurol Neurosurg Psychiatry 2000; 67:591–595.
14. Oakeshott P, Hunt GM. Long-term outcome in open spina bifida. Br J Gen Pract 2003; 53(493):632–636.
15. Hunt GM, Oakeshott P. Outcome in people with open spina bifida at age 35: prospective community based cohort study. BMJ 2003; 326(7403):1365–1366.
16. Tew B. The adolescent with spina bifida: academic achievement and employment prospects. Br J Spec Educ 1986; 13(1):22–26.
17. Tew B, Laurence KM, Jenkins V. Factors affecting employability among young adults with spina bifida and hydrocephalus. Z Kinderchir 1990; 45(suppl 1):34–36.
18. Hurley AD, Bell S. Educational and vocational outcome of adults with spina bifida in relationship to neuropsycholgical testing. Eur J Pediatric Surg 1994; 4(suppl 1): 17–18.
19. Castree BJ, Walker JH. The young adult with spina bifida. Br Med Clin Res Educ 1981; 283(6298):1040–1042.
20. Bomalaski MD, Teague JL, Brooks B. The long term impact of urological management on the quality of life of children with spina bifida. J Urol 1995; 154(2 Pt 2):778–781.
21. Loomis JW, Javornisky JG, Monahan JJ, Burke G, Lindsay A. Relations between family environment and adjustment outcomes in young adults with spina bifida. Dev Med Child Neurol 1997; 39(9):620–627.
22. Anderson CJ, Vogel LC. Employment outcomes of adults who sustained spinal cord injuries as children or adolescents. Arch Phys Med Rehabil 2002; 83(6):791–801.
23. Vogel LC, Klaas SJ, Lubicky JP, Anderson CJ. Long-term outcomes and life satisfaction of adults who had pediatric spinal cord injuries. Arch Phys Med Rehabil 1998; 79(12):1496–1503.
24. Anderson CJ, Vogel LC. Domain-specific satisfaction in adults with pediatric-onset spinal cord injuries. Spinal Cord 2003; 41(12):684–691.
25. Anderson CJ, Krajci KA, Vogel LC. Community integration among adults with spinal cord injuries sustained as children or adolescents. Dev Med Child Neurol 2003; 45(2):129–134.

26. Lonton AP, O'Sullivan AM, Loughlin AM. Spina bifida adults. Z Kinderchir 1983; 38(suppl 2):110–112.
27. Peterson PM, Rauen KK, Brown J, Cole J. Spina bifida: the transition to adulthood begins in infancy. Rehabil Nurs 1994; 19(4):229–238.
28. Schriner KF, Roessler RT, Johnson P. Identifying the employment concerns of people with spina bifida. J Appl Rehabil Couns 1993; 24(2):32–37.
29. Yelin E, Sonneborn D, Trupin L. The prevalence and impact of accommodations on the employment of persons 51–61 years of age with musculoskeletal conditions. Arthritis Care Res 2000; 13(3):168–176.
30. Diagnostic and Statistical Manual of Mental Disorders DSM-IV, 4th ed. Washington, DC: American Psychiatric Association, 1994.
31. Fletcher JM, Barnes M, Dennis M. Language development in children with spina bifida. Semin Pediatr Neurol 2002; 9(3):201–208.
32. Dennis M, Barnes M. Math and numeracy in young adults with spina bifida and hydrocephalus. Dev Neuropsychol 2002; 21(2):141–155.
33. Hommet C, Billiard C, Gillet P, et al. Neuropsychologic and adaptive functioning in adolescents and young adults shunted for congenital hydrocephalus. J Child Neurol 1999; 14:144–150.
34. Cadman D, Boyle M, Szatmari P, Offord DR. Chronic illness, disability, and mental and social well-being: findings of the Ontario Child Health Study. Pediatrics 1987; 79(5):805–813.
35. Holmbeck GN, Westhoven VC, Phillips WS, et al. A multimethod, multi-nformant, and multidimensional perspective on psychosocial adjustment in preadolescents with spina bifida. J Consult Clin Psychol 2003; 71(4):782–796.
36. Blum RW, Resnick MD, Nelson R, St Germaine A. Family and peer issues among adolescents with spina bifida and cerebral palsy. Pediatrics 1991; 88: 280–285.
37. DeLamater J, Friedrich WN. Human sexual development. J Sex Res 2002; 39(1):10–14.
38. Picco P, Lavia N, Leveratto L, et al. Central precocious puberty in children affected by myelomeningocele. Eur J Pediatr Surg 1995; 5:39–40.
39. Trollman R, Dorr HG, Strehl E, Katalinic A, Beyer R, Wenzel D. Growth and pubertal development in patients with meningomyelocele: a retrospective analysis. Acta Paediatr 1996; 85:76–80.
40. Hayden PW, Davenport SLH, Campbelle MM. Adolescents with myelodysplasia: impact of physical disability on emotional maturation. Pediatrics 1979; 1:53–59.
41. Thill ADW. The influence of pubertal timing on self-concept and depression in pre-adolescents with and without spina bifida [Dissertation Abstract]. Dissertation Abstracts International: Section B: the Sciences and Engineering. Vol. 63(6-B), January 2002, 3046. US: University Microfilms International.
42. Decter RM, Furness PD, Nguyen TA, McGowan M, Laudermilch C, Telenko A. Reproductive understanding, sexual functioning and testosterone levels in men with spina bifida. J Urol 1997; 157:1466–1468.
43. Diamond DA, Rickwood AM, Thomas DG. Penile erections in myelomeningocele patients. Br J Urol 1986; 58:434–435.
44. Hirayama A, Yamada K, Tanaka Y, et al. Evaluation of sexual function in adults with myelomeningocele. Hinyokika Kiyo 1995; 41:985–989.

45. Dik P, van Gool JD, de Jong TP. Urinary continence and erectile function after bladder neck sling suspension in male patients with spinal dysraphism. BJU Int 1999; 83:971–975.
46. Sandler AD, Worley G, Leroy EC, Stanley SD, Kalman S. Sexual function and erection capability among young men with spina bifida. Dev Med Child Neurol 1996; 38:823–829.
47. Sawyer SM, Roberts KV. Sexual and reproductive health in your people with spina bifida. Dev Med Child Neurol 1999; 41:671–675.
48. Verhoef M, Barf HA, Vroege JA, et al. The ASPINE Study: preliminary results on sex education, relationships and sexual functioning of Dutch adolescents with spina bifida. Eur J Pediatr Surg 2000; 10S:53–54.
49. Sipski ML, Alexander CJ, Rosen RC. The neurologic basis of sexual arousal and orgasm in women: effects of spinal cord injury. Ann Neurol 2001; 49:35–44.
50. Blackburn M, Bax MC, Morgan DJ. Sexuality disability and abuse. Research into practice? Eur J Pediatr Surg 1996; 6(suppl 1):45–46.
51. MacBriar BR. Self-concept of preadolescent and adolescent children with a meningomyelocele. Issues Compr Pediatr Nurs 1983; 6:1–4.
52. Murch RL, Cohen LH. Relationships among life stress, perceived family environment, and the psychological distress of spina bifida adolescents. J Pediatr Psychol 1989; 14:193–214.
53. Kazak AE, Clark MW. Stress in families of children with myelomeningocele. Dev Med Child Neurol 1986; 28:220–228.
54. King GA, Shultz IZ, Steel K, Gilpin M, Cathers T. Self-evaluation and self-concept of adolescents with physical disabilities. Am J Occup Ther 1993; 47:132–140.
55. Appleton PL, Minchom PE, Ellis NC, Elliott CE, Boll V, Jones P. The self-concept of young people with spina bifida: a population-based study. Dev Med Child Neurol 1994; 36:198–215.
56. Zurmohle UM, Homann T, Schroeter C, Rothgerber H, Hommel G, Ermert JA. Psychosocial adjustment of children with spina bifida. J Child Neurol 1998; 13:64–70.
57. Moore C, Kogan BA, Parekh A. Impact of urinary incontinence on self-concept in children with spina bifida. J Urol 2004; 171(4):1659–1662.
58. Aksnes G, Diseth TH, Helseth A, Edwin B, Stange M, Aafos G. Appendicostomy for antegrade enema: effects on somatic and psychosocial functioning in children with myelomeningocele. Pediatrics 2002; 109:484–489.
59. Resnick MD, Hutton L. Resiliency among physically disabled adolescents. Psychiatr Ann 1987; 17(12):796–800.
60. Kendler KS, Hettema JM, Butera F, Gardner CO, Prescott CA. Life event dimensions of loss, humiliation, entrapment, and danger in the prediction of onsets of major depression and generalized anxiety. Arch Gen Psychiatry 2003; 60(8): 789–796.
61. Holmbeck GN, Johnson SZ, Wills KE, et al. Observed and perceived parental overprotection in relation to psychosocial adjustment in preadolescents with a physical disability: the mediational role of behavioral autonomy. J Consult Clin Psychol 2002; 70(1):96–110.
62. Howe GW, Feinstein C, Reiss D, Molock S, Berger K. Adolescent adjustment to chronic physical disorders-I. Comparing neurological and non-neurological conditions. J Child Psychol Psychiatry 1993; 34(7):1153–1171.

63. Thompson RJ, Kronenberger WG, Johnson DF, Whiting K. The role of central nervous system functioning and family functioning in behavioral problems of children with myelodysplasia. J Dev Behav Pediatr 1989; 10(5):242–248.
64. Henningsen P, Zimmermann T, Sattel H. Medically unexplained physical symptoms, anxiety, and depression: a meta-analytic review. Psychosom Med 2003; 65(4): 528–533.
65. Arroll B, N Khin, N Kerse. Screening for depression in primary care with two verbally asked questions: cross sectional study. BMJ 2003; 327(7424):1144–1146.
66. Padua L, Rendeli C, Rabini A, Girardi E, Tonali P, Salvaggio E. Health-related quality of life and disability in young patients with spina bifida. Arch Phys Med Rehabil 2002; 83(10):1384–1388.
67. McAnarney ER, Pless IB, Satterwhite B, Friedman SB. Psychological problems of children with chronic juvenile arthritis. Pediatrics 1974; 53(4):523–528.
68. Minchom PE, Ellis NC, Appleton PL, et al. Impact of functional severity on self concept in young people with spina bifida. Arch Dis Child 1995; 73(1):48–52.
69. Westhoven VC. The longitudinal effect of perceived and observed family functioning on internalizing symptoms in young adolescents with spina bifida. [Dissertation Abstract] Dissertation Abstracts International: Section B: the Sciences and Engineering. Vol. 63(12-B), 2003, 6111. US: University Microfilms International.
70. Wallander JL, Varni JW. Social support and adjustment in chronically ill and handicapped children. Am J Community Psychol 1989; 17(2):185–201.
71. Lazarus RS, Lanier R. Stress-related transactions between person and environment. In: Pervin LS, Lewis M, eds. Perspectives in Interactional Psychology. New York: Plenum, 1978:311.
72. Luthar SS, Cicchetti D, Becker B. The construct of resilience: a critical evaluation and guidelines for future work. Child Dev 2000; 71(3):543–562.
73. Search Institute. Forty Developmental Assets. http://www.search-institute.org/assets/forty.htm; Accessed April 28, 2004.
74. Benson PL, Scales PC, Leffert N, Roehlkepartain EC. A Fragile Foundation: The State of Developmental Assets Among American Youth, Search Institute: Minneapolis, MN, 1999.
75. Murphey DA, Lamonda KH, Carney JK, Duncan P. Relationships of a brief measure of youth assets to health-promoting and risk behaviors. J Adolesc Health 2004; 34(3):184–191.
76. Palmer JS, Kaplan WE, Firlit CF. Erectile dysfunction in patients with spina bifida is a treatable condition. J Urol 2000; 164(3 Pt 2):958–961.
77. Denny S, Clark TC, Fleming T, Wall M. Emotional resilience: risk and protective factors for depression among alternative education students in New Zealand. Am J Orthopsychiatry 2004; 74(2):137–149.
78. Sherman RG, Berling BS, Oppenheimer S. Increasing community independence for adolescents with spina bifida. Adolescence 1985; 20(77):1–13.
79. Lollar DJ, Reinoehl JK, Leverette AT, Martin JC, Posid VA. Facilitating and assessing progress toward independence: SPARX. Z Kinderchir 1989; 44(suppl 1): 18–20.
80. King GA, Specht JA, Schultz I, Warr-Leeper G, Redekop W, Risebrough N. Social skills training for withdrawn unpopular children with physical disabilities: a preliminary evaluation. Rehabil Psychol 1997; 42(1):47–60.

81. Elksnin LK, Elksnin N. Introduction to the special issue. Exceptionality 2001; 9(1–2):19–32.
82. Gresham FM. Social skills assessment and instruction for students with emotional and behavioral disorders. In: Lane KL, Gresham FM, Shaughnessy TE, eds. Interventions for Children with or at Risk for Emotional and Behavioral Disorders. Boston: Allyn and Bacon, 2002:242–258.
83. Donald M, Dower J. Risk and protective factors for depressive symptomatology among a community sample of adolescents and young adults. Aust NZ J Public Health 2002; 26(6):555–262.
84. Pelkonen M, Marttunen M, Aro H. Risk for depression: a 6-year follow-up of Finnish adolescents. J Affect Disord. 2003; 77(1):41–51.
85. Katon W, Rutter C, Ludman EJ, et al. A randomized trial of relapse prevention of depression in primary care. Arch Gen Psychiatry 2001; 58(3):241–247.
86. Cornell Youth and Work Program. http://www.human.cornell.edu/youthwork/index.html; accessed April 28, 2004.
87. Adolescent Health Transition Project. http://depts.washington.edu/healthtr/; accessed April 28, 2004.
88. Porter S. Transition Planning for Adolescents with Special Health Care Needs and Disabilities: A Guide for Health Care Providers (2000). http://www.communityinclusion.org/transition/providerguide.html; accessed April 28, 2004.

# 9

# Review of Current Neurosurgical Issues

**Kerry R. Crone and Benjamin Ling**
*Department of Neurosurgery, Cincinnati Children's Hospital Medical Center, University of Cincinnati College of Medicine, Cincinnati, Ohio, U.S.A.*

## OVERVIEW

The general term neural tube defect refers to all defects that occur because of improper closure of the neural tube during development. Defects include improper development of both the anterior neuropore (of which the most dramatic result is anencephaly) and the posterior neuropore. Defects of the posterior neuropore that affect the spinal elements may be classified broadly as spinal dysraphism or spina bifida. This entity encompasses a spectrum of presentations from occult lesions that involve sinus tracts and lipomas to open lesions. In this chapter, we limit our discussion to the more commonly known open lesion myelomeningocele.

## SURGICAL HISTORY

The first recorded surgical treatment of spina bifida in Western literature dates back to the 1600s with the report of ligation of a myelomeningocele sac. With the refinement of surgical techniques at the turn of the 20th century, Fraser reported the first series of 131 surgically treated patients (1). In this series, only 63% of patients survived until discharge from the hospital and only 23% were still alive at follow-up (minimum six years). In the 1930s and 1940s, surgeons advocated delayed repair of the defect to allow for epithelialization of the neural placode (2), however, complications and death secondary to infection and hydrocephalus were common. With the advent of ventriculoperitoneal shunting in the 1950s, hydrocephalus became treatable and earlier repair of myelomeningoceles was possible with less likelihood of cerebrospinal fluid leakage breaking down the wound. During the next two decades, debate focused on patient selection for repair. Interventions typically took place shortly after birth and resulted in substantially higher long-term survival rates (3). By the 1980s, reports of patient series demonstrated 82% to 86% survival rates with follow-up of at least five years (4,5).

## ANATOMY AND PATHOLOGY

Patients with myelomeningoceles nearly always exhibit two other pathologic entities, that is, hydrocephalus and Chiari II malformation. Although these two problems may seem anatomically distinct from spina bifida, current developmental theories may explain how these pathologies actually relate to one another.

### Myelomeningocele

Understanding the principles of myelomeningocele repair necessitates familiarity with the anatomy of the defect. Myelomeningoceles can be located anywhere from the mid-thoracic to the sacral region and vary in diameter, ranging less than 1 cm to more than 5 cm. During fetal development, improper closure of the posterior neuropore results in an uncanalized spinal cord, an open dural tube, nonunion of the dorsal spinal elements, and a midline musculofascial defect. At presentation, a myelomeningocele may be described as a sac of variable size filled with spinal fluid with a peripheral margin of dystrophic skin (Fig. 1A). At the center of the lesion, the neural placode is a segment of spinal cord exposed to air that has not canalized. A groove, which is the remnant of the central canal of the spinal cord, runs longitudinally down the center of the placode. In cross-sectional view, nerve roots are seen exiting from the anterior

(A) (B)

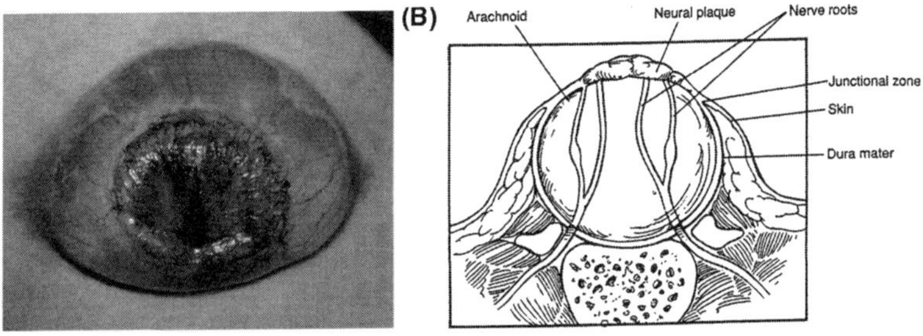


**Figure 1** Typical lumbar myelomeningocele. (**A**) Photograph shows the exposed neural placode at the center of the cerebrospinal-fluid-filled lesion. *Source*: Courtesy of Mayfield Clinic, Cincinnati, Ohio, U.S.A. (**B**) Cross-sectional view shows the relationships between the open neural placode, ventrally extending nerve roots, underlying dural layer, and surrounding skin. *Source*: From Ref. 26.

surface of the placode (Fig. 1B). A thin layer of tissue, called the junctional zone, surrounds the placode circumferentially; at its edges, this zone is attached to the surrounding skin. The dura splays outward and forms a bowl under the lesion; its edges fuse to the surrounding lumbosacral fascia.

Infants with myelomeningoceles generally present with neurological deficits at birth. Function depends to a large extent on the spinal level of the myelomeningocele. Defects located in the sacral region may affect only bowel and bladder function and not affect motor strength of the lower extremities. However, thoracic lesions may render the child paraplegic. Neurological function also depends on the amount of functional tissue remaining in the placode. Although quantification of functional tissue is difficult to estimate at the patient's bedside or in the operating room, surgeons performing a repair should assume that viable neurological tissue still exists in the placode. Evidence for this has been shown in a series of pathological examinations of spinal cords in eight stillborn fetuses with myelomeningoceles in which varying amounts of tissue loss were observed at the defect site (6). However, a large degree of normal development of the cord had occurred where ventral remnants of the cord remain.

A "two-hit hypothesis" has been proposed to explain this functional diminution of the placode. The initial dysfunction, which occurs from the embryologic defect, is worsened later by secondary insults that can include in-utero exposure of the placode to amniotic fluid, trauma to the placode against the uterine wall during gestation, and trauma during delivery (7). On the basis of this hypothesis, one rationale is to lessen or prevent these secondary "hits" by intrauterine repair of the myelomeningocele.

## Chiari II Malformation

A Chiari II malformation consists of a constellation of intracranial and cervical abnormalities, of which the most clinically relevant is the downward herniation of cerebellar and brainstem tissue below the foramen magnum that is seen in virtually all newborns with myelomeningoceles (Fig. 2). The proposed mechanism for this anomaly suggests that the myelomeningocele allows excessive outward drainage of spinal fluid through its defect during development. Because the spinal fluid column is in continuity with the intracranial cerebrospinal fluid compartments, this drainage early in development theoretically leads to a collapse of the rhombencephalic vesicle, which then results in a small posterior fossa. Growth of the cerebellum and brainstem within a small posterior fossa results in the downward herniation and caudal displacement of the cerebellar vermis and brainstem into the cervical spinal canal (8).

Generally 10% to 20% of infants will develop symptoms from the Chiari II malformation within the first three months of life. Symptoms may include dysphagia, apnea, stridor, aspiration, and extremity weakness. Clinical outcomes become more complicated in infants with symptomatic Chiari II malformations.

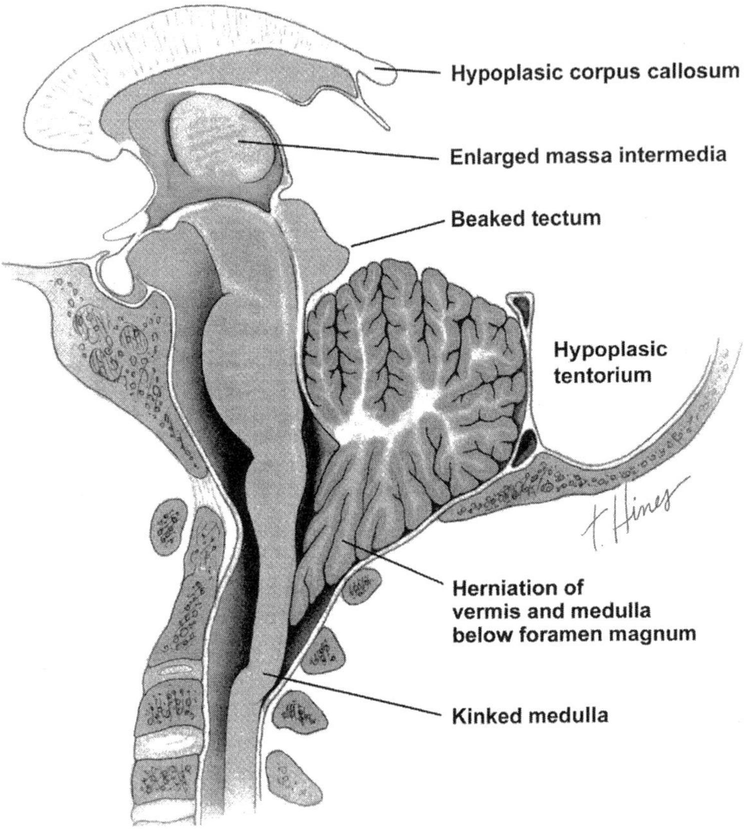


**Figure 2** Mid-sagittal section of a Chiari II malformation. Note the low-lying obex and cerebellar tonsils and vermis. *Source*: Courtesy of Mayfield Clinic, Cincinnati, Ohio, U.S.A.

Although the current operative mortality approaches 0% for neonates with a myelomeningocele and an asymptomatic Chiari II malformation, mortality rises up to 30% for those with a symptomatic Chiari II malformation (9). Surgical decompression, which entails a multilevel cervical laminectomy and probable duraplasty, should be performed early to minimize progression of these symptoms.

## Hydrocephalus

The term hydrocephalus refers to the enlargement of the ventricular system of the brain caused by the buildup of cerebrospinal fluid under pressure. Cerebrospinal fluid is produced by the choroid plexus in the lateral ventricles and flows through the foramina of Monro to the third ventricle. Flow of cerebrospinal fluid continues

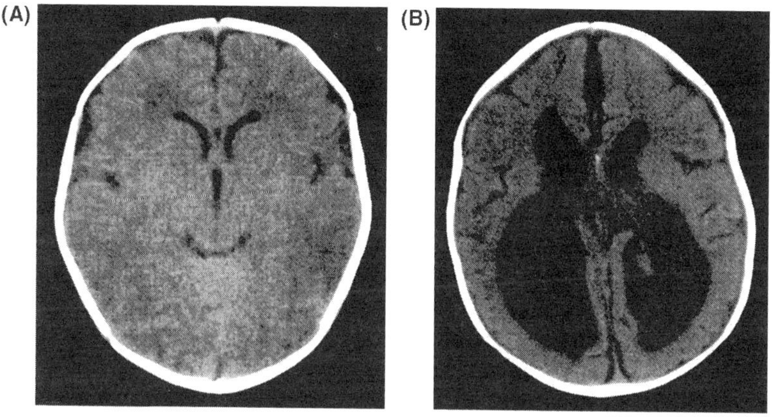


**Figure 3** CT scan compares normal ventricular size (**A**) with enlarged ventricles from hydrocephalus (**B**). *Source*: Courtesy of Mayfield Clinic, Cincinnati, Ohio, U.S.A.

out of the third ventricle through the aqueduct of Sylvius to the fourth ventricle and then out into the subarachnoid space where it is absorbed over the convexities of the brain through the arachnoid granulations. Hydrocephalus may be categorized broadly into two types as obstructive or communicating. Obstructive hydrocephalus occurs when a mass lesion or a congenital anomaly blocks or impedes cerebrospinal fluid flow along its pathways. Communicating hydrocephalus occurs when malabsorption of cerebrospinal fluid at the arachnoid granulations causes a uniform expansion of all cerebrospinal fluid spaces in the brain.

Routine ultrasound studies of the ventricular system have shown ventricular dilatation in 95% of neonates with myelomeningoceles (10) (Fig. 3). Although causes of the hydrocephalus remain unclear, both communicating and obstructive factors have been speculated to occur. Possible causes include aqueductal stenosis, fourth ventricular outlet obstruction due to a tight Chiari II malformation, or underdevelopment of the arachnoid granulations. Regardless of the cause, approximately 90% of infants with myelomeningoceles will require treatment of hydrocephalus within the first six weeks of life. In addition to accelerated head growth, symptoms of increased intracranial pressure caused by hydrocephalus may include irritability, lethargy, emesis, a bulging fontanelle, or distended scalp veins.

## SURGICAL TREATMENT

### Traditional Repair of Myelomeningocele

The exposed nature of delicate neural structures and open communication with the cerebrospinal fluid spaces generally necessitates closure of a myelomeningocele within the first 24 hours after birth to minimize further damage to the placode and prevent infection. The child should be hemodynamically stable to safely undergo repair. If a delay is necessary, some authors have reported satisfactory results waiting up to 72 hours for repair without an increase in complications (10). While awaiting repair, a dressing of sterile saline-soaked gauze covered by plastic wrap usually helps to prevent the desiccation of the placode from prolonged exposure to air. Administration of perioperative antibiotics is at the discretion of the surgeon. The practice at the senior author's (Kerry R. Crone) institution is administration of ampicillin and gentamycin shortly after birth until three days postoperatively.

The principle of surgical repair is reconstruction of the neural tube and its coverings to avoid meningitis and protect functioning neural elements. On the basis of the observation that more than one-third of children subsequently gain motor functions not previously detected, the placode should be considered functional even if the initial examination demonstrates no muscle activity below a certain spinal level (11). After an initial incision is made at the junction zone of the myelomeningocele, the placode is circumferentially dissected from the surrounding arachnoid adhesions. Reasonable efforts should be made to preserve any blood vessels encountered during this dissection because these likely supply neural elements.

Once the placode is freed, careful attention is given to ensure the edges of the placode are clean and without any epithelial remnants, which may give rise to an inclusion dermoid tumor if left within the closure. At this point, some surgeons reconstruct the neural tube by sewing the lateral edges of the placode together. Although this step is controversial, it decreases the surface area of the spinal cord that may adhere to or cause scarring of the surrounding dura, which could then result in cord tethering later in life (12). The dural layer is then identified, dissected free, and sewn together to reconstruct the dural tube around the neural elements. Lateral release of the lumbosacral fascia and musculature allows for another layer of closure in the midline over the defect. Finally the skin is undermined and closed (Fig. 4). In some patients with large myelomeningoceles, it is occasionally difficult to obtain a standard closure and a plastic surgeon is needed to assist in the closure.

## Intrauterine Repair

Studies that longitudinally followed the in-utero development of children with spina bifida suggest that the problems associated with myelomeningoceles (i.e., spinal cord dysfunction, Chiari II malformation, and hydrocephalus) were the delayed consequences of the original neural tube defect (8,13). In a theoretical sense, these problems might be minimized or even prevented if intervention occurred pre-emptively. Such was the philosophy behind the ideas and development of fetal neurosurgical techniques. Fetal surgery, which was originally developed in the 1980s, was used successfully in the treatment of severe congenital abnormalities, such as diaphragmatic hernias. In applying these techniques to

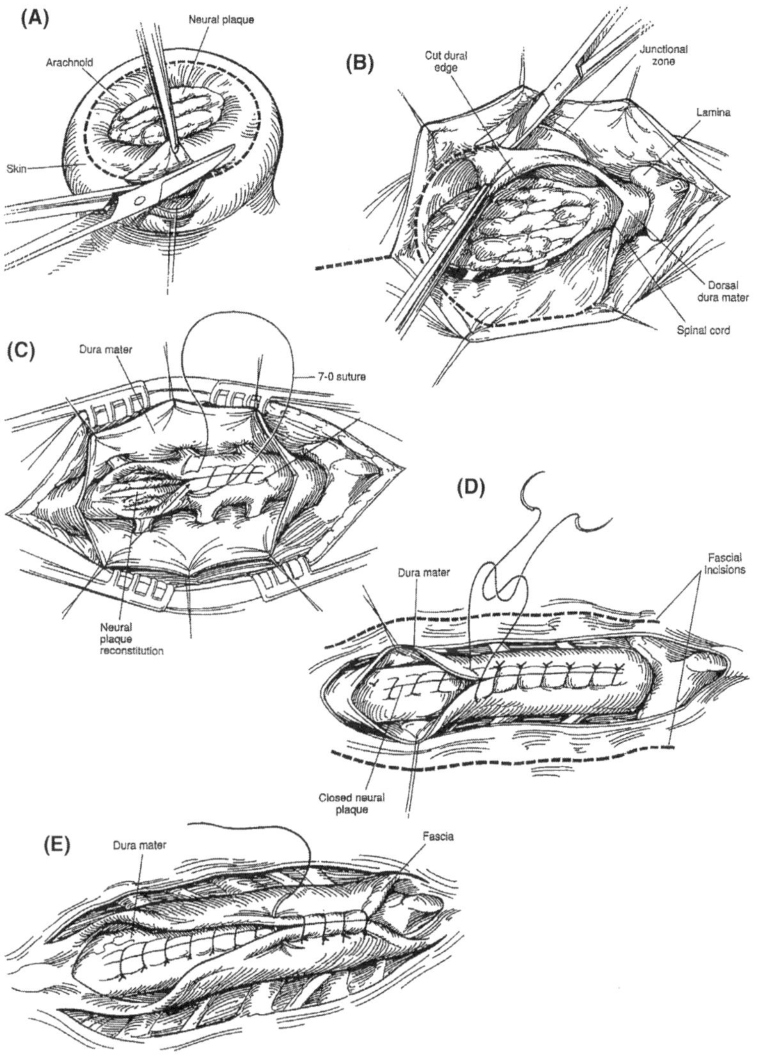


**Figure 4** Step-by-step example of a myelomeningocele repair where a multilayered closure is achieved. (**A**) Incision of the junctional zone and dissection of the placode. (**B**) Identification and dissection of dural layer. (**C**) Sewing together of lateral edges of the placode. (**D**) Closure of dural layer. (**E**) Incision and closure of surrounding lumbosacral fascial layer. *Source*: From Ref. 26.

neurosurgical diseases, surgeons first attempted to treat hydrocephalus in-utero with ventriculo-amniotic shunts; these shunts were soon abandoned because of poor outcomes (14). Intrauterine myelomeningocele repair was then described in 1997 and has been performed at three different U.S. institutions.

Fetuses that have undergone intrauterine repair range in age from 22 to 30 weeks gestation. The technique of intrauterine repair begins with a standard low transverse abdominal incision in the mother to mobilize the uterus. A hysterotomy is performed in the upper segment of the uterus (similar to the classic cesarean section), and the fetus is visualized. As surgery is performed through the hysterotomy, intrauterine fluid volume is maintained to prevent placental separation, contractions, and expulsion of the fetus. After the myelomeningocele defect has been identified, closure requires a different approach than that previously described because of fragility of the tissues. Sutton et al. described first dissection of the placode free, sewing of an allograft skin patch over top of the neural structures, and then mobilization and closure of the fetal skin (15). Bruner et al. described the technique as dissection of the placode free, identification, and freeing of the dural layer to sew over top the placode and nerve roots, and then a primary skin closure (16). Whereas the standard technique achieves a three-layer closure (dura, muscle and fascia, skin), only a two-layer closure is performed with intrauterine techniques. After closure, the uterine wall and maternal abdominal incision are closed in standard manner.

Although outcomes for fetal repair of myelomeningoceles do suggest some benefits, follow-up data are short term and all reports are from single institutions with nonrandomized patients. In 1999, Bruner et al. reported a decreased incidence of hindbrain herniation in 29 patients; specifically, only 38% of myelomeningoceles repaired by intrauterine techniques demonstrated cerebellar herniation compared with 95% in a historical control group repaired postnatally (15). The requirement for ventriculoperitoneal shunting was 59% in this group of 29 infants after in-utero repair compared with 91% in the control group. In a concurrent 1999 study, Sutton et al. also showed objective improvement by serial MRI imaging in hindbrain herniation in nine surviving patients and noted only four patients required shunting (14). A urologic study in six patients repaired by intrauterine technique showed no change in urodynamic patterns compared with infants who had undergone standard postnatal treatment (17). Lower extremity function also did not appear to improve in 37 patients who underwent in-utero repair compared with lesion-matched infants who underwent postnatal repair (18).

Until a multicenter, prospective, randomized trial is performed, the benefits of fetal surgery for myelomeningocele is unknown compared with standard postnatal closure. Premature labor and delivery are not insignificant risks, and long-term outcomes need to be addressed. At this time, a randomized trial has been designed and is currently underway.

## Cerebrospinal Fluid Diversion

Treatment options for hydrocephalus involve some manner of diversion of the accumulated cerebrospinal fluid. Ventricular shunting remains the most common treatment modality in which drainage of the lateral ventricle of the

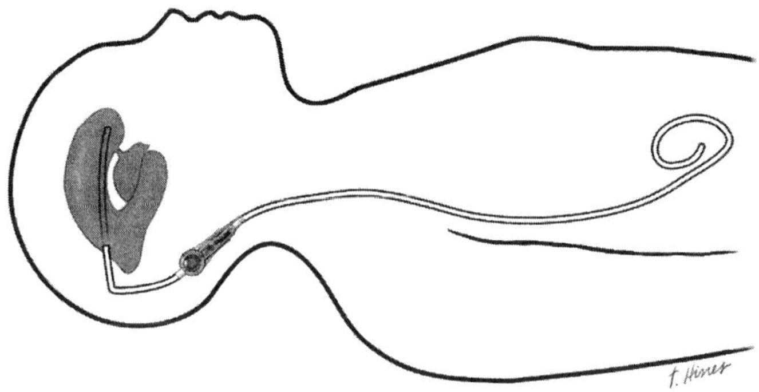


**Figure 5** Ventriculoperitoneal shunt with subcutaneously tunneled valve and tubing. *Source*: Courtesy of Mayfield Clinic, Cincinnati, Ohio, U.S.A.

brain is by a catheter that exits the skull and connects to a valve underneath the scalp. From there, the catheter is tunneled underneath the skin to drain into one of a number of different body cavities, typically the abdominal peritoneal cavity, thoracic pleural cavity, or right atrium of the heart (Fig. 5). However, shunt malfunction can be a frequent complication. Up to half of shunted myelomeningocele patients will require at least one shunt revision within the first year postoperatively (19). While an entire volume may be dedicated to the various types of shunt malfunction and their management, most may be attributed to a mechanical dysfunction or some type of flow alteration. Some of the more common malfunctions seen are occlusion of a proximal or distal catheter, valve malfunction, catheter breakage or disconnection, and over drainage or malabsorption of cerebrospinal fluid. Other shunting complications include infections and hardware erosions through the skin or other tissue planes.

The routes of ventricular cerebrospinal fluid flow that are particularly vulnerable to narrowing or obstruction are the cerebral aqueduct (which connects the third and the fourth ventricle) and the fourth ventricle outlets. If obstructive hydrocephalus is present because of flow impedance in these areas, consideration may be given to a third ventriculostomy. In this procedure, an endoscope is introduced through a frontal burr hole into the lateral ventricle. With guidance of the scope through the foramen of Monro into the third ventricle, creation of a small fenestration of the third ventricle floor can help to establish a communication between the third ventricle and the prepontine subarachnoid space (Fig. 6). This opening allows cerebrospinal fluid to bypass its usual route of outflow. With equilibration of flow and pressure between the ventricles and subarachnoid space, improved cerebrospinal fluid absorption occurs during the ensuing days to weeks so that the hydrocephalus eventually resolves. Although this procedure is advantageous because no permanent hardware is implanted as compared with a shunting procedure, there is a low incidence of the third ventriculostomy remaining open in infants with myelomeningocele. Older children tend to have a greater

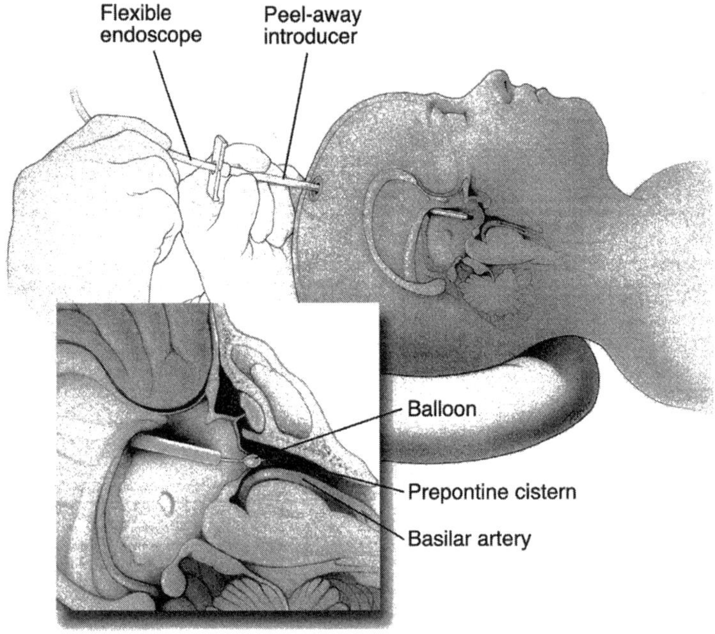


**Figure 6** During third ventriculostomy, a steerable endoscope is introduced through a burr hole and guided into the third ventricle through the foramen of Monro from the lateral ventricle. An inflatable balloon may be used to enlarge the fenestration in the ventricular floor and create an open communication to the prepontine subarachnoid space. *Source*: Courtesy of Mayfield Clinic, Cincinnati, Ohio, U.S.A.

chance of maintaining a successful third ventriculostomy. If their ventricular anatomy is favorable, this is a viable treatment option when children return at a later age with a malfunctioning shunt. With proper selection, 50% to 75% of patients with myelomeningocele may benefit from undergoing endoscopic third ventriculostomy (20).

## Tethered Cord Release

With any open surgical procedure, the physiological healing process involves deposition of scar tissue at the operative site. Children who have undergone myelomeningocele repair often form scar tissue at the site of the repaired placode, the sutured dura, and the overlying muscle and soft tissue layers. If the placode or adjacent nerve roots or both scar adhering to the dura or other surrounding structures, a tethered spinal cord may result. A normal spinal cord floats freely in cerebrospinal fluid and is loosely held in the dural sac by the exiting nerve roots, dentate ligaments, and filum terminale. A tethered spinal cord is defined as fixation of the cord, usually in an abnormally caudal position, to surrounding structures (e.g., dura, fascia, and skin). Growth or skeletal motion of the child then stretches and creates tension in the spinal cord and nerve roots that may cause motor and sensory dysfunction. In a tethered cord model in cats, Yamada et al. showed that a spinal cord under tension exhibited a metabolic and electrophysiologic susceptibility to hypoxic stress (21). Theoretically, continued stress eventually would lead to neuronal and axonal dysfunction caused by the structural damage from impaired metabolism.

A diagnosis of the tethered cord syndrome is made primarily on the basis of clinical signs and symptoms as well as the radiographic finding of a low conus medullaris. Manifestations include back pain, sensory disturbance, gait deterioration, increased lower extremity contractures, increasing foot deformities, progressive scoliosis, and worsening bowel and bladder function. In the literature, the incidence of tethered cord in patients after myelomeningocele repair ranges from 3% to 15%. Some authors suspect the incidence may be higher because of oversight by patients, caretakers, and healthcare workers (22). Early detection of tethered spinal cord is important because the longer the duration of symptoms and neurologic deficits, the less favorable the outcome despite detethering (23).

The goal of surgical treatment is to detach the area of scarred placode and nerve roots from the overlying dura or fascia and to minimize injury to the neural elements. However, incision and dissection of the scar during surgery can be difficult because tissue planes are often indiscernible. Various techniques advocated to detach the scarred cord from its attachments range from blunt dissection to sharp dissection with a laser (24). A dural patch is often used to create a larger, redundant dural sac, which may have less chance of scarring to the cord. Commercially made dural substitutes are touted as less likely to adhere to scar. However, patients remain at a high risk for retethering, despite the best intentions, with conservative estimates of 15% to 20% of patients scarring (25). The goal of surgery is to at least halt the progressive deformity and/or neurologic decline. Some improvement in function or reversal of deformity may be expected depending on the age of the patient and the extent and duration of neurological deficit.

## CONCLUSIONS

Neurosurgical care of patients with myelomeningoceles involves not only the initial closure of the defect but lifelong follow-up of associated conditions, such as hydrocephalus and tethered spinal cord. New innovations in surgical management are currently being investigated and treatment modalities continue to improve. With timely and careful follow-up, the neurosurgeon plays a vital role in maximizing the patient's functional outcome.

## REFERENCES

1. Fraser J. Spina bifida. Edinburgh Med J 1929; 36:284.
2. Ingraham F, Swan H. Spina bifida and cranium: I. A survey of five hundred forty-six cases. N Engl J Med 1943; 228:559.

3. Ames MD, Schut L. Results of treatment of 171 consecutive myelomeningoceles, 1963 to 1968. Pediatrics 1972; 50:466–470.
4. McLone DG, Dias L, Kaplan WE, Sommers ME. Concepts in the management of spina bifida. In Humphreys RP, ed. Concepts in Pediatric Neurosurgery. Basel, Switzerland: Karger, 1985:97–106.
5. Steinbok P, Irvine B, Cochrane DD, Irwin BJ. Long-term outcome and complications of children born with meningomyelocele. Childs Nerv Syst 1992; 8:92–96.
6. Hutchins GM, Meuli M, Meuli-Simmen C, Jordan MA, Heffez DS, Blakemore KJ. Acquired spinal cord injury in human fetuses with myelomeningocele. Pediatr Pathol Lab Med 1996; 16:701–712.
7. Meuli M, Meuli-Simmen C, Yingling CD, et al. The spinal cord lesion in human fetuses with myelomeningocele: implications for fetal surgery. J Pediatr Surg 1997; 32:448–452.
8. McLone DG, Naidich TP. Developmental morphology of the subarachnoid space, brain vasculature, and contiguous structures, and the cause of the Chiari II malformation. Am J Neuroradiol 1992; 13:463–482.
9. Park TS, Hoffman HJ, Hendrick EB, Humphreys RP. Experience with surgical decompression of the Arnold–Chiari malformation in young infants with myelomeningocele. Neurosurgery 1983; 13:147–152.
10. McLone D. Myelomeningocele. In: Youmans J, ed. Neurological Surgery, 4th ed. Philadelphia: W.B. Saunders, 1996:843–860.
11. McLone D. Results of treatment of children born with a myelomeningocele. Clin Neurosurg 1983; 30:407–412.
12. McLone D. Care of the neonate with a myelomeningocele. Neurosurg Clin North Am 1998; 9:111–120.
13. Osaka K, Tanimura T, Hirayama A, Matsumoto S. Myelomeningocele before birth. J Neurosurg 1978; 49:711–724.
14. Sutton LN, Sun P, Adzick NS. Fetal neurosurgery. Neurosurgery 2001; 48:124–144.
15. Sutton LN, Adzick NS, Bilaniuk LT, Johnson MP, Crombleholme TM, Flake AW. Improvement in hindbrain herniation demonstrated by serial fetal magnetic resonance imaging following fetal surgery for myelomeningocele. JAMA 1999; 282: 1826–1831.
16. Bruner JP, Tulipan N, Paschall RL, et al. Fetal surgery for myelomeningocele and the incidence of shunt-dependent hydrocephalus. JAMA 1999; 282:1819–1825.
17. Holmes NM, Nguyen HT, Harrison MR, Farmer DL, Baskin LS. Fetal intervention for myelomeningocele: effect on postnatal bladder function. J Urol 2001; 166: 2383–2386.
18. Tubbs RS, Chambers MR, Smyth MD, et al. Late gestational intrauterine myelomeningocele repair does not improve lower extremity function. Pediatr Neurosurg 2003; 38:128–132.
19. Caldarelli M, Di Rocco C, La Marca F. Shunt complications in the first postoperative year in children with meningomyelocele. Childs Nerv Syst 1996; 12:748–754.
20. Brockmeyer D, Abtin K, Carey L, Walker ML. Endoscopic third ventriculostomy: an outcome analysis. Pediatr Neurosurg 1998; 28:236–240.
21. Yamada S, Zinke DE, Sanders D. Pathophysiology of "tethered cord syndrome." J Neurosurg 1981; 54:494–503.
22. Phuong LK, Schoeberl KA, Raffel C. Natural history of tethered cord in patients with myelomeningocele. Neurosurgery 2002; 50:989–995.

23. Satar N, Bauer SB, Shefner J, Kelly MD, Darbey MM. The effects of delayed diagnosis and treatment in patients with an occult spinal dysraphism. J Urol 1995; 154:754–758.
24. Reigel DH. Tethered myelomeningocele. In: McLone D, ed. Pediatric Neurosurgery: Surgery of the Developing Nervous System. Philadelphia: W.B. Saunders Co, 2001:279–281.
25. Reigel DH, Ammerman RT, Rotenstein D. Health care of the adult with spina bifida. In: McLone D, ed. Pediatric Neurosurgery: Surgery of the Developing Nervous System. Philadelphia: W.B. Saunders Co, 2001:266–278.
26. Reigel DH. Myelomeningocele repair. In: McClone DG, ed. Pediatric Neurosurgery, 4th ed., Elsevier, 2001:261–265.

# 10

# New Orthopedic Trends

**Junichi Tamai**
*Division of Pediatric Orthopedic Surgery,*
*Cincinnati Children's Hospital Medical Center, Cincinnati, Ohio, U.S.A.*

**Jose Herrera-Soto**
*Arnold Palmer Hospital for Children, Orlando, Florida, U.S.A.*

**Alvin H. Crawford**
*Division of Pediatric Orthopedic Surgery,*
*Cincinnati Children's Hospital Medical Center, Cincinnati, Ohio, U.S.A.*

## INTRODUCTION

Orthopedic management of spina bifida patients continues to evolve. This chapter reviews recent trends in the management of spine, hip, and lower extremity deformities in children with myelomeningocele.

Refinements in instrumentation design and surgical technique have improved the outcomes of spine operations. Spine deformity correction allows the child with myelomeningocele to sit upright with minimal assistance of the upper extremities, freeing the hands to perform table-top activities. Improved sitting balance, better respiration, and easier access for gastrointestinal and urinary diversion are other benefits.

The patient's ambulatory status varies depending on the level of the lesion. Thoracic and high lumbar level lesion patients may be ambulatory during childhood but generally use wheelchairs by the time they are adolescents. Low lumbar level and sacral level patients may require assistive aids such as crutches, walkers, and ankle-foot orthoses (AFOs); however, they often continue to ambulate as adults.

Improvement in mobility, not ambulation, is the primary goal for the child with myelomeningocele. Lower extremity orthopedic operations must take this into consideration. Radiographic improvement does not always correlate with gains in functional outcome. In addition, spina bifida patients are prone to poor wound healing, greater risk for nonunion and pseudarthrosis, and surgical site infections. Because the underlying neurological condition does not improve with surgery, persistent or worsening muscle imbalance may alter operative results.

## SPINE DEFORMITY

Spinal deformities in the myelomeningocele population are common and complex, requiring a multidisciplinary team for management. Spinal deformities can be congenital or acquired later in life. About 15% of these deformities are congenital, including scoliosis due to vertebral malformations, congenital kyphosis related to posterior dysplasia, and intrathecal anomalies such as diastematomyelia. The congenital deformities need close monitoring and management. It may be necessary to prevent curve progression by arresting asymmetric growth. Deformities acquired later in life include idiopathic-like scoliosis, pelvic obliquity-related scoliosis, and neuromuscular, or paralytic, curves. Curves can also result from a tethered cord or hydrocephalus. Kyphosis and scoliosis are the two major types of spinal deformities in the myelomeningocele population.

### Kyphosis

#### Natural History for Kyphotic Spinal Deformity

Kyphosis is a spinal deformity present exclusively or primarily in the sagittal plane. Lateral view radiographs of the spine show this roundback deformity well. Up to 21% of myelomeningocele patients may have a kyphotic spinal deformity. Kyphosis is most common in patients with lower thoracic level of paralysis, although it can also be present in patients with upper thoracic and lower lumbar levels of paralysis (1). The natural history of kyphotic spine deformity is curve progression. Mintz et al. (2) compared the progression of congenital lumbar kyphosis in different groups of myelomeningocele patients. Patients who had initial radiographs taken at or before one year of age who had a kyphosis $>90^\circ$ progressed $12.1^\circ$/year. Patients who had initial radiographs taken after one year of age had progression rates between $6.4^\circ$ and $6.7^\circ$ a year, regardless of initial curve magnitude. Martin et al. (3) found that nonoperative treatment led to curve progression. At the initial visit, the average age was 1 year 11 months and the average curve magnitude was $70^\circ$. By the last visit, the average age was 19 years 7 months and the average curve magnitude was $106^\circ$.

#### Morbidity Associated with Kyphotic Spine Deformity

Kyphotic spine deformity has a considerable adverse effect on a number of bodily systems and functions. Kyphotic deformities result in thoracolumbar flexion with decreased trunk height (Fig. 1A). The space available for the lung can decrease,

**(A)**

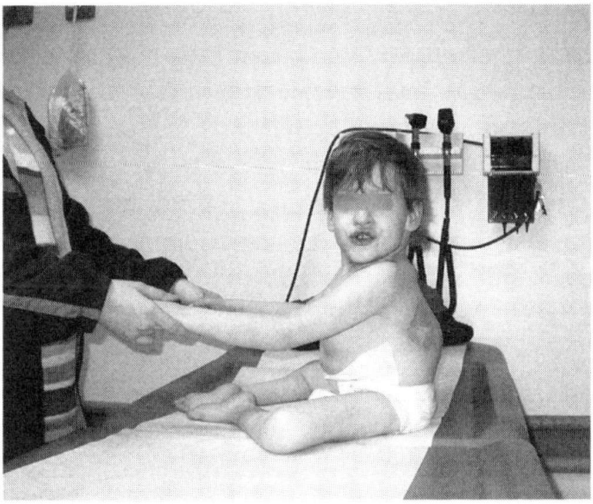

**(B)**

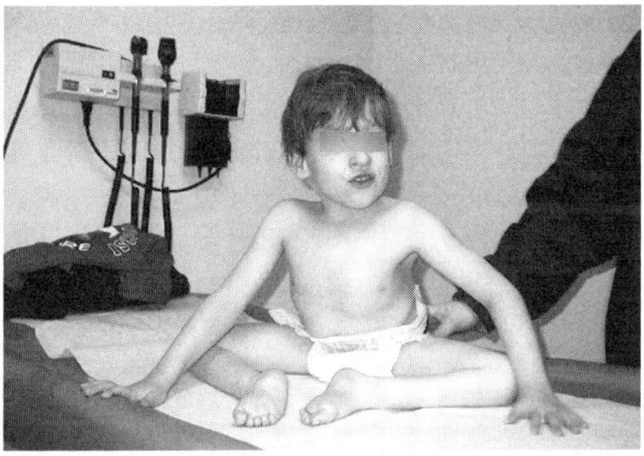

**(C)**

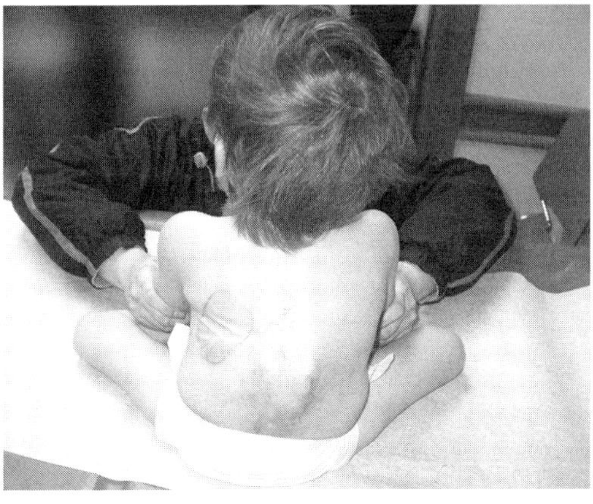

**Figure 1** (**A**) This five-year-old boy with a thoracic-level myelomeningocele has a kyphotic spinal deformity and a shortened trunk. (**B**) The patient uses his hands to support his forward-leaning trunk. Note his externally rotated hips. (**C**) Note the pressure sores over the kyphotic deformity.

resulting in thoracic insufficiency syndrome (4) and contributing to breathing problems. Compression of the chest against the thighs can also cause respiratory compromise from loss of diaphragmatic breathing, that is, secondary thoracic insufficiency syndrome (5). Clinically, these patients have a marionette sign, with synchronous bobbing of the head with respiration. Torso compression can also lead to increased abdominal pressure, resulting in eating difficulties and potential malnutrition. Because the hands are required to support the trunk in the kyphotic patient, they are not free to perform manual tasks (Fig. 1B). This can also make self-catheterization particularly difficult, if not impossible. Furthermore, the limited access to the anterior abdominal wall makes creating and caring for gastrointestinal and urinary diversions difficult. The spinal deformity may hinder transfers and ambulation with or without assistive devices. Pelvic obliquity may affect not only sitting balance, but also standing, due to a functional leg length discrepancy. Finally, prominences created by the spinal deformity and pelvic obliquity combined with lack of sensation predispose these patients to skin ulcerations over the kyphosis and the ischial tuberosities (Fig. 1C).

## Nonoperative Management of Kyphosis

Bracing for kyphotic deformity is ineffective in halting curve progression. Furthermore, bracing applies pressure on the insensate skin overlying the kyphotic deformity, promoting ulceration. Appropriate shaping of the wheelchair back pad is an important part of pressure sore prevention and management (3).

## Potential Benefits of Kyphosis Correction Surgery

Surgical stabilization of the spine achieves better truncal alignment, improved seating in the wheelchair, and elimination of skin pressure over the kyphotic spine segment. In addition, operative treatment improves respiratory function, frees the upper extremities for use, and leads to easier use of mobility aids, that is, wheelchairs, walkers, or forearm crutches. The improvement in posture can also help with efficacy in gastrointestinal and urinary diversion. Correction of pelvic obliquity may improve sitting balance and can minimize functional leg length discrepancy. A study of 39 myelomeningocele patients by Lintner and Lindseth (6) found that all the children and their families believed that the procedures were beneficial, despite some long-term loss of correction over an average follow-up of 11 years.

## Neonatal Kyphectomy

Kyphectomy involves resection of the sharply angled kyphotic spine segment followed by reconnection of the remainder of the spine with wires or sutures, forming a shorter but straighter spine. The orthopedic surgeon can perform the neonatal kyphectomy on the newborn child with myelomeningocele in conjunction with the dural sac closure performed by the neurosurgeon (Fig. 2A). In the

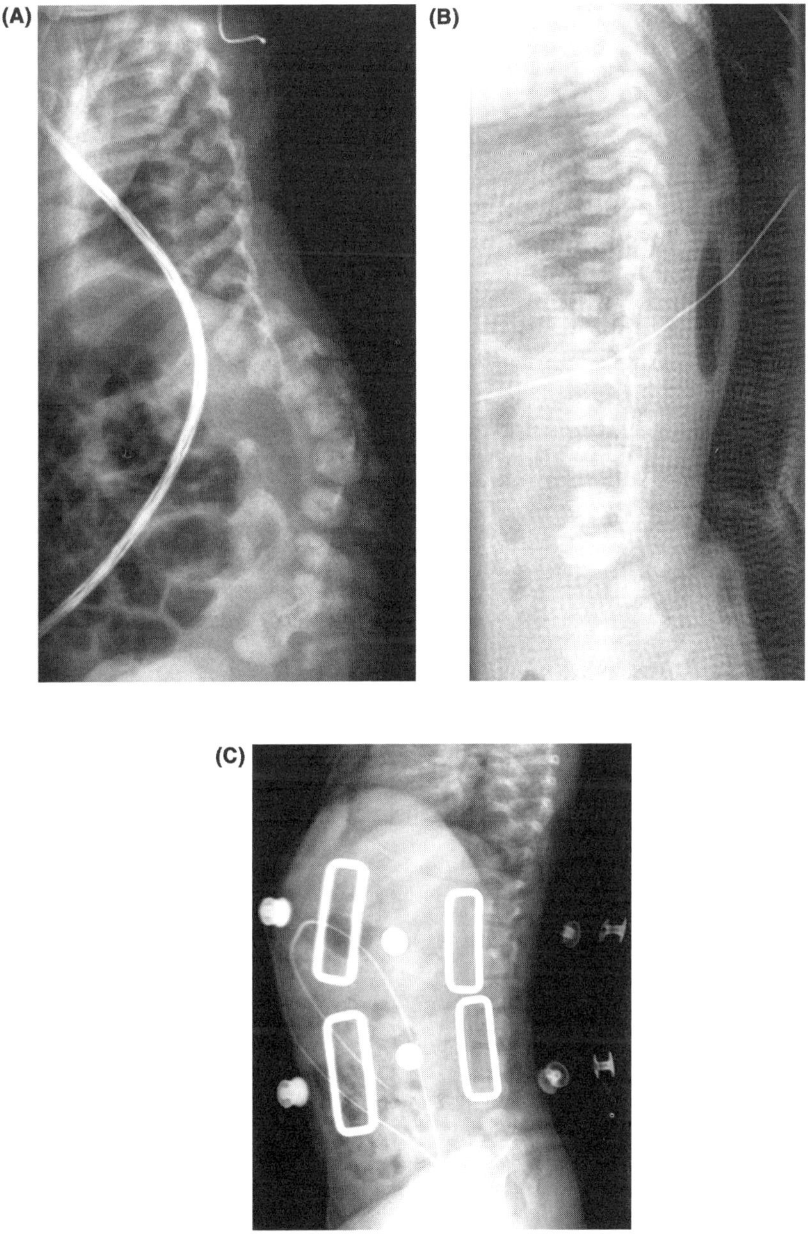


**Figure 2** (**A**) This newborn has a kyphotic deformity of the lumbar spine. (**B**) This patient underwent a neonatal kyphectomy and was placed in a cast to maintain the correction. (**C**) The correction is maintained in a hyperextension brace two years later. The patient will eventually develop a kyphotic deformity but it will be less severe than that of someone who had not undergone a kyphectomy as a newborn.

past, neonatal kyphectomy was associated with high peri-operative mortality due to excessive bleeding. Although only performed at selected centers, neonatal kyphectomy is safer now due to the development of mono- and bipolar electrocautery, which allows better control of sinusoidal bleeding. In our series (7), the average preoperative kyphotic angle was 67° and the average correction was 77°, creating some degree of lordosis. The average loss of correction, at an average follow-up of seven years and four months, was 55°, resulting in an average kyphosis of 45°. Some kyphosis eventually recurs despite the procedure, presumably due to persistent muscle imbalance between the front and back of the spinal column. However, the resulting curve is longer and the curve magnitude is smaller, making it less technically demanding to treat surgically later. After neonatal kyphectomy, the patient stays prone for the first three to four days for wound care and then goes into a well-padded pantaloon cast (Fig. 2B) in the "sky diver's" position. The patient later transitions to a hyperextension brace (Fig. 2C).

### Kyphectomy in Children

Children greater than three years of age are more commonly the candidates for kyphosis correction surgery. Several techniques are available. The most common method of treatment, described by Lintner and Lindseth (6), involves resection of the lordotic segment cephalad to the apical vertebra of the kyphotic deformity. They reported good long-term results. One center recently reported that the subtraction (decancellation) vertebrectomy technique with preservation of the dural sac was a safe and efficacious technique for correction and stabilization of kyphotic deformities in young patients with myelomeningocele (8). This technique involves removing the cancellous bone inside each vertebral body. The surgeons then manipulate the spine so that the emptied vertebral bodies flatten and realign in a manner that corrects the kyphosis. McCarthy (9) has described annulotomy and disk release as another technique to use in conjunction with the above methods.

In the past, surgeons used sutures or wires only at the kyphectomy site to stabilize the patients who underwent kyphectomies, then immobilized them in casts or braces for many months to achieve bony fusion (Fig. 3). More recently, surgeons have employed segmental spinal instrumentation, including rods and sublaminar wires or cables, to stabilize the thoracic spine above the kyphectomy site (Fig. 4A and B). This technique provides multiple points of fixation for the rods while allowing guided growth. In a young child, especially under 10 years of age, one limits the fusion to the pelvis or lumbar spine. Extraperiosteal exposure and preservation of the facet joints minimize the chance of a bony fusion along the thoracic spine. The sublaminar wires or cables will move up along the rods as the child's spine grows and may even move past the proximal end of the rods over time; this is known as the "Luque trolley" effect. In the child approaching skeletal maturity, fusion of the entire spine is the goal. Fusion consists of decortication, facetectomy, and bone grafting. For these patients, additional fixation points with cables, wires, and screws can help maintain deformity correction.

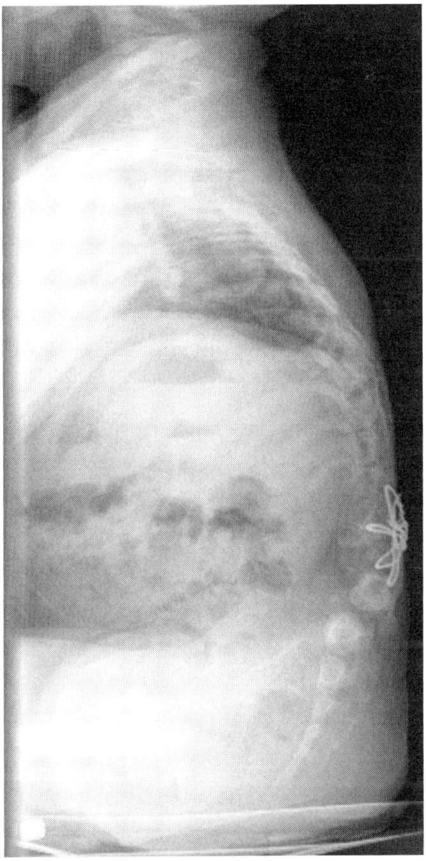

**Figure 3** This four-year-old girl with a thoracic-level myelomeningocele underwent a kyphectomy and fusion with instrumentation. The implants were prominent and therefore were removed. The kyphectomy site was stabilized with wires and a cast. This sitting radiograph out of the cast shows satisfactory alignment.

In kyphosis-correction surgery, secure pelvic fixation is imperative because the natural forward leaning posture of the kyphotic patient leads to great stress on the caudal portion of the instrumentation. Significant advances in pelvic fixation have improved spinal instrumentation for the myelomeningocele patient.

Although pelvic fixation in spine surgery for neuromuscular patients usually involves the ilium, osteopenia and the small size of the pelvis in the myeolodysplastic child make this ineffective. Often, the iliac tables are too thin to accommodate the distal ends of the rods. In addition, pelvic procedures may have left large holes, reducing the area for pelvic fixation. Furthermore, the iliac wings in these patients are relatively parallel to each other compared with other children, and thus are in poor position to serve as anchors. Even if

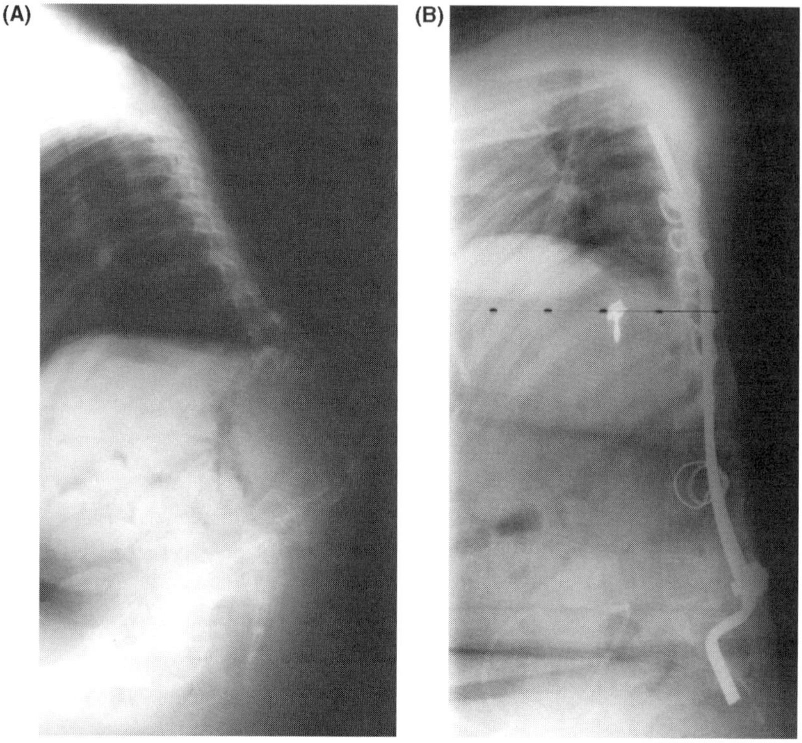


**Figure 4** (**A**) This nine-year-old girl with a thoracic-level myelomeningocele has a sharp kyphotic deformity. (**B**) The patient underwent kyphectomy and fusion with segmental spinal instrumentation. Note the use of sublaminar wires in the thoracic spine and the placement of the distal ends of the rods into the sacrum. The kyphosis correction was performed by removing a segment of the spine and reattaching the rest of the spine to achieve a straight profile.

the rods were placed properly between the inner and outer tables of the posterior ilium (Galveston technique), the direction of force for kyphosis reduction attempts tend to drive the rods back out of the pelvis (10).

After spinal fusion and instrumentation to the pelvis, the patient loses flexibility in the lumbosacral spine. When the patient changes position, the forces go through the pelvic fixation sites. As a result, the rods toggle back and forth in the ilium each time the patient moves, leading to a "windshield wiper" sign on the radiographs which implies loosening of the fixation.

The sacrum is a more reliable and stout structure for fixation than the ilium and, hence, is a better fixation point for myelomeningocele patients. In the Dunn–McCarthy technique, the lower portion of the rods are prebent into an S-shape and passed anterior to the sacral alae (11). Warner and Fackler introduced a modification of the original Dunn–McCarthy technique and

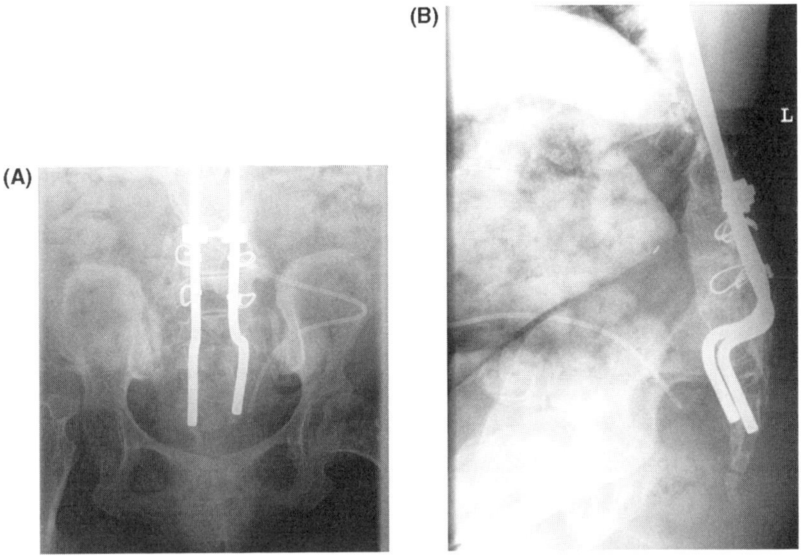


**Figure 5** (**A**) Warner and Fackler described a technique in which the distal ends of the rods are bent at right angles and inserted into the sacral foramina. (**B**) The lateral view shows the spatial relationship between the rods and the sacrum more clearly.

placed the bent distal end of the rod through the first sacral foramen. They bent the rods at right angles (Fig. 5A and B). This technique avoids injury to the visceral and vascular structures anterior to the spine because the rod placed through the right first sacral foramen is in the anatomic clear space anterior to the sacrum. The left rod lies posterior to the rectum. The distal tip of the bent rod hugs the anterior surface of the sacrum (12). McCall reported success with a modification of the above technique by making 20° to 40° bends, instead of right angles, depending on the sacral inclination. Nolden et al. (8) report using lumbosacral pedicle screw fixation with intrasacral distal rod insertion (Roger Jackson technique), in which they place rods directly into the body of the sacrum. Dubousset and coworkers (13) have reported good results with iliosacral screw/rod constructs.

In summary, several techniques achieve secure sacral fixation for kyphosis-correction surgery. Segmental spinal instrumentation with sacral fixation provides rigidity of construct, immediate and long-term deformity correction, low instrument profile, and obviates the need for long-term immobilization (14).

## Complications and Consequences of Kyphosis Correction

Ligation of the spinal cord and the dura at the same level during kyphosis-correction surgery can lead to life-threatening increase in intracranial pressure (15).

Refinements in this technique, involving ligation at different levels so that the cerebrospinal fluid can continue to circulate in the thecal sac, have significantly increased the safety of this procedure.

The assumption that the spinal cord below the level of the myelomeningocele lesion has no function may not be accurate. The safety of cordotomy (severing the spinal cord) during surgical correction of congenital kyphosis in myelomeningocele is debatable, particularly in regard to bladder function. Lalonde and Jarvis (16) reviewed 13 patients and concluded that there were no ill effects if the cordotomy were performed below the neurological level and there were no tethering. Other authors report cord resection as a routine part of the operation (6,10,12,17). However, Pontari et al. (18) reported four children with thoracic-level paraplegia and severe myelokyphosis who underwent distal spinal cord resection at the time of kyphectomy. All were continent before spinal cord resection and became incontinent afterward. Urodynamic studies confirmed lower urinary tract denervation. These authors recommend preoperative urodynamic evaluation and urological consultation and suggest preservation of the cord in selected patients with residual sacral function.

## Scoliosis

### Natural History of Scoliosis

Scoliosis is spinal deformity in the coronal plane. Anterior–posterior or posterior–anterior radiographic views of the spine show this deformity well (Fig. 6). The incidence of spinal deformity in the myelomeningocele population is higher with increasing age and level of neurological involvement (19). A recent study (20) found 52% of children with myelomeningocele and lipomeningocele aged 10 or older have scoliosis. In this group, the incidence of scoliosis was 90% in children with a thoracic neurological level or a last intact laminar arch (LILA) at the thoracic level. For those with an LILA below L4, the incidence was closer to 10%. Furthermore, the incidence of scoliosis in community ambulators is about a half that in nonambulators. The scoliosis curve progression is greatest before 15 years of age. Fifty-four percent of patients with curves 40° or greater progressed more than 5 degrees a year. The average progression was 12.5° for patients with curves $\geq$40° over the mean follow-up period of 4.3 years (21). In an ambulatory patient, progression of a scoliotic curve can make walking more difficult. In nonambulatory patients, pelvic obliquity causes sitting balance problems. Severe curvatures cause impairments similar to those seen in myelomeningocele patients with kyphosis.

### Nonoperative Management of Scoliosis

Bracing will benefit only a select group of spina bifida patients with scoliosis. Lindseth (22) suggests a trial of bracing for children younger than the age of seven years if the curve is supple and can be corrected. A Swedish report (23)

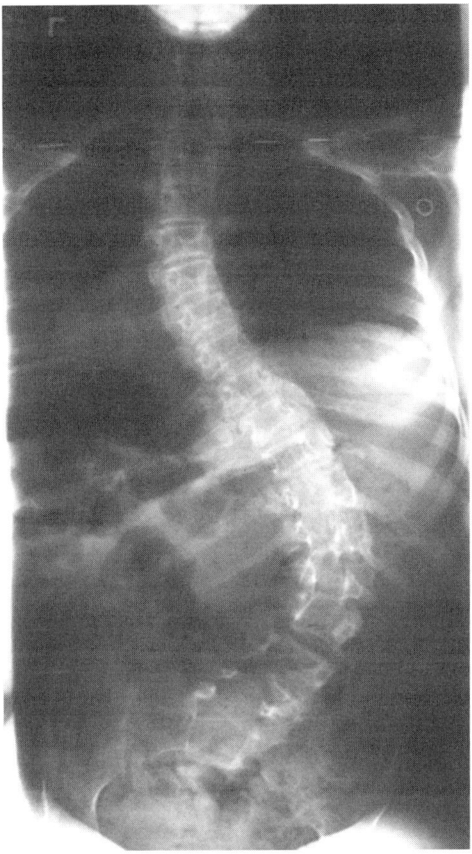

**Figure 6** This 15-year-old girl with a high-lumbar-level lesion has a progressive scoliotic deformity with associated pelvic obliquity. Note the missing posterior elements of the lumbar spine.

found that a Boston type underarm brace controlled scoliosis progression in patients with curves $\leq 45^\circ$. Curve progression was slowed in patients with larger initial curves. However, most other authors feel that bracing is not effective in halting curve progression (24–26). Bracing is mainly helpful for children with functional problems due to the spinal curvature. The brace can temporarily assist with sitting and standing posture. A pitfall of brace management of these patients is the development of skin ulcerations, usually in insensate areas. These children, therefore, should not wear braces to bed. In addition, the child's family needs to understand that bracing is a temporary measure, not a cure. Furthermore, any child with respiratory compromise will only have more difficulty breathing with the brace. Heavy-set children are another group who will not benefit from bracing. Obesity prevents the brace from applying corrective forces on the ribs.

There is no evidence to suggest that an exercise program or physical therapy will have a beneficial effect on scoliotic deformities associated with myelomeningocele (25).

## Morbidity Associated with Scoliosis

Unlike other scoliosis patients whose fusion levels are determined by the curve type, fusion and instrumentation for patients with myelomeningocele generally extend to the pelvis, regardless of curve type. Fusion to the pelvis may alter ambulatory capacity. Spinal cord tethering can be a factor in curve progression and therefore requires consideration by the clinician. Assessment by the neurosurgery team is imperative in the presence of clinical signs suggesting tethering, such as a decrease in ambulatory function, an increase in muscle spasticity or tightness, alterations in bladder function, and pain. Untethering may help reduce muscle spasticity and restore bladder and ambulatory function. However, it does not halt curve progression (27). Additional morbidity related to scoliosis and associated pelvic obliquity includes sitting balance impairment and difficulty in positioning in the wheelchair.

## Potential Benefits of Scoliosis Surgery

Deformity correction, fusion, and instrumentation of the scoliotic spine in myelomeningocele patients have benefits similar to that in patients with adolescent idiopathic scoliosis. A fused spine balanced in both the coronal and sagittal planes halts curve progression and improves cosmesis. As with kyphosis correction in spina bifida, benefits associated with scoliosis correction include leveling of the pelvis, decreased risks for pressure sores, freeing of the hands for manual activities, and better access for urinary diversion. Scoliosis surgery in patients with myelomeningocele also improves pulmonary function (28).

The work of Campbell et al. (5) has focused on children with severe spinal deformity and thoracic insufficiency syndrome. Campbell's work has been groundbreaking because of his recognition that the characteristics of the entire thoracic cage, including both the spine and the ribs, determine the patient's respiratory function. In their patients, some of whom have myelomeningocele, Campbell's group found that traditional curve correction and fusion of the spine are inadequate and sometimes detrimental to respiratory function. As a result, Campbell et al. developed a technique to lengthen and expand the constricted hemithorax. This technique involves opening wedge thoracostomy with primary longitudinal lengthening using a chest-wall distractor known as a vertical, expandable prosthetic titanium rib. Ultimately, Campbell's method allows growth of the thoracic spine and rib cage, thereby helping patients with thoracic insufficiency syndrome to breathe more easily.

A recent study by Wai et al. (29) challenges the commonly used indications to perform spine surgery on myelomeningocele patients. They found that only coronal imbalance was significantly related to any physical function outcome, of which sitting balance was the only one. No aspect of spinal deformity affected self-perception. Therefore, the authors suggest that the only potential benefit of spinal deformity surgery may be the improvement of sitting balance by correction of coronal deformity. The same group also advocates a child and family centered approach to the functional effects of scoliosis and other spinal deformity in myelomeningocele (30).

## Surgical Management of Scoliosis in Myelomeningocele

Surgical indications for spinal deformity in a child with myelomeningocele are (*i*) progressive deformity greater than approximately 50°, (*ii*) deformity $<50°$ that interferes with function or causes secondary problems, and, rarely, (*iii*) neurological dysfunction caused by the deformity (26). The surgery is challenging and is often performed by a surgical team consisting of a neurosurgeon and an orthopedic surgeon. The entire team must adhere to latex precautions (31–34).

The goal of the neurosurgical team is to address any abnormal functioning of the nervous system that may be contributing to the development or worsening of the deformity and to prevent neural axis injury from the deformity correction. The procedures most commonly recommended are shunt revision, spinal cord detethering, Chiari malformation decompression, and syrinx drainage.

The treatment goals for the orthopedic surgeon are to achieve a solidly fused, corrected, and balanced spine in both the coronal and sagittal planes over a level pelvis. The standard treatment for scoliosis is posterior spinal fusion with instrumentation. Spinal deformity correction can usually wait until the child is 10 years of age, since spinal fusion at an early age prevents further growth and results in a short trunk.

Before proceeding with a posterior spinal fusion and instrumentation with or without kyphectomy, the orthopedic surgeon must check on shunt function, the presence of a urinary tract infection, status of the weight-bearing skin over the buttocks and upper thighs, and health of skin over the spine segment to be manipulated.

Obtaining a solid fusion remains the most critical aspect of the operation. Previous scarring in the region from the myelomeningocele sac closure makes soft tissues dissection tedious and difficult. If a posterior longitudinal incision is required, the surgeon exposes the posterior elements of the spine by starting proximal to the dysraphic region. An inverted Y-shaped incision may help avoid the sac closure site, gain wide exposure of laterally splayed out posterior elements and the ilium, and minimize the risk of dural tears (26). Fusion to the upper thoracic spine prevents thoracic kyphosis above the fusion and improves spinal fixation. Posterior spinal fusion with segmental instrumentation supplemented with anterior spinal fusion with or without instrumentation may improve the results (35). Pedicular remnant wires and pedicle screws can provide fixation points in segments where the laminae are not present (Fig. 7). Fusion and instrumentation, generally, extend to the pelvis. Technical advances for pelvic fixation used for kyphosis correction also apply to scoliosis correction. Correction of pelvic obliquity with the Luque–Galveston technique has been effective for other neuromuscular patients. For the reasons stated in the Kyphosis section, the iliac fixation is not secure. The sacral bar technique addresses this by placing a bar transversely through the outer table of the ilium at the level of the S1 spinous process and posterior superior iliac spines. The surgeon then marries the bar to standard Cotrel–Dubousset-like rods (36). The Zeller modification of adding a nut to this construct minimizes backing out of the bar and loss of the fixation.

Some surgeons have challenged the necessity to fuse or instrument to the pelvis. They believe that mobility at the lumbosacral junction is important for ambulation and daily activity. Pre-existing hip contractures can cause more problems when the lumbosacral junction is immobilized. Technical advances involving pedicle screws have allowed surgeons to achieve stable fixation in dysplastic

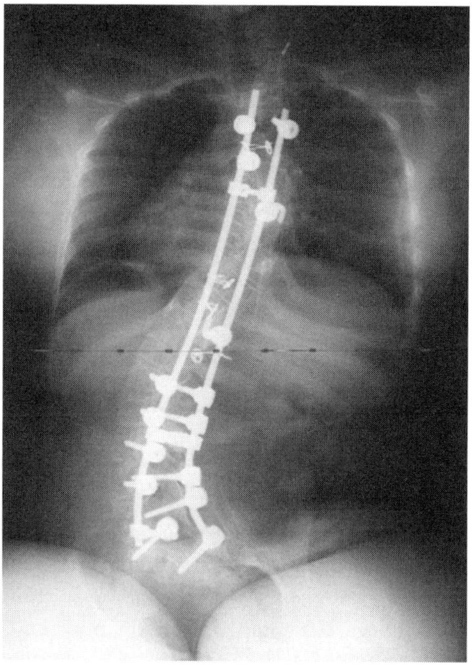

**Figure 7** Segmental spinal instrumentation used to stabilize this patient's scoliosis includes pedicle screws, laminar hooks, spinous process wires, and rods. Regardless of the exact combination of implants used, the advantage of using segmental instrumentation is having multiple fixation points along the spine.

vertebral levels, previously not possible (37). In an ambulatory patient with <10° of pelvic obliquity, Warner recommends stopping the fusion and instrumentation short of the pelvis. In nonambulatory patients with >10° of pelvic obliquity, Warner (38) suggests that fusion and instrumentation should extend to the pelvis. Other investigators have observed that spontaneous correction of pelvic obliquity can occur with instrumented fusion short of the sacrum (39).

Anterior-only fusion with instrumentation can effectively correct the deformity in a select group of spina bifida patients. The potential advantages are fewer fusion levels, lower blood loss, and avoidance of compromised posterior skin and poorly vascularized paraspinal muscles, resulting in decreased infection rates. The selection criteria include (*i*) thoracolumbar curve less than 75°, (*ii*) compensatory curves less than 40°, (*iii*) no increased kyphosis, and (*iv*) no syrinx (40). Limited anterior-only fusions in very young children with severe curves may delay definitive, more extensive fusion operations. Anterior approach to the spine is easier from the left side since it is near the aorta; approach from the right side is more dangerous since the vena cava is more easily injured than the aorta. Careful exposure is imperative to avoid injury to the ureter, which may be obscured by scarring from prior urologic procedures.

### Complications and Consequences of Spinal Deformity Surgery

Patients with myelomeningocele who undergo spine operations have a high complication rate in the peri-operative and postoperative period (41,42). Care by an experienced team of meticulous healthcare professionals is essential.

Spina bifida patients have a higher rate of pseudarthrosis (41). The posterior elements of the spine are highly dysplastic and may not provide adequate bony surface for bone grafting. Failure of proper fusion is the likely underlying problem in the presence of instrumentation failure, that is, rod breakage, screw loosening, or wire breakage (Fig. 8A and B). Combination of anterior fusion with posterior fusion with instrumentation has improved long-term deformity correction and has reduced the rate of pseudarthrosis.

Postoperative surgical site infection rate is higher in the myelomeningocele population compared with most other groups and can be very challenging to manage (Fig. 9). An infected instrumented spine will require multiple debridements. Surgeons usually do not remove the infected instrumentation until the spine has fused. After removal of the instrumentation, the spine fusion mass may lose some of the deformity correction achieved during the initial procedure.

In a well-fused spine, changes in the spinal mobility may alter the patient's skills in transfers and activities of daily living. The changes in posture and sitting position may give rise to a different distribution of pressure ulcers. Postoperative attention to skin care is critical.

Deformity correction at the expense of neurological function results in suboptimal functional outcome. The surgery may not maintain the patient's

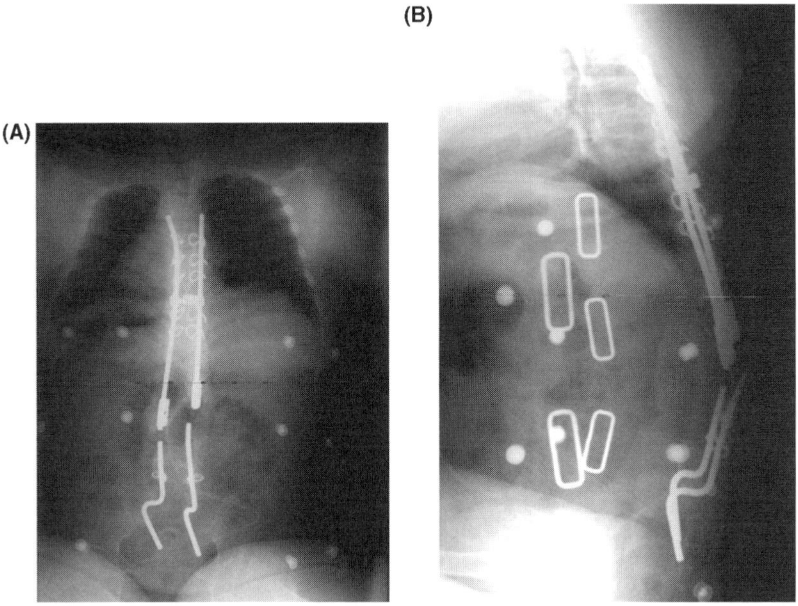


**Figure 8** (**A**) This patient underwent kyphectomy and fusion with instrumentation complicated by multiple breaks in the rods. She had the instrumentation revised only to have rod failure below the repair site. Implant failures occur with pseudarthrosis of the kyphectomy and fusion site. (**B**) The lateral view shows the patient leaning forward and the ends of the broken rods becoming prominent. The patient subsequently underwent a second revision instrumentation and fusion. The need for revisions is not unusual after spine surgery in myelomeningocele patients.

current level of neurological function but, in fact, may decrease it. Anterior-only fusion can result in loss of quadriceps function (40). Neurophysiological monitoring can help detect changes in spinal cord function during the operation.

Finally, younger patients who underwent posterior-only fusions are at risk for crankshaft phenomenon. Crankshaft phenomenon occurs when continued growth of the unfused anterior portion of the spine leads to rotational deformity.

## HIP DEFORMITY

### Hip Instability

Management recommendations for hip subluxations and dislocations in the myelomeningocele patient have been controversial and continue to evolve. One approach is to keep the hips "loose" and "out." A "loose" hip is flexible and allows motion without excessive force. A hip that is "out" is one left

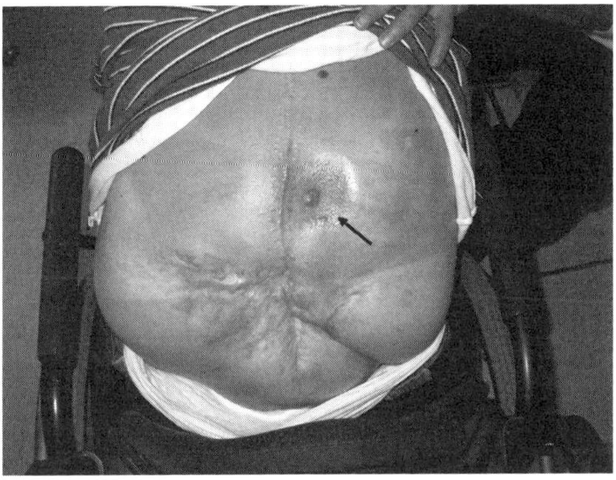

**Figure 9** This patient underwent kyphectomy and fusion with instrumentation. Note the dime-sized pustule on the right side of the midline back incision. This area drains periodically. This chronic infection of the spinal instrumentation can be suppressed with oral antibiotics until she achieves complete spinal fusion, at which time she can have the instrumentation removed.

subluxated or dislocated. The patients with dislocated but mobile hips can stand with a walker with customized adjustments (43). An alternative approach involves stabilizing subluxated or dislocated hips even if the treatment may cause hip stiffness, thereby predisposing the patient to fractures. The controversy exists because hip surgery does not always improve functional outcome for a myelomeningocele child with dislocated hips. Only selected patients benefit from the procedures and the selection criteria are not consistent.

## Etiology

Muscle imbalance is the major cause for hip deformity (44–46). Unopposed action of the hip flexors (iliopsoas) and adductor muscles against paralytic hip abductors and hip extensors leads to femoral head subluxation and/or dislocation and acetabular dysplasia. The sitting position also contributes to hip instability by exacerbating the muscle imbalances. The proximal femur may also show abnormalities, including coxa valga and increased femoral anteversion. Occasionally, an external rotatory component due to tight hip capsules and external rotators may exist.

## Patient Grouping

Level of spinal cord involvement and associated muscle imbalances in the myelomeningocele patient correlate with patterns of hip deformity and instability. Determining the prevalence of hip subluxations and dislocations can be difficult due to study population differences. The available studies vary in definitions of neurosegmental levels and patient groupings.

Available studies suggest that myelomeningocele patients with L3–L4 lesions have the highest prevalence of hip instability at birth. Carroll and Sharrard (47) found that the percentages of unstable hips in each neurosegmental group were as follows: thoracic level (20%), L1–L2 level (52%), L3–L4 level (64%), L5 level (18%), and sacral level (0%). In Beeker and Scheers' series, the distribution of unstable hips at birth in each neurosegmental group was similar: thoracic (10%), L1–L2 (41%), L3 (62%), L4 (19%), L5 (0%) (48). However, L3 level patients do not have an increase in the rate of hip instability after three years of age. In contrast, thoracic and upper-lumbar-level patients can continue to have an increase in hip instability after 10 years of age.

## Management in Neonatal Period

The Pavlik harness is not suitable for children with myelomeningocele. Although it is effective for developmental dysplasia of the hip in normal infants, the device worsens the hip instability in spina bifida children by pushing the femoral head posteriorly even though they lack adequate posterior acetabular wall coverage. Furthermore, placement in the frog-leg position with the Pavlik harness tends to further shorten the iliopsoas tendon, which is the major hip-deforming force.

## Surgical Management

Mobility, not ambulation, is the most important goal in the management of the myelomeningocele patient. Many parents want their children to walk, even if it is difficult and requires great effort. Their wishes do not always take into account the socialization needs of the patients—to keep up with their peer group. As long as they are independently mobile with assistive devices, spina bifida patients can keep up with the fully ambulatory peer group. This is more desirable than not being able to keep up, despite being ambulatory. It is essential for the physicians treating these patients to help families understand that hip dislocations do not affect the ability to ambulate in the low thoracic or high lumbar myelomeningocele patients (44,45,49,50); therefore, ambulation should not be the goal of hip surgery in these patients.

At one time, many surgeons aggressively treated spina bifida patients with subluxated or dislocated hips to restore normal anatomic alignment. However, as myelomeningocele patients began to survive longer, it became obvious that the long-term outcomes of hip stabilizing and reducing procedures were not as positive as previously thought. Currently, surgeons manage hip disorders in the myelomeningocele population based on the patient's neurosegmental level.

### Thoracic Level and High Lumbar Level

Patients with thoracic-level and high-lumbar-level lesions do not benefit from open reduction of unilateral or bilateral hip dislocations. Because the major surgical procedures for these issues, particularly osteotomies and open reductions of the hip, can cause hip stiffness, they may actually be harmful for these patients. Stiffness is detrimental to both ambulatory and hygiene activities. Furthermore, in combination with disuse osteopenia, joint stiffness predisposes these patients to fractures when caregivers and therapists manipulate the legs. Finally, Feiwell (51) found that patients undergoing extensive reductions and tendon transfers frequently redislocated. Therefore, the orthopedic treatment goals for thoracic and high-lumbar-level myelomeningocele patients are to obtain a straight spine, leveled pelvis, and loose, rather than stiff, hips.

### Low Lumbar Level

Management of hip instability in the myelomeningocele patient with a low-lumbar-level lesion is controversial. In general, surgical management of hip instability in this population is limited to selected ambulatory patients (usually older than two years) who use minimal orthotic equipment (below knee). Surgeons have subdivided this group by neurosegmental levels and by motor strength of different muscle groups to help guide treatment. Asher and Olson (52) advocated reduction of dislocated hips only in patients with intact L4–L5 motor control. In low-lumbar-level patients with intact quadriceps, medial hamstring, and anterior tibialis muscle function, the surgeons should reduce both unilateral and bilateral hip dislocations and augment them with pelvic or femoral osteotomies. However, patients with intact quadriceps but weak medial hamstrings and anterior tibialis muscles should be left alone if they have bilateral dislocations (Fig. 10); open reduction may be helpful if the hip dislocation is

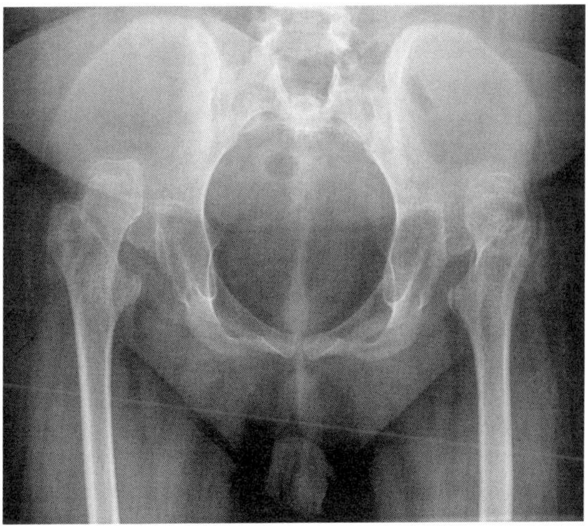

**Figure 10** This 14-year-old boy with a midlumbar-level myelomeningocele has bilateral hip dislocations. He has no hip pain. He uses a wheelchair for transportation and can perform transfers independently.

unilateral. There is a lack of consensus regarding the management of hip instability in patients with motor function at L3–L4 and functioning adductors.

Surgical treatment in this group is associated with a number of complications. Reduction of high-riding bilateral dislocations may be associated with hip stiffness. Loss of reduction may occur despite adequate surgical technique for a variety of reasons. Factors associated with loss of reduction include delay in surgical treatment and associated adaptive changes (44), spasticity, persistence of coxa valga, and pelvic obliquity. Pelvic obliquity due to significant leg length difference may cause the high hip to dislocate, despite adequate care. Long-term follow-up of Chiari pelvic osteotomy in myelomeningocele patients showed that the technique did not achieve hip stability (53).

### Sacral-Level Lesions

Sacral-level myelomeningocele patients with bilateral or unilateral hip dislocations benefit from surgical procedures to reduce the hips, similar to otherwise normal children with developmental hip dislocations.

Management of spina bifida patients with tendon transfers owes its roots to the treatment of patients with polio. A half-century ago, the polio patient was the paralytic model. First, Thompson and coworkers (54) described the transfer of the external oblique muscle to the greater trochanter in polio patients to improve abductor power and gait pattern. In 1952, Mustard described transfer of the iliopsoas tendon to the anterolateral greater trochanter to function as an abductor for the polio patient. Later, Sharrard (55) proposed transferring the polio patient's iliopsoas tendon to the posterolateral greater trochanter so that it could function as both a hip abductor and extensor. In a series of myelomeningocele patients, Phillips and Lindseth (56) described a triple transfer consisting of external oblique transfer to the greater trochanter, adductor transfer to the posterior ischium, and tensor fascia lata transfer to the gluteus maximus tendon. The authors reported improved gait, ambulatory independence, and fewer orthotic requirements in the majority of their patients. Another study also demonstrated good results with iliopsoas transfer and adductor release. The results of external oblique transfer with adductor transfer yielded excellent results without altering the flexor–extensor balance since the psoas remained intact. Late flexion contractures did not develop. Scoliosis and pelvic obliquity were absent in the external oblique transfer group (57).

### Summary

A recent consensus statement recommends hip reduction for bilateral hip dislocations in ambulatory low lumbar and sacral-level myelomeningocele patients. Thoracic and high lumbar patients who do not ambulate do not benefit from hip reduction surgery. Management of low lumbar patients who have unilateral dislocation continues to be controversial. If adequate quadriceps strength is present, an open reduction may be beneficial (26).

## SOFT-TISSUE HIP CONTRACTURES

Patients with higher lumbar levels of involvement tend to have flexion contractures. Midlumbar myelomeningocele (L3–L4) denotes stronger hip flexors and adductors with no extensor or abductor opposition. Therefore, these patients develop hip subluxation leading to later dislocation at about three to four years of age.

Rigid soft-tissue contractures require releases to allow above-the-hip bracing, basic care, and some ambulation when possible. Soft-tissue releases allow adequate hip extension, thereby facilitating brace wear. Elimination of the crouching posture also allows patients to fit into a stander, allowing them to be upright and bear weight. Bearing weight reduces the number of fractures by minimizing the development of osteopenia. Release of the adductor muscles is important to allow adequate hip abduction. These procedures are relatively minor and done bilaterally. The goal of the operations is a pair of loose hips in which contractures do not recur (45,50).

### Hip Flexion Contractures

Hip flexion contractures tend to occur most frequently in the myelomeningocele patients with thoracic and high-lumbar-level lesions. Prolonged sitting or unopposed pull of the iliopsoas, rectus femoris, and sartorius muscles are the likely causes. The treatment of flexion contracture begins at birth. Early physical therapy and parental involvement in the patient's rehabilitation are crucial. Stretching exercises should include the hip flexors and knee flexors, which tend to be tight concomitantly. Later in life, usually between two and three years of age, when upper extremity strength can be assessed, the physician can prescribe orthotics for the lower extremities. Good upper extremity function will be important when using walkers to ambulate with braces. Furthermore, the patients will require sufficient balance to achieve ambulatory capacity. Even patients lacking strong arms and good balance can benefit from being upright by using a parapodium.

Flexion contractures over 30° tend to prevent proper bracing and ambulatory capability. The deformity can also produce severe compensatory lumbar hyperextension, leading to increased upper extremity effort to balance the body. Surgical correction should include a tenotomy of the iliotibial band, iliopsoas, rectus, and sartorius. An anterior hip capsulotomy may be necessary (50). At the end of the procedure, a full correction of the flexion contracture is necessary to prevent recurrence. The recommended time for the procedure is just prior to the start of gait training. The deformity tends to recur if the procedure were performed too early. If the correction is not full after soft-tissue releases, Feiwell recommended performing proximal femur extension osteotomy of about 30° to 40° to correct the flexion deformity. The patient stays for four weeks in long leg casts with a cross bar (Petrie type) with some abduction and $>20°$ of internal rotation. As pain control allows, the patient lies either prone or supine with the hips extended. Limited sitting periods allow feeding and transportation. If the patient is very young at the time of the osteotomy, the natural remodeling of bone may decrease or eliminate the correction and the flexion deformity may return, necessitating repeated extension osteotomies.

### Hip External Rotation Contractures

Hip external rotation contractures are the least common hip deformity and typically result from lying supine with the hips flexed, abducted, and externally rotated. Attempts to prevent such contractures involve flexibility exercises and application of orthosis, which hold the hips in extension and adduction. Surgery is necessary only when patients have problems with brace fitting. These patients have tight posterior capsules and short hip external rotator muscles. Menelaus recommends posterior hip capsule release. Other authors recommend proximal femoral derotational osteotomy to internally rotate the entire lower extremity. The tight soft tissues are left intact. All of the patients who had osteotomies had marked gait improvement. Eighty-nine percent of theses patients had improvement of the deformity (58).

### Hip Adduction and Abduction Contractures

Hip subluxations and dislocations are associated with adduction contractures, most frequently in thoracic-level patients. Soft-tissue releases of the adductors allow $>45^\circ$ of abduction. Valgus osteotomies of the proximal femur can also correct adduction contractures in severely involved hips. Postoperative immobilization in a spica cast can protect the osteotomy while allowing the patient to stand, minimizing the risk of fractures by preventing disuse osteopenia. If fixation is strong, the patient can begin ambulation without immobilization. The patient benefits from rehabilitation programs, emphasizing range of motion and gait training. Night splints can help avoid recurrences.

Abduction contractures of the hip can result from contractures of the iliotibial band and the tensor fascia lata, causing pelvic obliquity and scoliosis. Treatment involves proximal release of the tensor fascia (Ober procedure) and/or division of the iliotibial band distally. Recalcitrant cases require femoral varus osteotomy.

## KNEE DEFORMITIES

Management of knee contractures in the myelomeningocele patients may be problematic. A release of one side of the joint may create a problem on the opposite side. Both sides of the joint may need releases in order to balance the co-spasticity. The surgeon may need to combine a rectus femoris release with release of the hamstrings, medially and/or laterally. There is considerable controversy.

The knee in a myelodysplastic patient should have the ability to flex to 90° to allow proper sitting and to decrease the incidence of fractures around the knee. Joint stiffness creates a lever arm that results in fractures of the osteopenic bone when these patients undergo physiotherapy by their therapists and caregivers. Daily stretching and therapy may prevent many of these contractures. Some believe, although it has not been proven, that therapy may delay loss of ambulation ability by maintaining contracture-free limbs.

## Knee Flexion Contractures

Knee flexion contractures are rarely present at birth. These contractures develop and worsen over time, especially in thoracic-level patients (59). Hip and ankle contractures, lack of ambulation, lack of motor function, and increased time spent in the sitting position all contribute to worsening of the contractures. Progression of knee flexion contractures can lead to loss of ambulatory ability. Flexion contractures are increasingly common in the older age group and early sitters have worse contractures than late sitters. Flexion contractures beyond 15° to 20° can interfere with brace fitting, preventing the child from being upright, regardless of how much ambulation would otherwise be possible. When severe, this deformity may pose difficulties in wheelchair positioning (Fig. 11A).

Numerous options are available for surgical treatment of knee flexion contractures. Simple hamstring-biceps tenotomy is not effective. Distal iliotibial band resection can help extend the knee. Hamstring tendon resection combined with posterior capsular release may be necessary. Dias advocates a radical flexor release through two longitudinal incisions. The medial incision allows resection of the semitendinosus, semimembranosus, gracilis, and sartorius tendons. Through the lateral incision, the surgeon resects the biceps and iliotibial band. Once the nerves and vessels are protected, surgery consists of detachment of the gastrocnemius muscles from the femoral condyles and an extensive capsulectomy. Division of the posterior cruciate ligament may be necessary to obtain full extension. No more than 5° of flexion should remain after the operation. Careful monitoring of the vascular status of the limb is imperative. A well-padded cylinder cast with the knee fully extended is appropriate if the preoperative flexion were less than 40°. If the preoperative flexion contracture were over 40°, some knee flexion is necessary to avoid vascular compromise. Cast changes every three days will gradually extend the knee. An above-the-knee night splint in full extension replaces the cast after 10 to 14 days (60). Supracondylar hyperextension correction of the distal femur can redirect the position of the lower extremity without risking the neurovascular structures in the popliteal fossa. Staple hemiepiphyseodesis of the anterior distal femoral physis in the growing child can gradually correct the flexion deformity by causing hyperextension at the distal femur. An alternative method involves a hyperextension osteotomy with internal

(A)
(B)
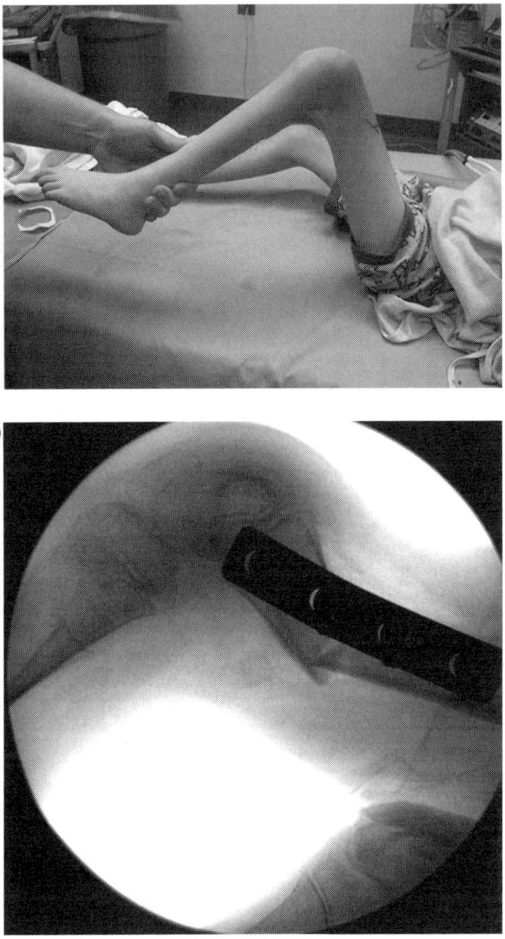

**Figure 11** (**A**) This nine-year-old boy with a high-lumbar-level lesion has a knee flexion contracture greater than 100°. He had several soft-tissue releases in the past. He had trouble sitting in his wheelchair and requested repositioning of his knee. (**B**) The patient underwent a shortening hyperextension osteotomy of his distal femur. The shortening was performed to minimize tension on the vascular structures behind his knee.

fixation (61). However, the deformity can recur due to remodeling of the bone (62).

## Knee Extension Contractures

Knee extension contractures are less common. A knee extension contracture can provide stability for standing or walking in a young child but can be socially unacceptable for an older patient. Sitting with an extended knee can be difficult when riding in a car, bus, or plane. Teratological hip dislocations and rigid clubfoot deformities often are present with this condition (60). Unlike knee flexion contractures, the majority of knee hyperextensions is present at birth. Use of serial casting can cause complications, such as pressure sores, bowing of the tibia, and fractures from forceful manipulations.

Current treatment consists of surgical tendon releases, preferably performed prior to ambulation. The primary indications for surgery include the inability to flex the knees for sitting purposes and achieve ambulation. Three methods are available for obtaining flexion. (*i*) An open V–Y lengthening of the quadriceps mechanism consists of incision of the quadriceps tendon in an inverted V fashion superior to the patella. Transverse division of the anterior capsule to the medial and lateral collateral ligaments allows flexion to 90° intraoperatively. Sutures hold the quadriceps at 45° of knee flexion. An above knee cast in 45° of flexion immobilizes the limb for two weeks. The patient then starts physical therapy to work on passive and active range of motion. An above knee night splint with 45° of flexion maintains correction (60,63). (*ii*) A percutaneous technique, similar to an Achilles tendon recession, may provide satisfactory results for the treatment of knee extension contractures in myelomeningocele patients during the neonatal period (64). This technique requires three stab wounds—a small incision in the midline of the distal thigh, two patellar breadths superior to the patella, which releases the fascia over the rectus tendon, and medial and lateral percutaneous incisions at the level of the patella to release the medial and lateral quadriceps and retinacula. After the operation, the patient is casted with the knee flexed to 90°. (*iii*) Division of the patellar tendon is another alternative, particularly for the patients with thoracic-level lesions. This is not suitable for all patients since 20% of patients may recover quadriceps function (65).

## Knee Instability

Almost all sacral and low-lumbar-level patients will be community ambulators during their teen years. Long-term outcome of adults with sacral-level myelomeningocele showed that 23% have knee pain (66). A review of 72 community ambulators found that 24% had knee symptoms (67). The average age of onset of symptoms was 28 years. All were also very active, and some presented with anteromedial or medial ligamentous laxity. All of the symptomatic low lumbar and one sacral individual had a characteristic abductor lurch with knee flexion and valgus deviation during stance. Only 14% of the nonsymptomatic group presented with this characteristic gait pattern. A fixed flexion contracture was not a significant stressor in the low lumbar group. However, 75% of symptomatic sacral patients had a small fixed flexion deformity without instability. The low lumbar patients developed mainly tibiofemoral arthrosis, whereas the sacral-level patients developed patellofemoral arthritis. About 24% of the community-ambulating patients developed arthrosis secondary to this abnormal gait pattern.

## TIBIAL TORSIONAL DEFORMITY

### Internal Tibial Torsion

The etiology of internal tibial torsion in myelomeningocele patients may be a combination of intrinsic internal tibial torsion and muscle imbalances. Excessive internal tibial torsion interferes with gait. Twister cables or twister straps can help externally rotate the feet enough to ease walking (68). A tibial derotational osteotomy corrects the deformity. Osteotomies in this region require judicious patient selection as nonunions are not uncommon. Gait and orthotic wear improves after correction.

### External Tibial Torsion

Myelomeningocele patients who ambulate can have external tibial torsion. In order to progress forward, the patient increasingly rotates the pelvis and applies valgus stress across the knee (69). Gait analysis showed that external tibial torsion with a thigh–foot-angle (TFA) $\geq 20^\circ$ in lumbosacral-level patients was associated increased valgus stress on the knee (70). Furthermore, one-third of these patients have associated ankle valgus (58). The combination of knee valgus and ankle valgus applies increased pressure on the medial malleoli, leading to pressure sores. This deformity, therefore, causes biomechanical stresses on the hips, knees, feet, and ankles. Solid AFOs improve knee extension during gait in patients with external tibial rotation $<20^\circ$. However, in patients with a greater rotational deformity, the brace cannot adequately control the altered ground-reaction forces. These patients are excellent candidates for derotational osteotomy of the tibia and fibula with fixation. Normalization of the TFA may minimize the risk of knee arthrosis. For patients with associated angular deformities, osteotomies with rigid fixation can correct both angulation and rotation. Healing of the osteotomies tends to take longer than that in neurologically intact patients.

## FOOT AND ANKLE DEFORMITY

### Valgus Deformity

Myelodysplasia patients with intact lower lumbar levels (L3–L5) tend to develop progressive hindfoot or valgus deformities. These deformities are not congenital and only develop later in life when the child becomes ambulatory and gains weight. The valgus deformity may be isolated at the ankle joint or combined with subtalar valgus. Valgus malalignment tends to worsen in ambulatory patients as they place stress with weight-bearing activities. The foot begins to flatten, evert, and externally rotate, leading to pressure sores at the medial or lateral malleoli and at the talonavicular joint. Braces do not adequately improve gait as they cannot correct or control the deformity sufficiently. In fact, braces may further predispose the child to pressure sores, particularly on the medial aspect of the foot and ankle.

A flatfoot deformity in myelomeningocele patients requires attention to both the ankle and the foot. Standing anteroposterior and lateral radiographs of the ankle and the foot can help localize the valgus deviation (Fig. 12A). For true ankle valgus, the weight-bearing films show the radiographic triad of a shortened fibula (high fibula station), lateral wedging of the distal tibial epiphysis, and lateral talar tilt (71). If ankle valgus exceeds 7°, surgical treatment may be helpful. Surgical recommendations vary by age. Children under eight years of age with nonfunctional triceps surae are candidates for an Achilles tenodesis to the distal fibula (72,73). This technique does not apply to patients with concomitant equinus or fixed calcaneus deformities. Furthermore, patients with functioning triceps surae should not undergo tenodesis.

Supramalleolar osteotomy with internal fixation continues to be an effective method to treat ankle valgus deformity in the patient with myelomeningocele. This technique involves osteotomies of the distal tibia and fibula. This procedure, however, is associated with several complications, including wound infections, nonunions, fractures, and tibia-fibular synostosis (74). The distal tibial wave osteotomy is a modification of the above technique (75). A novel transphyseal osteotomy of the distal tibia may be helpful for the child approaching skeletal maturity. This osteotomy cuts through and destroys the distal tibial growth plate, preventing any future deformity. The technique realigns the distal tibia and decreases the necessity for a fibular osteotomy (76). An effective but less invasive alternative is the percutaneous placement of a transphyseal medial malleolar screw (Fig. 12B). This can preferentially slow the growth on the medial aspect of the distal tibial physis and promote relative overgrowth of the lateral portion of the tibial physis, correcting the valgus malalignment (77). Correction averages 7° per year and the surgeon removes the implants to prevent overcorrection.

Hindfoot valgus deformity is more common in the lower-lumbar-level patients due to muscle imbalance. Surgery is necessary in the presence of severe deformity, pain, inability to brace, and ulcer formation. A triple arthrodesis is not appropriate on insensate feet, as it results in stiff feet prone to ulcerations and degenerative changes in adjacent joints. Medial displacement osteotomy corrects the hindfoot valgus while preserving motion at the subtalar joint. Of the 38 feet (27 patients) that underwent medial displacement osteotomy, four feet had recurrences. Three of them were associated with unrecognized ankle valgus that had been present before the operation and one recurred, despite adequate surgical indications (78).

(A)
(B)
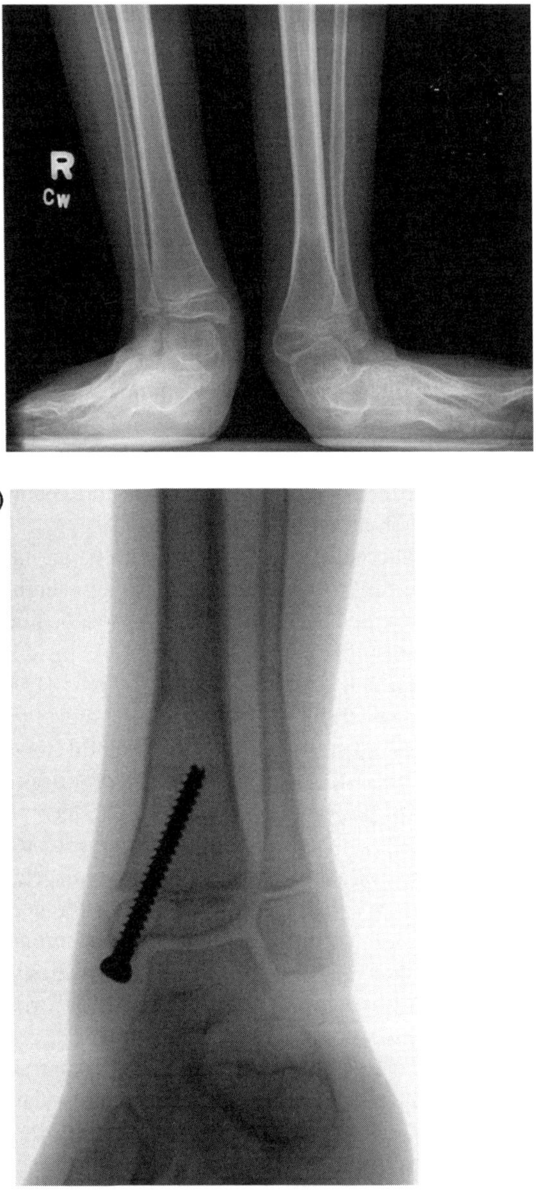


**Figure 12** (**A**) This standing radiograph of a nine-year-old girl with myelomeningocele shows a valgus deformity of the left ankle. The distal fibula physis, normally at the level of the ankle joint, is at the level of the distal tibial physis. The talus is markedly tilted. The right ankle, which is not in valgus, serves as a good comparison. Both feet have subtalar valgus deformities. (**B**) A fully threaded screw was placed through the medial malleolus of the left ankle to arrest the growth on the medial aspect of the ankle. The distal fibula and the lateral portion of the distal tibia will continue to grow. The valgus deformity of the ankle will slowly correct.

## FOOT AND ANKLE DEFORMITY

### Congenital and Developmental Foot Deformities

Foot abnormalities are the most common abnormalities in the myelomeningocele population, affecting 90% of these children. Muscle imbalances around the foot and ankle cause these deformities. Unopposed muscle forces in utero affect the cartilaginous growth of the midtarsal bones and the hindfoot, leading to bony deformities. Sharrard and Grosfield (79) showed that intrauterine paralysis is the major player in birth deformities. Intrauterine posture adds to the deforming forces.

Management of foot deformities can be challenging because these patients lack normal sensation of the foot. Some have no sensation. Skin breakdown can become a significant issue when wearing orthoses. Proper foot care education is critical. Physical therapists and caregivers can help to keep the foot supple with regular stretches so that the patients can bear weight on the soles of their feet. Ambulatory patients need treatment to keep their feet supple, plantigrade, and braceable in order to walk with minimal restrictions. Nonambulatory patients need treatment if the deformities affect shoe wear and foot positioning in the wheelchair.

### Talipes Equinovarus

Forty percent of all spina bifida patients are born with a clubfoot deformity (Fig. 13). Clubfoot deformity treatment in the spina bifida population differs from that of the idiopathic congenital clubfoot. Contractures or the retained activity of the tibialis muscles combined with the functional absence or weakness

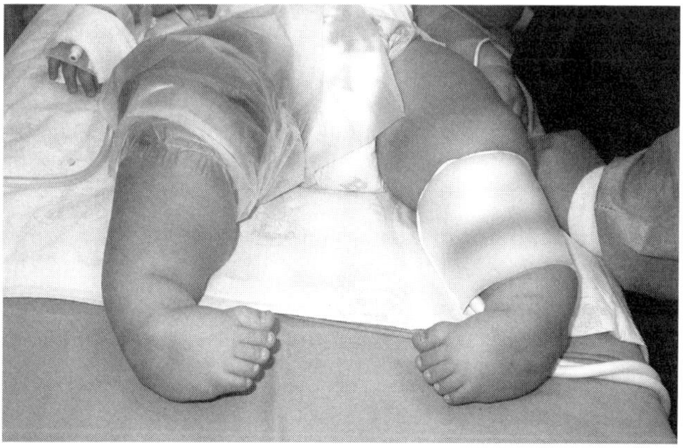

**Figure 13** This infant with a low-lumbar-level myelomeningocele has rigid, severe bilateral clubfoot deformities. Also note the thick thighs and calves commonly seen in this group.

of the peroneal muscles may be the etiology of this condition. In addition, spasticity, intrauterine malposture, fibrotic contractures, and weight bearing are possible causative factors for this deformity (80).

A course of serial casting and manipulation followed by percutaneous heel cord tenotomy and casting should be considered. Complications such as pressure sores, skin ulcerations, recurrence, difficulties in nursing, and sepsis with subsequent amputations can occur in spite of precautions (81). Though the deformity in this group is more resistant to nonsurgical treatment and has a greater tendency to recur, the casting can help stretch the soft tissues and skin to facilitate the definitive surgical treatment (82).

Radical soft-tissue release is the mainstay of deformity correction. The transverse Cincinnati incision allows the surgeon an excellent view of the patho-anatomy (83). A posteromedial release for an idiopathic clubfoot patient consists of lengthening and reattachment of tendons. In spina bifida patients, a mere lengthening of the tendons leads to recurrence of the deformity. Therefore, the surgeon performs a radical release by resecting about 2.5 cm of each tendon, minimizing the chance that the tendons will heal to each other. A supple, plantigrade, and braceable foot is the goal of surgery. Good foot position helps to preserve or achieve ambulation with minimal limitations. The reduction and stabilization of the hindfoot are critical parts of the correction (82). Metatarsal and cuboid osteotomies may help correct the adduction deformity. Rigid deformity in the older child (Fig. 14A–F), untreated or treated, may benefit from salvage procedures such as talectomy (84–86) or triple arthrodesis. Technical factors may influence the distribution of ground reaction forces on the plantar surface of the foot after talectomy (87). Tight intrinsic muscles can cause clawed toes. Plantar fascia release and metatarsal-phalangeal (MTP) tenotomies can solve this problem. Cast immobilization and bracing are imperative to achieve and maintain satisfactory results.

Poor clinical outcomes occur most commonly in the thoracic-level patient, despite the fact that this patient population does not have sensation or motor function of the lower extremities. Factors that may explain the higher incidence of complications include intra-uterine or postnatal malposture, upper motor neuron spasticity, affected articular surfaces, and abnormal fibrous tissue present in myelodysplastic clubfeet.

The most common residual deformity after clubfoot surgery in myelomeningocele patients is forefoot adduction (85). Bracing and later surgery may be necessary to correct this deformity. Several authors recommend lateral column shortening to correct this deformity. Functional level of involvement did not correlate with the final outcome.

## Equinus Deformity

Equinus contractures place the foot in a plantarflexed position, interfering with shoe wear and brace fitting (Fig. 15). The equinus deformity may have several etiologies. An active sacral reflex of the unopposed Achilles tendon

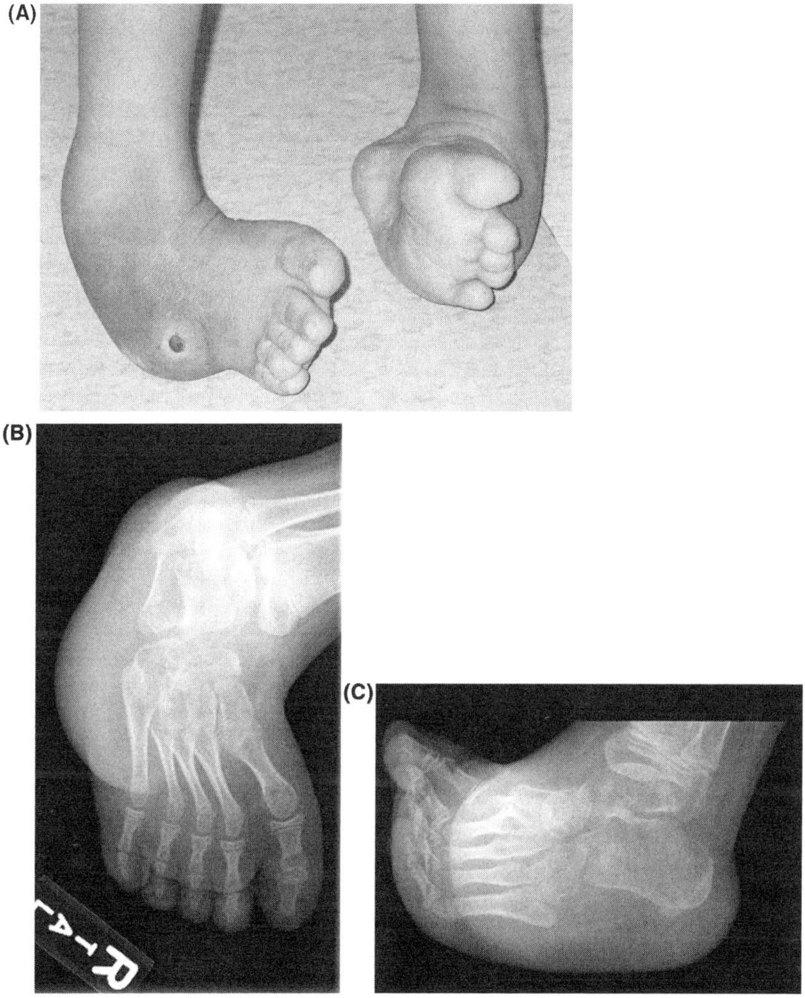


**Figure 14** (*Continued on next page*) (**A**) This nine-year-old girl with a low-lumbar-level myelomeningocele was never previously treated for her bilateral clubfoot deformities. She walked on the sides of her feet. Note the pressure sore over the thickened skin on the dorsolateral aspect of her right foot. She had no pain from the sore due to poor foot sensation. (**B**) Anterior–posterior radiograph of her foot shows the adductus deformity. The soft-tissue shadow shows the thickened skin over the lateral aspect of her foot. (**C**) The lateral view of her foot in maximum dorsiflexion shows the fixed equinus and cavus deformities of her foot. (**D**) The patient underwent radical soft-tissue release, talectomy, closing wedge cuboid osteotomy, and an extension osteotomy of the first metatarsal through a Cincinnati incision. (**E**) The smooth metatarsal pin was removed at four weeks after the operation. The threaded Steinmann pins in the hindfoot were removed at about eight weeks. The patient was kept nonweightbearing until the pins were removed. Note the disuse osteopenia. The patient was begun on graduated weightbearing in braces. (**F**) Both feet were corrected using the Cincinnati incision. Her feet are plantigrade and braceable.

(D)
(E)
(F)

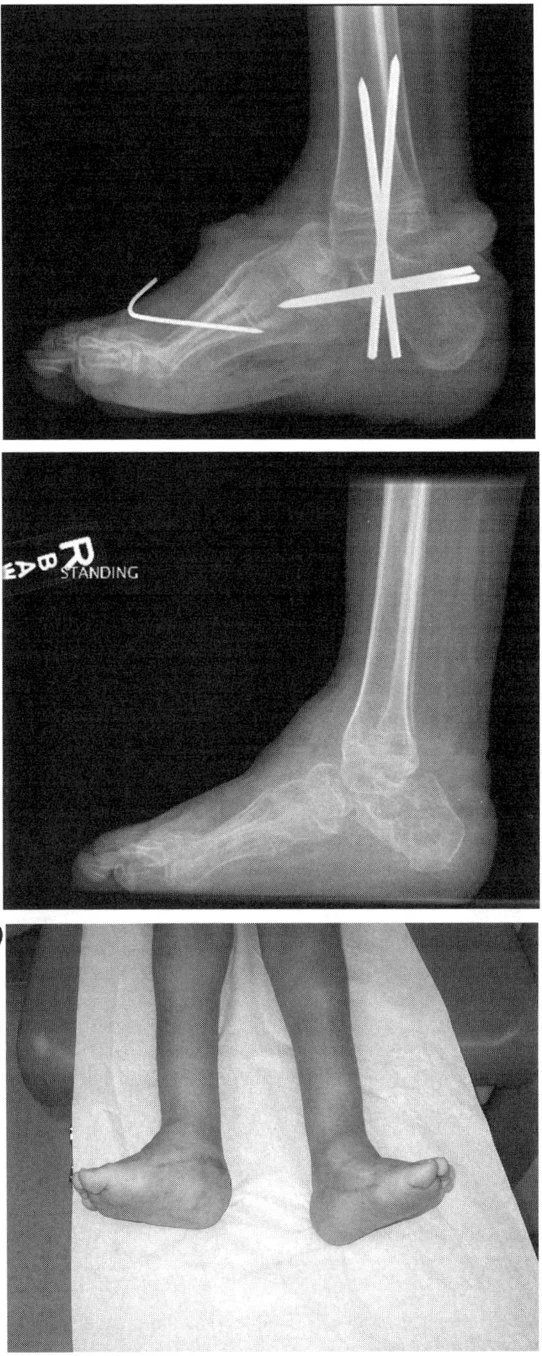


**Figure 14** *(Continued)*

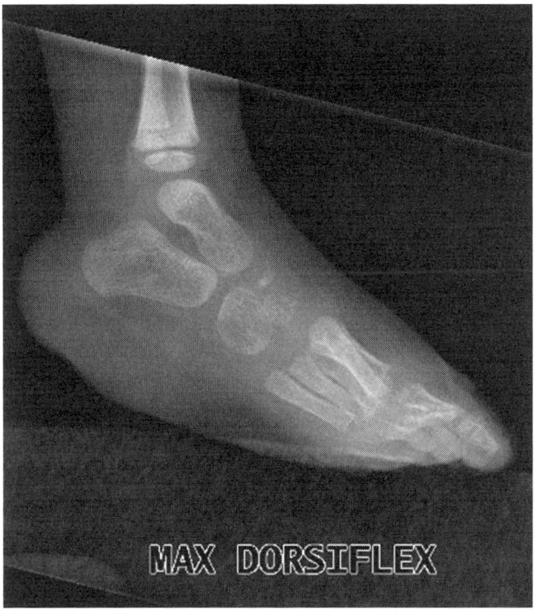


**Figure 15** This three-year-old girl with a high-lumbar-level myelomeningocele lesion has an equinus contracture. The entire foot is pointing down, despite an effort to push the foot into dorsiflexion.

and long-toe flexors can pull the heel such that the foot stays in a plantarflexed position. Also, the unopposed effects of gravity can elicit plantarflexion of the flaccid foot in children with thoracic-level involvement. A percutaneous heel cord tenotomy followed by casting and orthotic wear is effective. In ambulatory patients, a three-level percutaneous heel cord lengthening may be adequate for an isolated equinus deformity. Excessive lengthening of the heel cord can result in an iatrogenic calcaneus deformity.

Manipulations and serial casting may be appropriate for early and less severe deformities initially. A potential pitfall of this method is creation of an iatrogenic rocker-bottom deformity resulting from dorsiflexion of the midtarsal joints instead of the ankle. In cases refractory to conservative care or late cases where fixed deformities are present, either a posterior release or a radical excision of more than 2 cm of the tendon can prevent recurrence (88). Afterwards, an AFO can maintain correction.

After correction of the equinus deformity, some patients demonstrate toe flexion deformities due to tightening of the flexor hallucis longus and digitorum longus. This can cause pressure sores on the tips of the toes when the child ambulates, eventually leading to osteomyelitis of the toes. Tenotomies of the flexors at the plantar aspect or at the posterior ankle area (79) can prevent the toe flexion deformities and the associated problems.

## Vertical Talus

A planovalgus deformity of the foot may be the result of a vertical talus (Fig. 16A). The hallmark of this foot deformity is dorsal dislocation of the navicular bone on the talar head. Dorsal dislocation or subluxation of the calcaneocuboid joint may be present in severely rigid feet (80). Unlike the congenital vertical talus, the kind seen in spina bifida appears to develop over time. Patients with L5 and sacral-level lesions are most likely to develop this rare deformity due to weakness or paralysis of the posterior tibialis. Lateral radiograph of the ankle placed in maximum plantarflexion can differentiate the vertical talus deformity from an oblique talus deformity. In a true vertical talus foot, the talonavicular joint remains dislocated in plantarflexion. Manipulation and serial casting may partially correct the soft-tissue contractures. Surgical correction consists of radical soft-tissue release and reduction of the talus for young patients (Fig. 16B and C). For older patients, a talectomy may be more suitable.

## Calcaneus Deformity

A calcaneus deformity results from paralysis of L5-S1. Active ankle dorsiflexors combined with paretic plantarflexors tilt the calcaneus so the posterior end points towards the plantar aspect of the foot. If left untreated, the deformity tends to progress and bracing becomes difficult. The absence of sensation can lead to a heel pressure sore with subsequent ulcerations and osteomyelitis. Some of these children require partial calcanectomy or even amputation to control infectious dissemination.

An effective treatment for calcaneus deformity is posterior transfer of the anterior tibial tendon to the calcaneus through a window in the interosseous membrane with anterior capsulotomy and lengthening of the other dorsiflexors (89,90). The goals of the procedure have evolved. In the past, surgeons attempted to substitute the function of the absent triceps surae with tendon transfers. Banta et al. (90) reported decreased ankle dorsiflexion moments during ambulation as well as a decreased knee flexion in stance, especially with continued use of orthoses. Fernandez-Feliberti et al. (89) found that all patients with ulcerations preoperatively did not exhibit recurrence of the ulceration. Gait analysis showed that continued bracing is necessary to provide a more normal appearing and energy-efficient gait. Thus, a plantigrade and braceable foot is a realistic goal (91). Successful outcome is associated with transfer of an anterior tibialis muscle with voluntary control. Poor results in patients younger than four years of age may be related to difficulty in assessing voluntary muscle function in this group (92). Late surgical correction leads to failure due to bony changes. These older patients may benefit from osteotomies of the calcaneus and other tarsal bones, combined with soft-tissue releases. In a patient with active dorsiflexors, a posterior dorsal wedge calcaneal osteotomy combined with posterior transfer of the dorsiflexors has been beneficial.

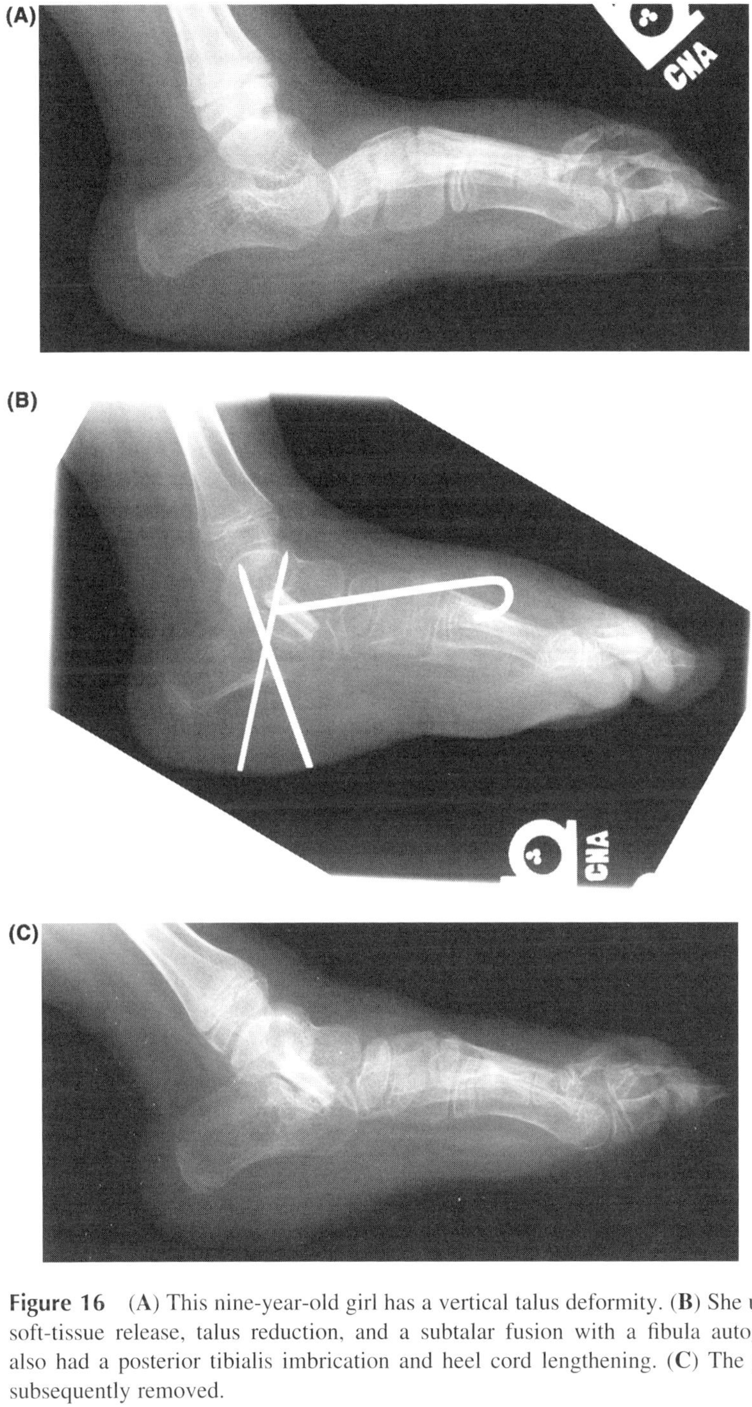


**Figure 16** (**A**) This nine-year-old girl has a vertical talus deformity. (**B**) She underwent soft-tissue release, talus reduction, and a subtalar fusion with a fibula autograft. She also had a posterior tibialis imbrication and heel cord lengthening. (**C**) The pins were subsequently removed.

### Pes Cavus

Pes cavus deformity refers to forefoot equinus with an exaggerated arch (Fig. 17). In the myelomeningocele population, it is most commonly seen in the adolescent patient. Plantar pressure ulcerations occur at either the calcaneus or the metatarsal head regions. Patients developing progressive pes cavus deformities may have spinal cord tethering or other intraspinal anomalies and therefore should undergo neurosurgical evaluation, especially if the cavus deformity is unilateral. Orthopedic treatment involves closing dorsal wedge osteotomies at the apex of the deformity and plantar fascia release. Loss of the intrinsic musculature can result in toe cock-up deformity, which includes fixed flexion contractures at the interphalangeal joints and hyperextension of the MTP joints. Extensor hallucis longus lengthening with tenodesis of the long-toe flexors to the proximal phalanx and dorsal MTP capsulotomies may be helpful. Internal fixation of the joints for at least four weeks is necessary to maintain correction (88).

## FRACTURE CARE

Fracture recognition in the spina bifida patient can be challenging. A febrile child with erythema and swelling over an extremity most likely has a fracture, not an infection.

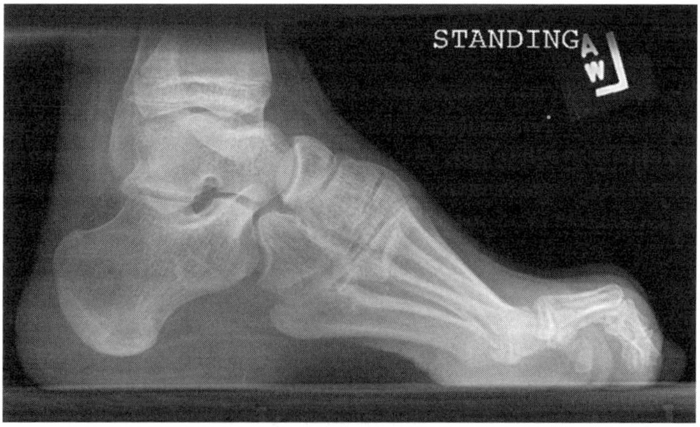


**Figure 17** This 12-year-old patient has a cavus deformity. Note the exaggerated arch. The dorsum of the foot has a "ski slope" appearance characterized by forefoot equinus and hyperextension of the metatarso-phalangeal joints and flexion of the interphalangeal joints. Furthermore, there is apparent flattening of the talus due to the oblique view of the ankle. The adductus deformity of the foot is inferred from this radiograph. The lateral view of the forefoot is combined with an oblique view of the ankle. A true lateral view of the ankle will show that the dome of the talus is rounded.

Laboratory studies often do not distinguish a fracture from an infection as there is elevation of the white blood cell count and the erythrocyte sedimentation rate (93). Bones of nonambulatory patients are so osteopenic that minimal trauma, such as diaper changes, may cause a fracture. In addition, the lack of sensation in the involved extremity not only results in delayed presentation, but also makes clinical examination difficult.

## Risk Groups

Fractures in the myelomeningocele population warrant special attention (94,95). A major risk factor is a recent operative procedure, with subsequent disuse osteopenia due to immobilization or bedrest. In addition, disuse osteopenia is very common in thoracic-level patients because they generally are not ambulators. Loss of shock absorption can also increase the risk of fractures as in a patient after a foot arthrodesis. Presence of contractures can increase the risk of fractures, particularly in the newborns with thoracic-level and high-lumbar-level involvement who have contractures above and below the bone (96).

## Fracture Management

Unlike some patient populations who have poor fracture healing, myelomeningocele patients tend to form abundant callus at the fracture site, much like closed head injury patients (Fig. 18). The etiology for the abundant callus is not known.

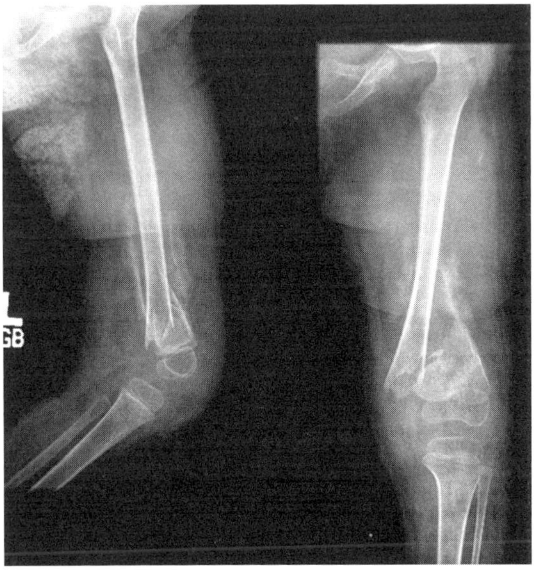

**Figure 18** Note the exuberant callus formation at the distal femur fracture site one week after injury.

Soft padding is adequate to treat fractures in newborns with spina bifida. For the older nonambulatory patient with a lower extremity fracture, treatment may consist of a combination of casting, splinting, and soft padding. In these patients, surgeons avoid prolonged hard cast immobilization because it may contribute to increased disuse osteopenia. In addition, the end of the cast may serve as a fulcrum for another fracture. For older ambulatory patients with lower extremity diaphyseal and metaphyseal fractures, formal casting is appropriate and lasts about four weeks. Once the fracture site stabilizes, weight-bearing activity in the cast will minimize the development of osteopenia. In general, upper extremity fractures are treated with hard cast immobilization in both the ambulatory and nonambulatory spina bifida patient.

### Physeal Fractures

A subgroup of patients suffer from physeal injuries rather than diaphyseal or metaphyseal fractures. Physeal injuries occur in less than 10% of patients with spina bifida. Myelomeningocele patients who sustain physeal fractures are mostly pubertal and have low-lumbar-level lesions (94,97). These physeal injuries are generally due to repetitive activity during ambulation. Cuxart also noted that physeal injuries most commonly occurred in flail regions below the neurological level of involvement. Therefore, patients and their relatives often do not recollect a history of trauma. However, in Cuxart's series, the majority of patients admitted to ambulating at home without their assistive devices. Also, a history of vigorous stretching of a joint contracture followed by swelling and an apparent improvement of motion may represent not a resolution of the contracture, but instead a transphyseal fracture. These patients demonstrate swelling and local warmth at presentation, which suggests the diagnosis of fracture, but unlike diaphyseal and metaphyseal fractures, they do not typically present with systemic fever or abnormal laboratory results.

The majority of physeal fractures in the myelomeningocele population are Salter–Harris type I epiphysiolysis. Radiographs show widening and irregularity of the growth plate. In cases where there is no obvious fracture of a long bone, radiographic stress views can help to rule out a physeal type of injury. Treatment of these fractures involves casting for about eight weeks until the radiographic appearance improves and the physeal widening resolves. Growth arrest may be seen after resolution of distal femoral physeal injuries.

## ORTHOSES

Ninety-five percent of children with myelodysplasia will require orthotic support.

### Thoracic Level and Upper Lumbar Level

In early childhood, a parapodium or a standing frame can support children with thoracic and upper-lumbar-level lesions in the upright position. This improves

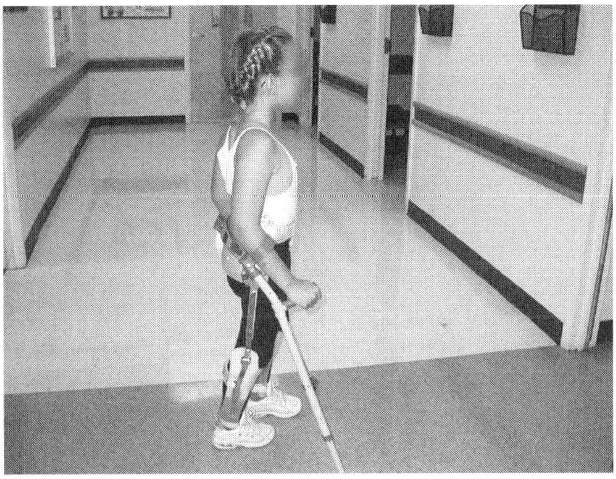

**Figure 19** This 10-year-old girl with a thoracic-level myelomeningocele uses forearm crutches and reciprocating gait orthoses.

interaction with the environment by allowing patients to view the world from a normal height and freeing up the hands for manual tasks. The majority of these patients will also require hip orthoses. Upper-lumbar-level children have similar orthotic needs as the thoracic-level patients. They tend to demonstrate a swing-through gait. The reciprocating gait orthosis (RGO) allows alternating gait (Fig. 19). When using an orthotic device, adequate joint flexibility allows proper locomotion. Hip flexor power is not a prerequisite but aids in commencing the swing phase. Compared to using hip–knee–ankle–foot-orthoses (HKAFOs), using RGOs creates a more normal gait and allows patients to ambulate longer distances (98,99). Energy requirements, measured by oxygen consumption and heart rates, are also lower for the HKAFO group. Rate of repair and gait training requirements are similar with both types of orthoses. Eventually, almost all thoracic-level and upper-lumbar-level patients use wheelchairs, regardless of the type of orthoses chosen.

## Lower Lumbar Level and Sacral Level

Patients with lower lumbar lesions lack adequate plantar flexors; resultant difficulty in pushing off during the gait cycle leads to a calcaneus gait. Because of the muscle imbalances, the foot develops a calcaneus deformity. These patients have altered plantarflexion/knee-extension coupling mechanisms: the weak plantar flexors increase the flexion moment at the knee and the dorsiflexion moment at the ankle, leading to a crouching gait.

AFO use is almost universal in the low lumbar and sacral groups. Braces control the ankle, subtalar, and midtarsal joints and prevent primary and recurring deformities. The solid AFOs compensate for triceps surae weakness (Fig. 20). The orthosis prevents the ankle from excessive dorsiflexion during stance

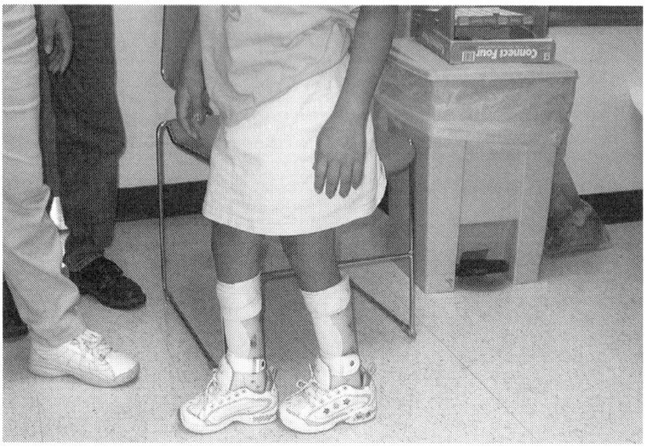

**Figure 20** This patient is wearing solid ankle-foot orthoses (AFOs). Special sneakers that are deep enough to accommodate AFOs are available.

phase and prevents crouching, improving the appearance of gait (100). Floor-reaction AFOs compensate for the weak plantarflexors by supporting the anterior tibia. This minimizes crouching during ambulation by preventing anterior tibial translation and relieving the quadriceps. Patients with sacral-level lesions do not need wheelchairs but may benefit from crutches for long-distance ambulation. The use of crutches does not alter the speed, but does improve hip kinematics and reduce hip joint stresses. Walking short distances without crutches does not significantly alter joint integrity (69).

## GAIT IN THE MYELOMENINGOCELE PATIENT

Myelomeningocele children begin independent walking at a later age than their normal peers. Those with more proximal levels of neurological involvement walk even later than those with more distal lesions. Children unable to ambulate by age four are unlikely to ever walk (101).

### Classification of Ambulation

The ability to ambulate is divided into four functional categories: community, household, nonfunctional, and nonambulators (102). Community ambulators are capable of ambulating full-time, except for prolonged intervals. Community ambulators may use aids like crutches and/or braces. The household ambulator is capable of ambulating at home with aids, but needs the assistance of a wheelchair in the community. They are capable of performing transfers from bed to chair with minimal assistance if any. Nonfunctional ambulators use wheelchairs and cannot depend on ambulation for mobility due to its enormous energy requirements. However, nonfunctional ambulators can walk during physical therapy sessions. Nonambulators are fully wheelchair-dependent; they may be able to transfer from bed to chair.

The most important factor in ambulatory capacity is the level of spinal involvement (52). Almost all of the patients with good quadriceps function (L4 or lower) are community ambulators (101). Motor power within the level of involvement also is a factor in walking capability (103). Additional factors affecting ambulatory capacity include weight, family environment, intelligence, patient motivation, spasticity, the presence of severe spinal abnormality, and the amount of pelvic obliquity (52,102,104). To ambulate, the child with spina bifida must have good balance, minimal joint contractures, plantigrade feet, and adequate hip and knee function. The effect of knee contractures on ambulation is discussed in the previous section. For patients with hydrocephalus, proper shunt function is critical for walking ability because increased intracranial pressure affects upper extremity and cognitive function. Powerful upper extremities and reasonable intelligence are necessary to handle ambulatory-assistive devices.

## Loss of Ambulation

The ambulatory capacity of many children with spina bifida diminishes with age due to increase in size and weight, making it difficult for them to ambulate without excessive energy expenditure. Fortunately, society has made wheelchair use more accessible and acceptable. The majority of the patients will lose the ability to ambulate between the ages of 10 and 15, a time of rapid growth and development when weight gain makes bracing difficult (103). Studies have shown that only about 4% of children with either a thoracic or a high lumbar level of involvement will continue to ambulate beyond adolescence. The importance of ambulatory capacity in thoracic-level children is controversial. Since the majority of thoracic and high-lumbar-level children become wheelchair-dependent early in life, some authors have recommended early use of wheelchairs. Others have advocated doing aggressive physical therapy and bracing to train the patients, feeling that these not only help to minimize the risk of obesity, develop strength, improve bone density, and prevent contractures, but also give patients a sense of accomplishment (65). In contrast to thoracic and high-lumbar-level spina bifida patients, one study of spina bifida patients surviving beyond age 20 found that 95% of the midlumbar-level patients were still ambulating (49). Similarly, children with low lumbar and sacral lesions usually remain community ambulators, although some require the use of orthoses. (105).

In addition to neurosegmental level, a number of other factors have been correlated with loss of ambulation in the myelomeningocele population. Specifically, poor sitting balance is predictive of future nonambulatory status. In a study of 206 patients with spina bifida, no patient with severe or moderate lack of sitting balance was a community ambulator (101). In addition, the presence of weakness, spasticity, and upper extremity dysfunction are related to the loss of ambulatory ability. Samuelsson and Skoog found that

Arnold–Chiari malformations and hydromyelia are responsible for losing functional levels and walking ability (106). In addition, fractures may also be a determining factor in loss of locomotion. Furthermore, it has been shown that scoliosis is highly correlated with ambulation, such that the higher the degree of curvature, the more likely the patient is to lose ambulatory ability. In Samuelsson and Skoog's study, all patients with curves $>30^\circ$ became nonambulators.

Hip flexion contractures have also been shown to affect maintenance of ambulation: contractures $>20^\circ$ have been correlated with nonambulatory status (106,107). In contrast, hip instability has not been implicated as a significant impairment to ambulation. Barden et al. (49) found that, among myelomeningocele patients greater than 20 years old, those with dislocated hips were able to ambulate freely without pain.

### Gait Analysis and Energy Expenditure

In order for the children with spina bifida to ambulate, they must compensate for muscle weakness and imbalance. This leads to abnormal gait patterns involving the hip, knee, and ankle. A weak gastroc–soleus complex has been shown to have a major role in gait pathology. Patients with weakness of the gastroc–soleus complex tend to adopt a calcaneus alignment at the ankle. This in turn causes the ground-reaction forces to pass posterior to the knee, causing an increased flexion moment. The weak or absent plantar flexors cannot compensate and the leg tends to externally rotate, creating valgus stresses to the knee. It has been shown that the use of AFOs can increase speed and decrease energy consumption and oxygen cost for the ambulating myelomeningocele patient (108).

## UPPER EXTREMITY INVOLVEMENT IN MYELODYSPLASIA

Because myelomeningocele is not only a spinal cord disease but also a central nervous system disease, upper extremity function may also be affected in children with spina bifida (109–111). As a result, patients with myelomeningocele may require both hands to perform manual tasks usually performed with one hand by a normal child. The presence or absence of upper extremity spasticity is the most important factor in predicting upper extremity dysfunction in the spina bifida population. For children with hydrocephalus, studies have shown that increasing number of shunt revisions correlates with worsened upper extremity function (110). The association between neurological level of involvement and upper limb function has been debated. Mazur et al. (110) found that patients with thoracic level of involvement were 4.5 times more prone to have abnormal dominant hand function than those with sacral involvement. Other investigators found no variation in upper limb function according to neurological level involvement (111,112).

## REFERENCES


1. Carstens C, Koch H, Brocai DR, Niethard FU. Development of pathological lumbar kyphosis in myelomeningocele. J Bone Joint Surg Br 1996; 78(6):945–950.
2. Mintz LJ, Sarwark JF, Dias LS, Schafer MF. The natural history of congenital kyphosis in myelomeningocele. A review of 51 children. Spine 1991; 16(suppl 8):S348–S350.
3. Martin J Jr, Kumar SJ, Guille JT, Ger D, Gibbs M. Congenital kyphosis in myelomeningocele: results following operative and nonoperative treatment. J Pediatr Orthop 1994; 14(3):323–328.
4. Campbell RM Jr, Smith MD, Mayes TC, et al. The characteristics of thoracic insufficiency syndrome associated with fused ribs and congenital scoliosis. J Bone Joint Surg Am 2003; 85-A(3):399–408.
5. Campbell RM Jr, Smith MD, Mayes TC, et al. The effect of opening wedge thoracostomy on thoracic insufficiency syndrome associated with fused ribs and congenital scoliosis. J Bone Joint Surg Am 2004; 86-A(8):1659–1674.
6. Lintner SA, Lindseth RE. Kyphotic deformity in patients who have a myelomeningocele. Operative treatment and long-term follow-up. J Bone Joint Surg Am 1994; 76(9):1301–1307.
7. Crawford AH, Strub WM, Lewis R, et al. Neonatal kyphectomy in the patient with myelomeningocele. Spine 2003; 28(3):260–266.
8. Nolden MT, Sarwark JF, Vora A, Grayhack JJ. A kyphectomy technique with reduced perioperative morbidity for myelomeningocele kyphosis. Spine 2002; 27(16):1807–1813.
9. McCarthy RE. Kyphosis: surgical management. In: Sarwark JF, Lubicky JP, eds. Caring for the Child with Spina Bifida. Rosemont, IL: The American Academy of Orthopaedic Surgeons, 2001:223–237.
10. Heydemann JS, Gillespie R. Management of myelomeningocele kyphosis in the older child by kyphectomy and segmental spinal instrumentation. Spine 1987; 12(1):37–41.
11. McCarthy RE, Dunn H, McCullough FL. Luque fixation to the sacral ala using the Dunn–McCarthy modification. Spine 1989; 14(3):281–283.
12. Warner WC Jr, Fackler CD. Comparison of two instrumentation techniques in treatment of lumbar kyphosis in myelodysplasia. J Pediatr Orthop 1993; 13(6):704–708.
13. Miladi LT, Ghanem IB, Draoui MM, Zeller RD, Dubousset JF. Iliosacral screw fixation for pelvic obliquity in neuromuscular scoliosis. A long-term follow-up study. Spine 1997; 22(15):1722–1729.
14. McCall RE. Modified luque instrumentation after myelomeningocele kyphectomy. Spine 1998; 23(12):1406–1411.
15. Winston K, Hall J, Johnson D, Micheli L. Acute elevation of intracranial pressure following transection of non-functional spinal cord. Clin Orthop Relat Res 1977; 128:41–44.
16. Lalonde F, Jarvis J. Congenital kyphosis in myelomeningocele. The effect of cordotomy on bladder function. J Bone Joint Surg Br 1999; 81(2):245–249.
17. Niall DM, Dowling FE, Fogarty EE, Moore DP, Goldberg C. Kyphectomy in children with myelomeningocele: a long-term outcome study. J Pediatr Orthop 2004; 24(1):37–44.
18. Pontari MA, Bauer SB, Hall JE, Emans JB. Adverse urologic consequences of spinal cord resection at the time of kyphectomy: value of preoperative urodynamic evaluation. J Pediatr Orthop 1998; 18(6):820–823.

19. Muller EB, Nordwall A. Prevalence of scoliosis in children with myelomeningocele in western Sweden. Spine 1992; 17(9):1097–1102.
20. Trivedi J, Thomson JD, Slakey JB, Banta JV, Jones PW. Clinical and radiographic predictors of scoliosis in patients with myelomeningocele. J Bone Joint Surg Am 2002; 84-A(8):1389–1394.
21. Muller EB, Nordwall A, Oden A. Progression of scoliosis in children with myelomeningocele. Spine 1994; 19(2):147–150.
22. Lindseth RE. Myelomeningocele. In: Morrisey RT, Weinstein SL, eds. Lovell and Winter's Pediatric Orthopaedics. 5th ed. Philadelphia: Lippincott Williams & Wilkins, 2001:601–632.
23. Muller EB, Nordwall A. Brace treatment of scoliosis in children with myelomeningocele. Spine 1994; 19(2):151–155.
24. Olafsson Y, Saraste H, Al-Dabbagh Z. Brace treatment in neuromuscular spine deformity. J Pediatr Orthop 1999; 19(3):376–379.
25. Richards BS. Nonsurgical management of the myelomeningocele spine. In: Sarwark JF, Lubicky JP, eds. Caring for the Child with Spina Bifida. Rosemont, IL: The American Academy of Orthopaedic Surgeons, 2001:181–188.
26. Lubicky JP. The surgical treatment of spinal deformities in myelomeningocele. In: Sarwark JF, Lubicky JP, eds. Caring for the Child with Spina Bifida. 1st ed. Rosemont, IL: The American Academy of Orthopaedics, 2001:171–180.
27. Pierz K, Banta J, Thomson J, Gahm N, Hartford J. The effect of tethered cord release on scoliosis in myelomeningocele. J Pediatr Orthop 2000; 20(3):362–365.
28. Carstens C, Paul K, Niethard FU, Pfeil J. Effect of scoliosis surgery on pulmonary function in patients with myelomeningocele. J Pediatr Orthop 1991; 11(4):459–464.
29. Wai EK, Young NL, Feldman BM, Badley EM, Wright JG. The relationship between function, self-perception, and spinal deformity: implications for treatment of scoliosis in children with spina bifida. J Pediatr Orthop 2005; 25(1):64–69.
30. Wai EK, Owen J, Fehlings D, Wright JG. Assessing physical disability in children with spina bifida and scoliosis. J Pediatr Orthop 2000; 20(6):765–770.
31. Tosi LL, Slater JE, Shaer C, Mostello LA. Latex allergy in spina bifida patients: prevalence and surgical implications. J Pediatr Orthop 1993; 13(6):709–712.
32. Dormans JP, Templeton J, Schreiner MS, Delfico AJ. Intraoperative latex anaphylaxis in children: classification and prophylaxis of patients at risk. J Pediatr Orthop 1997; 17(5):622–625.
33. Dormans JP, Templeton JJ, Edmonds C, Davidson RS, Drummond DS. Intraoperative anaphylaxis due to exposure to latex (natural rubber) in children. J Bone Joint Surg Am 1994; 76(11):1688–1691.
34. Birmingham PK, Dsida RM, Grayhack JJ, et al. Do latex precautions in children with myelodysplasia reduce intraoperative allergic reactions? J Pediatr Orthop 1996; 16(6):799–802.
35. Osebold WR. Stability of myelomeningocele spines treated with the mayfield two-stage anterior and posterior fusion technique. Spine 2000; 25(11):1344–1351.
36. Widmann RF, Hresko MT, Hall JE. Lumbosacral fusion in children and adolescents using the modified sacral bar technique. Clin Orthop Relat Res 1999; 364:85–91.
37. Rodgers WB, Williams MS, Schwend RM, Emans JB. Spinal deformity in myelodysplasia. Correction with posterior pedicle screw instrumentation. Spine 1997; 22(20):2435–2443.

38. Warner WC Jr. Surgical management of scoliosis. In: Sarwark JF, Lubicky JP, eds. Caring for the Child with Spina Bifida. Rosemont, IL: The American Academy of Orthopaedic Surgeons, 2001:189–198.
39. Wild A, Haak H, Kumar M, Krauspe R. Is sacral instrumentation mandatory to address pelvic obliquity in neuromuscular thoracolumbar scoliosis due to myelomeningocele? Spine 2001; 26(14):E325–E329.
40. Sponseller PD, Young AT, Sarwark JF, Lim R. Anterior only fusion for scoliosis in patients with myelomeningocele. Clin Orthop Relat Res 1999; 364:117–124.
41. Banta JV. Combined anterior and posterior fusion for spinal deformity in myelomeningocele. Spine 1990; 15(9):946–952.
42. Banit DM, Iwinski HJ Jr, Talwalkar V, Johnson M. Posterior spinal fusion in paralytic scoliosis and myelomeningocele. J Pediatr Orthop 2001; 21(1):117–125.
43. Heeg M, Broughton NS, Menelaus MB. Bilateral dislocation of the hip in spina bifida: a long-term follow-up study. J Pediatr Orthop 1998; 18(4):434–436.
44. Rueda J, Carroll NC. Hip instability in patients with myelomeningocele. J Bone Joint Surg Br 1972; 54(3):422–431.
45. Menelaus M. Orthopaedic management in children with myelomeningocele: a plea for realistic goals. Dev Med Child Neurol 1976; 18(suppl 37):3–11.
46. Drennan JC. Current concepts in myelomeningocele. In: Zuckerman JD, ed. Instructional Course Lectures. Rosemont, IL: American Academy of Orthopaedic Surgeons, 1999:543–550.
47. Carroll NC, Sharrard WJ. Long-term follow-up of posterior iliopsoas transplantation for paralytic dislocation of the hip. J Bone Joint Surg Am 1972; 54(3):551–560.
48. Beeker TW, Scheers MM. The hip joint in spina bifida accompanied by myelomeningocele: a review of the cases of a spina bifida team. Neuro-Orthop 1986;2:87–94.
49. Barden GA, Meyer LC, Stelling FH 3rd. Myelodysplastics—fate of those followed for twenty years or more. J Bone Joint Surg Am 1975; 57(5):643–647.
50. Dias L. Hip deformities in myelomeningocele. In: Tullos HS, ed. Instructional Course Lectures. Vol. 40. Park Ridge, IL: American Academy of Orthopaedic Surgeons, 1991:281–286.
51. Feiwell E. Surgery of the hip in myelomeningocele as related to adult goals. Clin Orthop Relat Res 1980; 148:87–93.
52. Asher M, Olson J. Factors affecting the ambulatory status of patients with spina bifida cystica. J Bone Joint Surg Am 1983; 65(3):350–356.
53. Mannor DA, Weinstein SL, Dietz FR. Long-term follow-up of Chiari pelvic osteotomy in myelomeningocele. J Pediatr Orthop 1996; 16(6):769–773.
54. Thomas LI, Thompson TC, Straub LR. Transplantation of the external oblique muscle for abductor paralysis. J Bone Joint Surg Am 1950; 32A(1):207–217, illustration.
55. Sharrard WJ. Posterior iliopsoas transplantation in the treatment of paralytic dislocation of the hip. J Bone Joint Surg Br 1964; 46:426–444.
56. Phillips DP, Lindseth RE. Ambulation after transfer of adductors, external oblique, and tensor fascia lata in myelomeningocele. J Pediatr Orthop 1992; 12(6):712–717.
57. Yngve DA, Lindseth RE. Effectiveness of muscle transfers in myelomeningocele hips measured by radiographic indices. J Pediatr Orthop 1982; 2(2):121–125.
58. Dias LS, Jasty MJ, Collins P. Rotational deformities of the lower limb in myelomeningocele. Evaluation and treatment. J Bone Joint Surg Am 1984; 66(2): 215–223.

59. Wright JG, Menelaus MB, Broughton NS, Shurtleff D. Natural history of knee contractures in myelomeningocele. J Pediatr Orthop 1991; 11(6):725–730.
60. Dias LS. Surgical management of knee contractures in myelomeningocele. J Pediatr Orthop 1982; 2(2):127–131.
61. DelBello DA, Watts HG. Distal femoral extension osteotomy for knee flexion contracture in patients with arthrogryposis. J Pediatr Orthop 1996; 16(1): 122–126.
62. Zimmerman MH, Smith CF, Oppenheim WL. Supracondylar femoral extension osteotomies in the treatment of fixed flexion deformity of the knee. Clin Orthop Relat Res 1982; 171:87–93.
63. Aprin H, Kilfoyle RM. Extension contracture of the knees in patients with meningomyelocele. Clin Orthop Relat Res 1979; 144:260–263.
64. Roy DR, Crawford AH. Percutaneous quadriceps recession: a technique for management of congenital hyperextension deformities of the knee in the neonate. J Pediatr Orthop 1989; 9(6):717–719.
65. Greene WB. Treatment of hip and knee problems in myelomeningocele. In: Zuckerman JD, ed. Instructional Course Lectures Vol. 48. Rosemont, IL: American Academy of Orthopaedic Surgeons, 1999:563–574.
66. Selber P, Dias L. Sacral-level myelomeningocele: long-term outcome in adults. J Pediatr Orthop 1998; 18(4):423–427.
67. Williams JJ, Graham GP, Dunne KB, Menelaus MB. Late knee problems in myelomeningocele. J Pediatr Orthop 1993; 13(6):701–703.
68. Dias LS. Management of tibial torsion. In: Sarwark JF, Lubicky JP, eds. Caring for the Child with Spina Bifida. Rosemont, IL: The American Academy of Orthopaedic Surgeons, 2001:151–153.
69. Vankoski S, Moore C, Statler KD, Sarwark JF, Dias L. The influence of forearm crutches on pelvic and hip kinematics in children with myelomeningocele: don't throw away the crutches. Dev Med Child Neurol 1997; 39(9):614–619.
70. Lim R, Dias L, Vankoski S, Moore C, Marinello M, Sarwark J. Valgus knee stress in lumbosacral myelomeningocele: a gait-analysis evaluation. J Pediatr Orthop 1998; 18(4):428–433.
71. Malhotra D, Puri R, Owen R. Valgus deformity of the ankle in children with spina bifida aperta. J Bone Joint Surg Br 1984; 66(3):381–385.
72. Dias LS. Ankle valgus in children with myelomeningocele. Dev Med Child Neurol 1978; 20(5):627–633.
73. Stevens PM, Toomey E. Fibular-Achilles tenodesis for paralytic ankle valgus. J Pediatr Orthop 1988; 8(2):169–175.
74. Abraham E, Lubicky JP, Songer MN, Millar EA. Supramalleolar osteotomy for ankle valgus in myelomeningocele. J Pediatr Orthop 1996; 16(6):774–781.
75. Kumar SJ, Keret D, MacEwen GD. Corrective cosmetic supramalleolar osteotomy for valgus deformity of the ankle joint: a report of two cases. J Pediatr Orthop 1990; 10(1):124–127.
76. Lubicky JP, Altiok H. Transphyseal osteotomy of the distal tibia for correction of valgus/varus deformities of the ankle. J Pediatr Orthop 2001; 21(1):80–88.
77. Davids JR, Valadie AL, Ferguson RL, Bray EW 3rd, Allen BL Jr. Surgical management of ankle valgus in children: use of a transphyseal medial malleolar screw. J Pediatr Orthop 1997; 17(1):3–8.

78. Torosian CM, Dias LS. Surgical treatment of severe hindfoot valgus by medial displacement osteotomy of the os calcis in children with myelomeningocele. J Pediatr Orthop 2000; 20(2):226–229.
79. Sharrard WJ, Grosfield I. The management of deformity and paralysis of the foot in myelomeningocele. J Bone Joint Surg Br 1968; 50(3):456–465.
80. Dias L. Myelomeningocele and intraspinal lipoma. In: Sponseller PD, ed. Orthopaedic Knowledge Update: Pediatrics 2. Rosemont, IL: American Academy of Orthopaedic Surgeons, 2002:249–264.
81. Flynn JM, Herrera-Soto JA, Ramirez NF, Fernandez-Feliberti R, Vilella F, Guzman J. Clubfoot release in myelodysplasia. J Pediatr Orthop B 2004; 13(4): 259–262.
82. de Carvalho Neto J, Dias LS, Gabrieli AP. Congenital talipes equinovarus in spina bifida: treatment and results. J Pediatr Orthop 1996; 16(6):782–785.
83. Crawford AH, Marxen JL, Osterfeld DL. The Cincinnati incision: a comprehensive approach for surgical procedures of the foot and ankle in childhood. J Bone Joint Surg Am 1982; 64(9):1355–1358.
84. Trumble T, Banta JV, Raycroft JF, Curtis BH. Talectomy for equinovarus deformity in myelodysplasia. J Bone Joint Surg Am 1985; 67(1):21–29.
85. Dias LS, Stern LS. Talectomy in the treatment of resistant talipes equinovarus deformity in myelomeningocele and arthrogryposis. J Pediatr Orthop 1987; 7(1):39–41.
86. Segal LS, Mann DC, Feiwell E, Hoffer MM. Equinovarus deformity in arthrogryposis and myelomeningocele: evaluation of primary talectomy. Foot Ankle 1989; 10(1):12–16.
87. Sherk HH, Marchinski LJ, Clancy M, Melchonni J. Ground reaction forces on the plantar surface of the foot after talectomy in the myelomeningocele. J Pediatr Orthop 1989; 9(3):269–275.
88. Drennan J. Foot deformities in myelomeningocele. In: Tullos HS, ed. Instructional Course Lectures. Vol. 40. Park Ridge, IL: American Academy of Orthopaedic Surgeons, 1991:287–291.
89. Fernandez-Feliberti R, Fernandez SA, Colon C, Ramirez N, Alegria M, Cintron K. Transfer of the tibialis anterior for calcaneus deformity in myelodysplasia. J Bone Joint Surg Am 1992; 74(7):1038–1041.
90. Banta JV, Sutherland DH, Wyatt M. Anterior tibial transfer to the os calcis with Achilles tenodesis for calcaneal deformity in myelomeningocele. J Pediatr Orthop 1981; 1(2):125–130.
91. Stott NS, Zionts LE, Gronley JK, Perry J. Tibialis anterior transfer for calcaneal deformity: a postoperative gait analysis. J Pediatr Orthop 1996; 16(6):792–798.
92. Georgiadis GM, Aronson DD. Posterior transfer of the anterior tibial tendon in children who have a myelomeningocele. J Bone Joint Surg Am 1990; 72(3): 392–398.
93. Townsend PF, Cowell HR, Steg NL. Lower extremity fractures simulating infection in myelomeningocele. Clin Orthop Relat Res 1979; 144:255–259.
94. Cuxart A, Iborra J, Melendez M, Pages E. Physeal injuries in myelomeningocele patients. Paraplegia 1992; 30(11):791–794.
95. Reikeras O, Hellum C. Fractures in children with myelomeningocele. Arch Orthop Trauma Surg 1981; 98(1):25–28.

96. Boytim MJ, Davidson RS, Charney E, Melchionni JB. Neonatal fractures in myelomeningocele patients. J Pediatr Orthop 1991; 11(1):28–30.
97. Kumar SJ, Cowell HR, Townsend P. Physeal, metaphyseal, and diaphyseal injuries of the lower extremities in children with myelomeningocele. J Pediatr Orthop 1984; 4(1):25–27.
98. McCall RE, Schmidt WT. Clinical experience with the reciprocal gait orthosis in myelodysplasia. J Pediatr Orthop 1986; 6(2):157–161.
99. Katz DE, Haideri N, Song K, Wyrick P. Comparative study of conventional hip–knee–ankle–foot orthoses versus reciprocating-gait orthoses for children with high-level paraparesis. J Pediatr Orthop 1997; 17(3):377–386.
100. Duffy CM, Hill AE, Cosgrove AP, Corry IS, Mollan RA, Graham HK. Three-dimensional gait analysis in spina bifida. J Pediatr Orthop 1996; 16(6):786–791.
101. Swank M, Dias L. Myelomeningocele: a review of the orthopaedic aspects of 206 patients treated from birth with no selection criteria. Dev Med Child Neurol 1992; 34(12):1047–1052.
102. Hoffer MM, Feiwell E, Perry R, Perry J, Bonnett C. Functional ambulation in patients with myelomeningocele. J Bone Joint Surg Am 1973; 55(1):137–148.
103. De Souza LJ, Carroll N. Ambulation of the braced myelomeningocele patient. J Bone Joint Surg Am 1976; 58(8):1112–1118.
104. Bartonek A, Saraste H. Factors influencing ambulation in myelomeningocele: a cross-sectional study. Dev Med Child Neurol 2001; 43(4):253–260.
105. Bowman RM, McLone DG, Grant JA, Tomita T, Ito JA. Spina bifida outcome: a 25-year prospective. Pediatr Neurosurg 2001; 34(3):114–120.
106. Samuelsson L, Skoog M. Ambulation in patients with myelomeningocele: a multivariate statistical analysis. J Pediatr Orthop 1988; 8(5):569–575.
107. Bartonek A, Saraste H, Samuelsson L, Skoog M. Ambulation in patients with myelomeningocele: a 12-year follow-up. J Pediatr Orthop 1999; 19(2):202–206.
108. Vankoski SJ, Kelp-Lenane C. Gait patterns in children with myelomeningocele. In: Sarwark JF, Lubicky JP, eds. Caring for the Child with Spina Bifida. Rosemont, IL: The American Academy of Orthopaedic Surgeons, 2001:269–282.
109. Mazur JM, Stillwell A, Menelaus M. The significance of spasticity in the upper and lower limbs in myelomeningocele. J Bone Joint Surg Br 1986; 68(2):213–217.
110. Mazur JM, Menelaus MB, Hudson I, Stillwell A. Hand function in patients with spina bifida cystica. J Pediatr Orthop 1986; 6(4):442–447.
111. Turner A. Hand function in children with myelomeningocele. J Bone Joint Surg Br 1985; 67(2):268–272.
112. Minns R. Upper limb function in spina bifida. Z Kinderchir 1977; 22(4):493–506.

# 11

# New Urological Trends

**Kazuyuki Nishinaka and Curtis A. Sheldon**
*Division of Urology, Cincinnati Children's Hospital Medical Center, Cincinnati, Ohio, U.S.A.*

## INTRODUCTION

Myelodysplasia is a common variant of neural tube defects, occurring in 1:1000 live births in the United States and estimated to affect 300,000 children worldwide. Approximately 20% of children have associated congenital anomalies. Despite new surgical advances and in utero procedures, children with neural tube defects have a variety of complex and challenging orthopedic, neurosurgical, and urological problems that require careful assessment and lifelong management to reduce disability and improve quality of life.

Congenital abnormalities of the spinal cord, or myelodysplasia, account for the great majority of neurogenic bladder dysfunctions seen in children. They consist of a heterogeneous group of developmental anomalies that include occult spina bifida, meningocele, myelomeningocele, lipomeningocele, primary tethered cord, diastematomyelia, intradural lipoma, dermoid cyst, syringomyelia, and sacral agenesis. These anomalies are associated with distortion of the developing neural tissues, with subsequent damage to the spinal cord. Closed spinal defect may be heralded at birth by an overlying skin lesion, such as a skin dimple, hairy tuft, a lipoma, or a limb deformity resulting from the associated neurological abnormalities. However, such defects might not be recognized until the onset of urinary incontinence, urinary tract infection (UTI), gait abnormalities, and inability of squat or other orthopedic problems in later childhood in association with the growth of the spine or increased morbility.

## Anatomy and Physiology of Voiding

The urinary bladder has two functions: storage and elimination of urine. Normal storage depends on a high degree of bladder compliance and a competent sphincter mechanism. Normal elimination requires coordination between the bladder and external sphincter.

Voiding is a function of spinal reflexes that are facilitated and inhibited by higher brain centers. Three sets of peripheral nerves are involved: sacral parasympathetic, thoracolumbar sympathetic, and sacral somatic nerves. Afferent nerve fibers from the bladder, urethra, and sphincters enter the thalamus and convey impulses to the parietal cerebral cortex. Contraction of the detrusor muscle occurs secondary to parasympathetic excitation, causing the bladder to contract. Sensory nerves leave the bladder and enter the spinal column through the pelvic nerves and sacral plexus (sacral parasympathetic, S2-4). The pudendal nerve that originates in the first two sacral columns through the pelvic nerves and sacral plexus (sacral somatic nerves) of the spinal column innervates the external sphincter. Sympathetic nerve fibers from the lumbar region (thoracolumbar sympathetic, T10-L12) cause the bladder to relax. During filling, sympathetic impulses assist in bladder volume accommodation and increase smooth muscle tone in the trigone and proximal urethral areas. This enables the bladder to expand under low pressure while assisting with continence by increasing outflow resistance. Somatic stimulation of the external sphincter maintains its closure, thus increasing outflow resistance. As the bladder reaches its capacity, numerous micturition contractions may occur as a result of the stretch reflex, although these can be inhibited in the normal situation. There is a decrease in urethral pressure that precedes the increase in bladder pressure during normal voiding, suggesting that urethral relaxation is the first step in micturition. There is a feedback mechanism such that the initial contraction activates receptors to increase afferent impulses and bladder contractions. The increase in frequency and intensity of the contractions is sustained for approximately one minute and then the muscle returns to a basal tone. This cycle will re-occur until the bladder is emptied, with increasing strength and frequency of the contraction.

Abnormal functioning of neurogenic bladders depends on the type and level of neurological injury but often includes uninhibited contractions, uncoordinated function of the detrusor muscle and the pelvic muscles, poor bladder compliance, inadequate urethral closure, or hyper-reflexia (defined as uninhibited bladder contractions in the face of a known neurological lesion).

## Myelodysplasia

The degree of neurological deficit in myelomeningocele is related to the level of the lesion, although level is often not predictive of bladder behavior. Lesions below the second sacral vertebra do not usually involve orthopedic problems. Spinal defects at or above the upper sacral area result in more significant orthopedic, neurological, and urological deficits that include neurogenic bowel and bladder. Lesions higher in the cord with preservation of reflex sacral function can result in detrusor–sphincter dyscoordination.

In 18% to 40% of children with myelodysplasia, there is a risk for latex and ethylene oxide allergies. Possible explanations for the sensitization include exposure from multiple surgical procedures or repeated catheterizations. The allergic response varies from allergic rhinitis, vasodilatation, edema, hives, rash, and wheezing to anaphylaxis. The response occurs when the child's skin comes in contact with latex products, although surgical contact and respiratory exposure have also been known to result in allergic reactions. Potential sources of medical latex exposure include gloves, tape, catheters, latex ports used in intravenous tubing, rubber tourniquets, vial stoppers, wheelchair wheels, Ambu bags, and stethoscopes (1). In a study comparing children with spina bifida with children undergoing multiple surgical procedures, Porri et al. (2,3) found that children with a history of multiple surgical procedures (more than six) were also at high risk for latex sensitization.

## Tethered Cord Syndrome

Tethered cord syndrome can occur with a variety of dysraphic conditions. This syndrome occurs when the spinal cord is abnormally caught between immovable structures such as scar tissue or lipomatous material at the caudal or cranial end of the cord. Consequently, the normally relaxed spinal cord is pulled and stretched as the child bends, moves, and grows. The resulting unnatural forces damage the blood vessels, nerve cells, and nerve fibers, or alternatively, result in ischemic changes to the cord. Cutaneous findings of spinal dysraphism and tethered cord syndrome as a part of an occult spina bifida may include lumbosacral cutaneous hemangiomas, hypertrichosis dermal sinus, subcutaneous lipoma, and skin appendages. Approximately 75% of patients with this syndrome have neurological changes such as radicular pain, weakness, asymmetric hyporeflexia, spasticity, sensory changes, and bowel/bladder dysfunction. The lower motor neuron symptoms may be caused by compression of the cord compared with upper motor neuron symptoms that are related to ischemic damage caused by the tethered cord. Orthopedic changes associated with tethered cord syndrome include foot deformities, limb length discrepancies, atrophy of the legs, gait disturbances, limb pain, and scoliosis. Bone abnormalities found in patients with tethered cord syndrome include bifid vertebrae, laminar defects, hemivertebrae, sacral aplasia, sacral agenesis, and multiple segmentation errors. New onset of urinary or bowel incontinence or changes in urodynamics with or without UTI may be urological indications of this syndrome.

The most common cause of progressive neurological, urological, and orthopedic deterioration is congenital tethering of a lipomeningocele (4). Timing of surgical intervention remains controversial if the patient is asymptomatic; however, most authors recommend early untethering to prevent neurological deterioration. Frequent assessment of neurological and urological function is required throughout the child's life to assess for recurrence of the tethered cord. A variety of modalities are used, including clinical assessment, radiological examination, and urodynamic testing.

Tethered cord syndrome can be primary (resulting from a form of spina bifida occulta) or secondary to previous closure of a dysraphic defect. In a study conducted by Tarcan et al, the urological outcomes of newborns with intially normal urodynamic studies and spina bifida were evaluated (5). They found a 32% risk of urologic deterioration related to spinal cord tethering by age six. Children with myelodysplasia are at risk for tethered cord resulting from postoperative adhesions or infection after the initial closure of the defect. Tethered cord may occur within weeks of closure of the defect or several years later until after pubertal growth is complete (secondary). Clinical manifestations are the result of ischemic changes or tension on the cord and often include a subtle change in bowel or bladder function. The usual treatment is surgical release of the tethered cord, but this does not always reverse the urological problems, and it may worsen the symptoms or create new problems. Generally, the shorter the duration of urological symptoms (infection, urgency, and incontinence), the more likely the child will stabilize or improve in the long term.

## Sacral Agenesis and Caudal Regression Syndrome

Sacral agenesis is described as congenital absence of the whole or of part of the sacral vertebrae S2–S5. When associated with anorectal malformations (anal atresia and rectovaginal fistula), a presacral mass, and hemisacrum, the triad of anomalies is known as Currarino syndrome and is localized on chromosome 7q36. Caudal regression is characterized by premature termination of the vertebral column (6,7). Embryologically, the vertebral column and genitourinary systems are formed simultaneously from mesodermal tissue before eight weeks of gestation. Approximately 15% to 25% of mothers of these children have insulin-dependent diabetes and have a 250 times increased risk of caudal regression than those without diabetes. There is variability in expression of the disease, with a high incidence of renal/urinary tract problems.

Frequently, children with involvement of the coccyx alone and/or the last two sacral segments are asymptomatic. Sacral agenesis generally represents a fairly fixed neurological deficit, as opposed to spina bifida. Further evaluation is required if neurological deterioration is noted (8,9).

## Detrusor–Sphincteric Dyssynergia

Detrusor–sphincteric dyssynergia (DSD) is a major problem in children with myelomeningocele and occurs when the external sphincter fails to relax or actually increases its activity during the voiding contraction. Some degree of detrusor–sphincteric incoordination, which is associated with a high voiding pressure and interruption of flow but with no impairment of overall bladder emptying, can be seen even in healthy infants during the first year of life (10–16). However, in children with neurogenic bladder, DSD manifests in a much more pronounced manner and together with pelvic floor overactivity may produce significant functional outflow obstruction, leading to elevated intravesical pressure, upper tract dilatation, high-pressure vesico-ureteral reflux (VUR), and incomplete bladder emptying. This obstruction, in turn, predisposes to recurrent UTI, and together, the adverse hydrodynamic factors and infections can cause substantial damage to the upper tract within a relatively short period of time. When bladder outlet resistance is chronically increased because of sphincteric dyssynergia, bladder compliance is likely to decrease as a result of detrusor overactivity and progressive collagen deposition, which can occur alone or in combination (17). This results in a small, contracted, poorly compliant bladder with contiguously elevated intravesical pressures during both filling and emptying. The decreased compliance not only may lead to increasing incontinence but also may produce a considerable degree of functional obstruction to upper tract drainage, and hence can be of crucial importance in the predisposition to renal functional impairment. Bladder emptying may be maintained by progressive compensatory detrusor hypertrophy and overactivity until the detrusor muscle becomes fatigued and bladder decompensation occurs. The bladder then loses its contractility, increases substantially in capacity, and fails to empty. Urinary retention occurs, and the resulting residual urine predisposes to recurrent infections if artificial emptying by clean intermittent catheterization (CIC) is not implemented. The combination of high intravesical pressures, VUR, and UTI allows transmission of both the elevated pressures and the pathogenic bacteria to the upper tract and heralds progressive renal deterioration.

Protection of kidney function in children with neurogenic bladder therefore depends on the successful maintenance of good bladder compliance to allow filling at a low pressure and satisfactory bladder emptying. Early urodynamic studies are necessary to identify babies who are at risk for upper tract deterioration as a result of functional intravesical obstruction from DSD or poor bladder compliance due to detrusor hypertonicity or often a combination of both.

## Sphincter and Pelvic Floor Inactivity

The main problem in patients with inactivity of the external sphincter and pelvic floor musculature is urinary incontinence. The amount and frequency of leakage are determined by the activity of the detrusor and the residual outlet resistance. If there is coexisting detrusor overactivity, then frequent leakage is expected with unstable detrusor contractions, resulting in a marked decrease in the functional bladder capacity. Alternatively, if sphincteric inactivity is combined with detrusor inactivity, then overflow urinary incontinence with continuous dribbling occurs. Because of the poor outlet resistance, urine leakage tends to appear in response to any detrusor contraction or elevation in intravesical pressure, thereby maintaining the pressure inside the bladder at a low level. Consequently, high-pressure VUR and recurrent UTI are not commonly seen and damage to the upper tracts is not an immediate hazard.

Management for external sphincteric inactivity in combination with detrusor inactivity should start with means to enhance regular and complete bladder emptying, usually by CIC (18). Frequently, this measure alone helps to substantially ameliorate the urinary incontinence problem to a more socially acceptable level, particularly if the bladder capacity is adequate. Manual expression of urine by suprapubic pressure (Credé's method) is not satisfactory because the bladder neck tends to be displaced caudally, resulting in kinking of the proximal urethra and incomplete bladder emptying. If complete dryness cannot be achieved by CIC alone, various surgical procedures to enhance the bladder outlet resistance, such as injection or formal reconstruction of the bladder neck, insertion of an artificial sphincter, bladder neck suspension, and so on, can be considered with or without concomitant bladder augmentation depending on whether the bladder capacity is sufficient.

Children with external sphincteric inactivity in combination with detrusor overactivity can be managed first with pharmacological manipulation, for example, anticholinergics, to reduce the unstable contractions. Again, commonly, this alone may lead to an increase in functional bladder capacity, in conjunction with a significant reduction in urinary leakage. Failing this, other measures to increase the bladder capacity, for example, bladder augmentation, may be necessary in combination with surgical procedures to enhance bladder outlet resistance after the child has acquired the proper techniques for CIC. The aim is to convert the bladder from a poorly compliant, small-capacity system to a more complaint system with adequate storage capacity and good outlet resistance.

## Neurogenic Bladder and Vesico-Ureteral Reflux

VUR occurs in approximately 30% of newborns with neurogenic bladders secondary to myelodysplasia (19). It has been noted that an elevation in intravesical pressures associated with neurogenic bladder magnifies the potential damage that may result from reflux by providing the hydrodynamic force needed to drive the pathogenic bacteria into the kidney parenchyma, thereby inducing pyelonephritis and renal scarring (20). Urodynamic studies have indicated that high pressures in decompensated bladders, especially in children with a combination of sphincter and detrusor overactivity, initiate and perpetuate the high-pressure reflux. It has been postulated that the high intravesical pressures may contribute to weakening of the detrusor musculature support at the ureterovesical junction, which is crucial for the normal antireflux mechanism. Inefficient bladder emptying with substantial postmicturition residuals also predisposes to recurrent UTI and further aggravates the damage to the upper tract (21). Steinhardt et al. (22) reported significant reduction in glomerular filtration rate occurring at high bladder pressures in myelodysplastic children.

It becomes clear, therefore, that VUR occurring in children with neurogenic bladder is largely secondary to the adverse urodynamic factors, rather than a primary event. Treatment should therefore be focused mainly on the underlying bladder dysfunction rather than on stopping the reflux.

## UROLOGICAL EVALUATION

A baseline renal and bladder ultrasound and radiographic voiding cystourethrogram are recommended shortly after birth. All infants should have a determination of postvoid residual (PVR) prior to discharge. Ultrasound (Table 1) is repeated every four months during the first two years of life, twice annually during the age of two to five years, every nine months between 5 and 10 years of age, and then on a yearly basis, but may be repeated earlier if recurrent UTI, hydronephrosis, or urinary incontinence develops. This test serves as a baseline as well as providing a regular indicator of the health of the upper tracts and state of the bladder. Less-frequent ultrasonography is reasonable if urodynamic findings suggest a low risk for renal deterioration. Because the risk of renal injury is the greatest and most devastating during the first two years of life, children in this age range are managed differently. It is pertinent to note that the neurological function of the bladder may silently change with time. This risk is, again, the greatest in younger children necessitating closer surveillance (Table 1) and greater emphasis on prophylaxis (Table 2).

Most children under two years of age should receive prophylactic antibiotics. Amoxicillin is administered until the child is over three to four months postconceptual age or greater than one month after resolution of hyperbilirubinemia, if present. Thereafter, suppression consists of either trimethoprim–sulfamethoxazole or Furadantin/Macrodantin (Table 2). Macrodantin capsules

**Table 1** Routine Imaging Surveillance at Cincinnati Children's Hospital Medical Center

| Age (yr) | Ultrasound | VCUG |
|---|---|---|
| 0–2 | q 4 mo | q 8 mo |
| 2–5 | q 6 mo | q 12 mo |
| 5–10 | q 9 mo | q 18 mo |
| >10 | q 12 mo | q 24 mo |

*Note*: Newborns with myelomeningocele receive a renal ultrasound and a radiographic voiding cystourethrography as soon as medically stable. All infants have a determination of postvoid residual prior to discharge. Because the risk of renal injury is the greatest and most devastating during the first two years of life, children in this age range are managed differently. It is pertinent to note that the neurological function of the bladder may silently change with time. This risk is, again, the greatest in younger children necessitating closer surveillance and greater emphasis on prophylaxis.

**Table 2** Suppressive Antibiotics

| Agent | Supplied | Dosage (po) |
|---|---|---|
| Amoxicillin | 125 mg/5 mL | 12.5 mg/kg/day |
| Trimethoprim–sulfamethoxazole | 40 mg/200 mg/5 mL, 80 mg/400 mg/tab | 2 mg/10 mg/kg/day |
| Nitrofurantoin/Macrodantin | 25 mg/5 mL, 25 mg/cap | 2 mg/kg/day |

may be opened and the crystalline contents sprinkled on the child's food to provide a very effective and palatable preparation. Recurrent high-risk infection not controlled by single or double prophylaxis may be treated with daily or alternative day intravesical gentamicin instillation under meticulous surveillance (Table 3).

The purpose of urodynamic testing in the newborn is to evaluate bladder pressures and identify bladders that put the upper tracts at risk for deterioration. Later studies are used to guide clinical management of urinary incontinence. The majority of children with myelodysplasia have urodynamic abnormalities that require close urological evaluation and follow-up. Approximately 6.5% to 12% of newborns will have abnormal urodynamic parameters (5,23,24).

Although some advocate expectant management with serial renal ultrasounds, others advocate initial urodynamic studies within the first one to two months of life. Urodynamic studies include a neurological evaluation of the perineal region, cystometrography, and external electromyography (EMG) of

**Table 3** Gentamicin Bladder Irrigation Protocol at Cincinnati Children's Hospital Medical Center

| Solution | 120 mg gentamicin in 250 mL normal saline |
|---|---|
| Dose | Treatment: 30 mL of gentamicin solution twice a day for 7 days<br>Maintenance: 30 mL of gentamicin solution at bedtime |
| Frequency | Daily/every other day/other |
| Duration | 3 mo/6 mo/other |
| Monitoring | All: baseline BUN/creatinine<br>Treatment therapy: BUN, creatinine, random gentamicin level after third dose and day 8<br>Maintenance therapy<br>High risk (patients with renal insufficiency, renal scarring, prior bladder augmentation): obtain BUN, creatinine, random gentamicin level twice/week for 2 wk, then once/week for 2 wk, then every 2 wk for duration of therapy<br>Low risk (all other patients): obtain BUN, creatinine, random gentamicin level once/week for 2 wk, then every 2 wk for 2 wk, then once/month for duration of therapy |

the pelvic diaphragm. Urodynamic findings in children with myelomeningocele include uninhibited bladder contractions, bladder areflexia, decreased compliance, and DSD. Fluorourodynamics allow simultaneous voiding cystourethrography, which otherwise should be performed to rule out reflux. Recently, urodynamic studies of children undergoing neural tube repair at approximately 27 weeks of gestation were compared with those of children undergoing repair in the neonatal period. No difference was found the incidence of uninhibited bladder contractions, hypotonia or bladder compliance (25). It is unclear whether early intervention will affect long-term continence.

Cystometrography is performed with a 5 to 7 Fr. dual lumen catheter inserted transurethrally into the bladder. Normal saline is infused into the bladder at a rate approximating 10% of expected bladder volume per minute. Total intravesical and detrusor pressures are differentiated by subtracting abdominal pressure obtained by means of rectal balloon. Detrusor pressure is monitored during the filling phase, with simultaneous documentation of EMG activity of the external urethral sphincter. Parameters assessed during urodynamics include bladder capacity, compliance, detrusor contractility, and maximum bladder capacity with leak point pressure. The functional or safe bladder capacity is defined as the volume of liquid held at pressures below 40 cm $H_2O$. Likewise, a dangerous leak point pressure for children who empty spontaneously is greater than 40 cm $H_2O$. This is based on classic studies by McGuire (26), who showed that upper tract deterioration was unlikely if pressures were kept below this level most of the time.

The goal of urological care is to prevent urinary tract deterioration and to promote urinary continence at the appropriate age. Intervention may include a combination of anticholinergic medication and CIC, as well as surgical procedures to increase or decrease bladder outlet resistance and increase bladder compliance. The mechanisms of urinary incontinence are diverse and include overflow evacuation caused by detrusor instability and a nonrefluxing sphincter, limited storage capacity caused by hyper-reflexia and poor compliance, and low urethral resistance from sphincter denervation (27).

## NONSURGICAL MANAGEMENT IN NEUROGENIC BLADDER WITH SPINA BIFIDA

### Introduction

A few decades ago, urinary diversion, usually with an ileal conduit, was the ultimate outcome for most children with spina bifida. The revolutionary institution of CIC has changed the algorithm totally. Furthermore, many new drugs have been developed during the past decade and have decreased the need for surgery.

The outcome of the upper urinary tract is related to the combination of the detrusor and sphincteric function. Hyper-reflexic detrusor has a detrimental effect on the upper urinary tract only when the sphincter fails to relax simultaneously, a situation called DSD as described earlier. When the sphincter is weak or areflexic, the kidneys are protected, but in this situation urinary incontinence becomes a problem. On the basis of these basic concepts, the objectives of therapy for neurogenic bladder dysfunction are well defined: protecting the kidneys from progressive damage by reducing the intravesical pressure during both filling and emptying, and improving the quality of life by providing urinary continence. Therapy is individualized, e.g., to reduce high intravesical pressure in a patient with detrusor hyper-reflexia or CIC in a child who cannot empty his/her bladder adequately. CIC and oral pharmacological agents are the first-line treatment in most patients with bladder dysfunction and urinary incontinence regardless of the etiology. The early institution of therapy seems very beneficial. Highly selected patients may also benefit from new forms of anticholinergic agents as well as biofeedback. Surgical therapy should be reserved for cases that are totally unresponsive to conservative therapies.

## Initiation of Clean Intermittent Catheterization in Infants with Myelodysplasia

It is well known in spinal cord injuries that there is a spinal-shock period that lasts typically 6 to 12 weeks, characterized by an areflexic bladder and urinary retention. After this, the detrusor may be hyper-reflexic or areflexic, and coordination or dyssynergia with the urethral sphincter occurs depending on the level of spinal cord injury. It is likely that closure of the neural tube defect causes spinal shock, as in children with myelomeningocele. Baskin et al. (28) found five out of 35 patients in whom an areflexic bladder matured to a hyper-reflexic bladder over the first few months of life. In a more recent study, Stoneking et al. (29) confirmed this finding. In a retrospective analysis of 54 children who underwent myelomeningocele repair, nearly all patients required CIC for urinary retention after surgery (29). In 74%, this lasted less than two weeks, but in 26% the effect was seen for up to six weeks after surgery (29). Baskin et al. (28) obtained excellent results in preventing upper urinary tract changes with an aggressive program of anticholinergic agents combined with CIC. In contrast, after the period of spinal shock, Stoneking et al. (29) observed their patients and ultimately 38% of children needed CIC or vesicostomy before toilet training. This suggests that preventive institution of therapy could be beneficial. In a retrospective analysis of 46 children treated before or after one year of age, Wu et al. (30) reported confirmatory results. There was a significantly lower rate of bladder augmentation in the group treated early. In addition, the early institution of CIC also seems to have psychological benefits, with an apparent improvement in family compliance and the ability to assist the child in coping with their disease and with CIC. In a similar comparison of prophylactic treatment to observation in a high-risk group of 45 patients with myelodysplasia, the group treated early again had a decreased rate of augmentation cystoplasty (17% vs. 41%) and improved bladder function (31). These data suggest a beneficial effect of early evaluation and therapy, especially in high-risk groups. Initial evaluation should include renal/bladder ultrasound and urodynamic study. The urodynamic study is crucial because the intravesical pressure and the coordination of the detrusor with the external sphincter are good predictors of future renal and bladder function (32). If sophisticated urodynamic studies are not possible, a relatively simple leak point pressure has been shown to be predictive of upper tract outcome (26). A leak point pressure higher than 40 cm $H_2O$ will result in a high rate of upper tract changes. Both anticholinergic therapy and CIC should be instituted in this group in order to avoid damage secondary to high intravesical pressures.

## Clean Intermittent Catheterization

Thirty years of worldwide experience has made CIC the primary choice for bladder emptying in the treatment of children with neurogenic bladder dysfunction. Although there are some concerns about the risk of infection and patient/family compliance, CIC remains the best method to empty areflexic bladders with maximum efficacy and minimal side effects. In a recent study of the risks of infection, two techniques of intermittent catheterization were compared in patients with myelomeningocele (33). One group of patients used new sterile catheters for each catheterization and were compared to the other group who used a reusable clean catheter for each catheterization. Both groups were followed for four months and the results showed that bacteriuria was present in almost 75% of patients, but there was no difference in its frequency with either regimen. Only two symptomatic UTIs were seen in each group in a total of 158 urine samples. These data show that the use of sterile catheters is an unnecessary expense for most patients and confirm that CIC with a reusable catheter is an excellent method of bladder emptying in this patient group.

Stagnated urine that results from bladder hypotonia, elevated sphincteric pressure, or DSD is a frequent finding in children with a neurogenic bladder. The result is recurrent UTI and potential renal damage. Differentiating UTI from colonization in an asymptomatic patient with a neurogenic bladder is quite difficult. Children with positive urine cultures are not actively treated with antimicrobial therapy in the absence of symptoms. The following symptoms may or may not be present: temperature higher than 38°C, pyuria ($>10$ white blood cell count/high power field), bacteriuria greater than $10^5$ colony-forming units, unusually cloudy urine, abdominal pain, emesis, malodorous urine, diarrhea, or more frequent incontinence. Szucs et al. (34) examined the urine in asymptomatic children with spina bifida managed with CIC. The findings suggest that asymptomatic patients with spina bifida who have bacteriuria and elevated interleukin-8 levels have a true infection rather than colonization.

## Anticholinergic Therapy

Patients with an areflexic detrusor and a high PVR urine are the best candidates for CIC therapy. Patients with hyper-reflexic detrusor require conversion to a lower pressure detrusor. Although this can be performed surgically, the preference is to do this by nonoperative means whenever possible.

Oxybutynin chloride is a well-known anticholinergic and antispasmodic agent. Its efficacy on clinical and urodynamic parameters has been documented in infants and neonates (28,35). In a study of 41 children with myelomeningocele and detrusor hyper-reflexia (36), who were evaluated urodynamically before and within three months after the initiation of combined therapy, oxybutynin significantly increased the maximal bladder capacity and decreased the detrusor pressure at maximal capacity. Continence was improved also in 70% of children over six years of age who were incontinent before therapy.

The major problem with oxybutynin is the high rate of side effects. Dry mouth, constipation, and heat intolerance may be seen in almost one-third of patients and are the main reason for dropout. Because of the pharmacokinetics of the drug, oxybutynin should be administered three to four times a day, which results in reduced patient compliance. To overcome this problem, a slow-release form of the drug has been developed. Studies in adults have demonstrated the same success rate with better tolerability with the slow-release formulation (37), and Youdim et al. (38) studied retrospectively the efficacy and safety of the extended-release oxybutynin in children with bladder dysfunction (neurogenic or urge incontinence without neurological abnormalities). They confirmed that treatment with extended-release oxybutynin was effective and well tolerated. This formulation is suggested for any children who require anticholinergic medications and can swallow a pill.

Another promising drug is tolterodine tartrate. Like oxybutynin, it is a muscarinic receptor antagonist, and its efficacy in treating the overactive bladder has been demonstrated in adults (39). Compared with oxybutynin, its selectivity for the bladder is similar, but it is eight times less potent at the antimuscarinic receptor in the parotid gland (40–42), suggesting that it will cause less dry mouth. In a study of 22 children (0.1 mg/kg) with detrusor hyper-reflexia (21 myelomeningocele and one spinal cord trauma), Goessl et al. (43) used tolterodine as either a replacement therapy for oxybutynin or an initial therapy (43). Tolterodine was found to be equal to oxybutynin in efficacy and had fewer adverse effects in the group that had previously been treated with oxybutynin. Although not directly applicable to patients with neurogenic dysfunction, in a study of 33 children with overactive bladder (urgency, frequency, and urge incontinence), different dosages of oral tolterodine demonstrated linear pharmacokinetics and excellent efficacy in decreasing voiding frequencies and incontinence episodes (44). Only two patients discontinued the treatment because of adverse effects. A new form of extended-release tolterodine has been introduced recently. It should have equal efficacy and fewer side effects.

### Intravesical Agents

Another alternative to reduce side effects is the intravesical administration of oxybutynin. Many different preparations have been described, and there are therefore many discrepancies in results, particularly patient compliance (45). One popular method consists of the dissolution of a 5 mg tablet of oxybutynin chloride in 30 mL sterile saline and the instillation of this suspension into the bladder via a catheter. The daily dosage and frequency of intravesical instillation remain controversial, but most authors recommend using the medication three times a day. It has been demonstrated that intravesical oxybutynin chloride is absorbed rapidly, and greater serum levels are obtained than after oral administration (46). In a study that compared the side effects, Ferrara et al. (47) demonstrated that intravesical administration was safer and better tolerated than oral oxybutynin chloride. However, out of 34 children, six still had side effects such as drowsiness, hallucinations, and cognitive changes. In contrast, out of 67 children who underwent treatment with oral oxybutynin, 11 discontinued the therapy because of side effects. Di Stasi et al. (48,49) looked at the plasma levels of oxybutynin and its metabolic *N*-desetyl oxybutynin after oral administration, intravesical instillation (passive diffusion), and intravesical instillation combined with electric current (electromotive administration). The authors found that electromotive administration increased the intravesical uptake of the oxybutynin, resulting in an improvement in urodynamic parameters compared with oral administration or passive diffusion. They concluded that some part of the intravesical oxybutynin (3 of 15 mg in their study) must be sequestered in the urothelium during intravesical instillation, and electric current might be useful for refractory cases.

Another new medication that has been shown to be effective in the treatment of patients with overactive bladder is resiniferatoxin. It acts via desensitization of unmyelinated C fibers (afferent nerves of the bladder). Whether this mechanism of action will be effective in patients with spina bifida is questionable. There is a single case report in the literature on the use of resiniferatoxin in a child with myelomeningocele (50). A nine-year-old boy with low bladder compliance and grade II bilateral VUR failed both oral and intravesical oxybutynin. Resiniferatoxin was tried intravesically. Three months after one instillation, the boy was without evidence of reflux and had improved bladder complacence. Because the results in adults with overactive bladder are promising, this medication has significant potential for use in children with spina bifida, but many more studies are needed to determine the efficacy and safety of the drug in this population.

## Intravesical Injection Therapy

Since the 1980s, botulinum-A toxin (BTX) has been used for the treatment of various conditions such as strabismus, dystonia, and spasticity and other disorders that cause inappropriate striated muscle contraction. It is a selective blocker of acetylcholine release at the neuromuscular junction. In urology, it was first studied in adult patients with spinal cord lesions that resulted in either DSD (51) or detrusor hyper-reflexia (52,53). Promising results in temporarily paralyzing the sphincter in the adult population have led the investigators to study the efficacy of BTX in the bladders of children with high intravesical pressure. In a prospective study of a highly selected group (54,55), BTX was injected under anesthesia at 30 to 40 sites into the bladder wall of 17 children. All had intravesical pressures greater than 40 cm $H_2O$, despite a high dosage of anticholinergic medication. A repeat urodynamic study two to four weeks after the injection showed a significant increase in maximal bladder capacity and detrusor compliance. Although there was a decrease in incontinence episodes, this difference was not statistically significant. No side effect was noted except one child who showed increased PVR urine.

### Biofeedback

Biofeedback therapy is an alternative treatment to CIC and anticholinergic agents for children who have voiding dysfunction and are unable to relax their pelvic floor during voiding (56,57). The basic technique involves learning to contract and relax the pelvic floor muscles using visual and auditory monitors of electromyographic activity. This technique is very labor-intensive, and motivation and patient cooperation are very important for successful treatment. A recent study suggested combining a noninvasive urodynamic method with various psychological techniques (such as externalizing the problem, empowerment, and homework), to overcome the difficulties with conventional treatment (58). A total of 77 children with DSD were treated, and after a relatively short follow-up period (mean of 8.6 months), 61% had improvement in both urinary symptoms and urodynamic parameters. Experience in myelomeningocele patients is very limited. Only one out of six girls with spina bifida has improvement after biofeedback, probably because there were so few healthy nerves remaining. It appears that biofeedback has great potential in children with nonneurological voiding dysfunction, but limited efficacy in children with myelomeningocele.

## SURGICAL MANAGEMENT IN NEUROGENIC BLADDER WITH SPINA BIFIDA

### Introduction

Reconstruction of the urinary tract in children with myelomeningocele continues to evolve. The main problems facing the pediatric urologists relate to preservation of the anatomical and functional integrity of the kidneys and the achievement of urinary continence.

Surgery for neurogenic bladder can be done to promote safe bladder pressures, urinary continence, or both. Goals related to urinary continence include creating a high-volume, low-pressure bladder and obtaining adequate outlet resistance. Preoperative evaluation includes urodynamic testing, laboratory studies, and radiographic studies to assess for bladder compliance, bladder outlet resistance, existing bladder capacity, electrolyte abnormalities, renal impairment, and anatomic abnormalities of the upper and lower urinary tract (59–61). The family and child should be assessed for the ability to comply with CIC if they are required to continue this procedure in the postoperative period.

### Reducing Leak Point Pressure

In the infant with high intravesical pressure and upper tract changes, initial management is anticholinergic medication and intermittent catheterization. When this fails, surgical approaches may be considered. Although bladder pressures can be decreased through the use of bladder augmentation, most would consider this treatment to be overly aggressive for infants and young children. The focus is generally on decreasing the leak point pressure, which can be accomplished by creating an alternate exit route for urine (vesicostomy) or by decreasing the resistance at the level of sphincters (urethral dilation).

### Vesicostomy

This procedure involves exteriorizing a portion of the native bladder to the skin, forming a direct urinary conduit. A retrospective study identified 23 patients with myelodysplasia who had undergone cutaneous vesicostomies for various reasons: hydronephrosis, recurrent UTI, developmental delay, VUR, and failure to perform intermittent catheterization. Hydronephrosis resolved in 100% of patients. Although surgical reconstruction of the urinary tract is the preferred method for treating elevated intravesical bladder pressures and preserving renal function after failure of medical therapy, temporary vesicostomy diversion is a successful technique to prevent recurrent UTI and preserve renal function in selected patients (62).

### Urethral Dilation

The use of external urethral sphincter dilation for the management of patients with myelodysplasia who have elevated leak point pressures and/or poor bladder compliance has been in practice for more than 30 years. A recent retrospective review of 25 patients who underwent this procedure demonstrated that this method improved urodynamic parameters and prevented upper urinary tract damage in a selected group of patients (27). The authors found that patients with significantly abnormal urodynamic parameters and uninhibited detrusor contractions were less likely to respond to this treatment.

### Bladder Augmentation

Surgical enlargement of the urinary bladder continues to be the mainstay of reconstruction for those children with reduced functional bladder capacity and compliance who do not respond to pharmacological manipulation (Table 4). The bladder is augmented to improve its function as a low-pressure reservoir

**Table 4** Bladder Augmentation

| Augmentation type | Advantages | Disadvantages | Applications |
| --- | --- | --- | --- |
| None | Lowest risk of complication | Renal injury if bladder noncompliant | Whenever possible |
| Autoaugmentation | No metabolic consequences<br>May be performed extra-peritoneally | Augmentation surface not amenable to ureteral/MNU implant<br>Risk of perforation<br>Limited clinical experience | Sufficient native bladder surface for implant<br>Near-normal bladder capacity |
| Ureterocystoplasty | No metabolic consequences<br>May be performed extra-peritoneally | Augmentation surface not amenable to ureteral/MNU implant<br>Requires presence of a large dilated ureter | Sufficient native bladder surface for implant |
| Seromuscular augment | No metabolic consequences | Augmentation surface less amenable to ureteral/MNU implant<br>Long-term compliance benefits questionable | Sufficient native bladder surface for implant<br>Near-normal bladder capacity |
| Ileocystoplasty | Technically simple | Augmentation surface less amenable to ureteral/MNU implant<br>Acidosis/mucous/stone<br>Infection | Sufficient native bladder surface for implant<br>Stomach unavailable |
| Colocystoplasty | Ureteral/MNU implant possible<br>Technically simple | Acidosis/mucous/stone<br>Infection | Stomach unavailable |
| Gastrocystoplasty | Avoids acidosis/mucous/stone (infection)<br>Ureteral/MNU implant readily performed | Hematuria/dysuria<br>Rare alkalosis | Wide application |

in an attempt to achieve continence or protect the kidneys. In the modern management, the incidence of endstage renal disease is rare in myelodysplastic children.

Preoperative urodynamic studies are mandatory before surgery to correct urinary incontinence is undertaken. Not only is it imperative to assess bladder capacity and compliance but also to evaluate the bladder outlet. Augmentation alone will not provide continence if the outlet resistance is low. In our practice, the choice of intestinal segments is individualized according to their renal function or concomitant procedures.

## Autoaugmentation

Snow et al. (63) described an alternative approach to gastrointestinal (GI) augmentation that involved excision and blunt dissection of the detrusor muscle from the underlying mucosa (Fig. 1). A large bladder diverticulum that

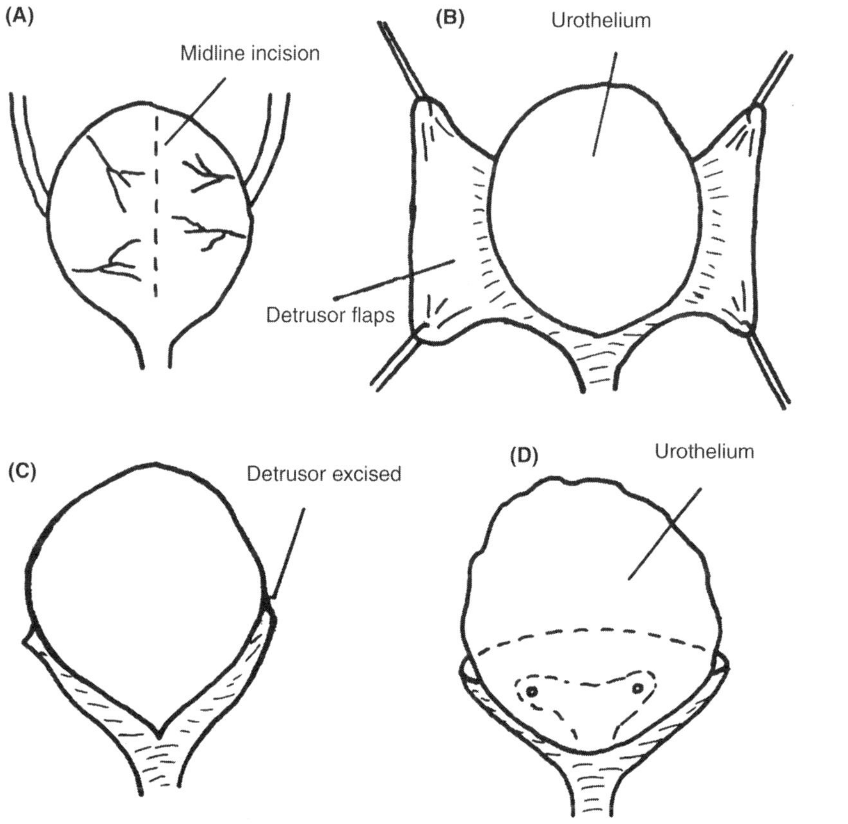


**Figure 1** Autoaugmentation. (**A** and **B**) The bladder is incised in the midline. (**C** and **D**) The detrusor musculature is excised, leaving the mucosa protruding as a wide-mouthed diverticulum.

improves compliance and decreases intravesical pressures is created (64,65). In this approach, the entire procedure can be performed extraperitoneally. Eliminating the use of intestinal segments avoids the risk of bowel obstruction, metabolic complications, and mucus production and decreases the risk of malignancy, stone formation, and UTI. This procedure does not increase bladder capacity to the extent of an intestinal augmentation, and therefore the ideal patient should have a reasonable bladder capacity with a poorly compliant bladder. Preliminary long-term results in a small series of patients demonstrated poor outcomes in 7 of 11 patients, who required a second procedure with enterocystoplasty (66). Careful evaluation of the appropriate candidate is necessary to ensure success with autoaugmentation.

### Ureterocystoplasty

The procedure involves taking a massively dilated ureter, incising it vertically, and attaching it to the bladder to form a spherical container (Fig. 2) (67). This results in increased bladder capacity and improved continence (68). Unfortunately, this technique is limited to a selected group of patients who have a large hydroureter and a nonfunctioning kidney. Given the early institution of anticholinergics and CIC in most myelodysplastic patients, this scenario is not often encountered. The benefits of using native urothelium in both autoaugmentation and ureterocystoplasty include the lack of mucus production that minimizes the risk of forming stones and developing infections, decreased rates of malignant transformation, and reduced metabolic complications compared with GI augmentations (68).

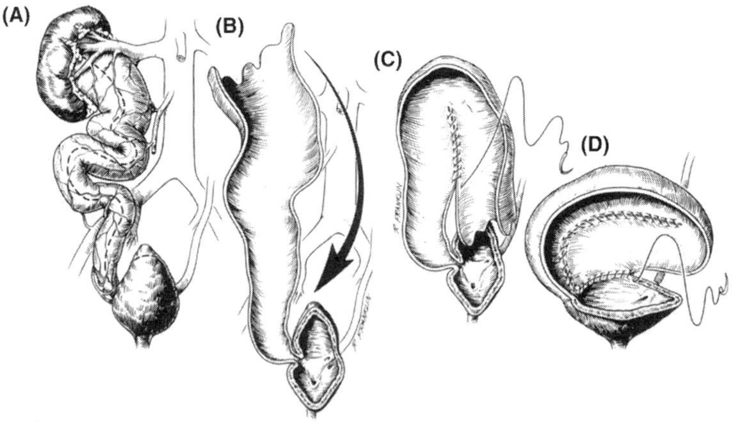


**Figure 2** Ureterocystoplasty. (**A**) Incision for detubularization of dilated ureter and pelvis and for bivalving of native bladder for ureteral cystoplasty. (**B**) The nonfunctioning kidney is removed and the ureteral blood supply is preserved. (**C** and **D**) The ureter remains attached to the bladder and is configured into a U-shaped patch that is anastomosed to the bladder.

## Enterocystoplasty

The most common form of bladder augmentation uses a segment of the GI tract as a patch on the bladder. Ileum, sigmoid, cecum, and stomach have all been used. Jejunum is avoided because of the high likelihood of metabolic consequences (69,70). As part of the procedure, the native bladder must be bivalved aggressively or incised in a stellate pattern to avoid creating a large bladder diverticulum following placement of the intestinal segment on the bladder (71). In general, a 15 to 25 cm segment of ileum or colon is isolated, detubularized, and reconfigured into a U, S, or W shape and sewn onto the bivalved native bladder, creating a spherical reservoir (72–74).

## Ileocystoplasty

The most common type of augmentation performed is ileocystoplasty (Fig. 3). This procedure involves isolation of ileum at least 10 to 15 cm proximal to the ileocecal valve to preserve the function of the distal terminal ileum (bile salt reabsorption and production of vitamin B12). As described previously, the segment of ileum is detubularized, reconfigured into a U, S, or W shape, and sewn to the bivalved bladder, forming a spherical-shaped reservoir. One disadvantage of

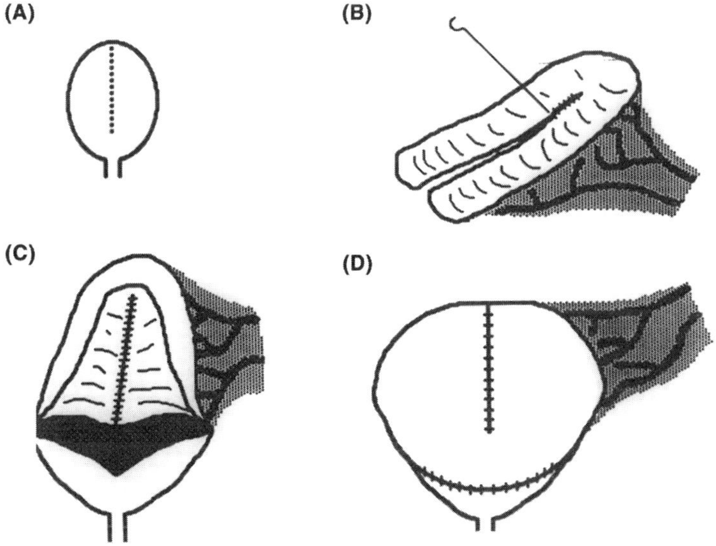


**Figure 3** Ileocystoplasty. (**A**) The native bladder is bivalved. (**B**) The detubularized segment is folded and anastomosed to form a U-shaped flap. The reconfiguration can be done in a U, S, or W-type fashion or folded as a cup patch. (**C** and **D**) The U-shaped flap is anastomosed to the bivalved bladder beginning in the midline posteriorly.

this approach is that the longer distance from the ileal segment to the bladder may rarely result in tension on the bladder anastomosis (61).

## Sigmoid Cystoplasty

The approach and technical aspects of this procedure are similar to those for ileocystoplasty. The sigmoid colon is often large, redundant, and in close approximation to the bladder, making it an excellent segment for augmentation. The position of the sigmoid facilitates the anastomosis to the bladder; however, higher rates of mucus production and higher enteric contraction rates have been reported (61).

## Gastrocystoplasty

In patients with renal insufficiency, short gut syndrome, or irradiated bowel, the use of the stomach is a preferred alternative for augmentation (75). A wedge-shaped piece of stomach is isolated and its blood supply is preserved; it is mobilized through the transverse colon mesentery and sewn to the bladder (Fig. 4) (76). This alternative has several advantages. (*i*) The stomach lacks the ability to absorb hydrogen ion and therefore will not cause metabolic acidosis. (*ii*) The gastric mucosa is deficient in mucous-secreting glands. The absence of mucous, the predominant nidus of stone formation in augmented bladder, coupled with the ability of the stomach to secrete acid, a natural inhibitor of bacterial colonization, almost eliminates the risk of stone formation.

Although some metabolic abnormalities associated with gastrocystoplasty, including hypochloremic metabolic alkalosis are reported (77), in our practice,

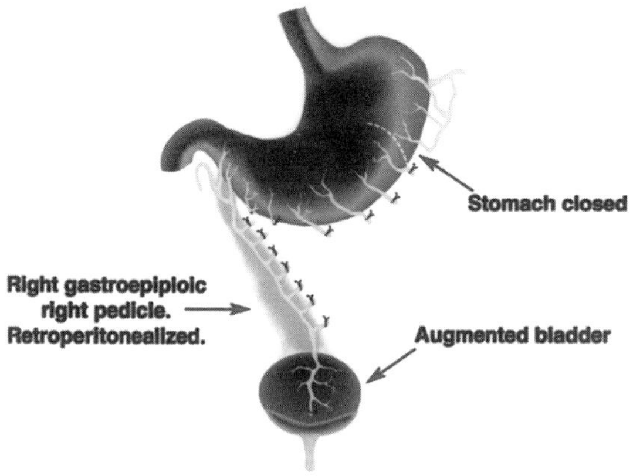


**Figure 4** Gastrocystoplasty. Rhomboid-shaped stomach wedge is resected from the greater curvature. The right gastroepiploic artery is used as the vascular pedicle and is ligated distal to the wedge so that the segment can be easily placed into the pelvis. The gastric wedge is then anastomosed to the bladder.

the metabolic alkalosis has never been encountered. Another potential consequence is the hematuria–dysuria syndrome, which might occur in up to one-third of the patients undergoing a gastric augmentation, but its exact etiology is unknown.

At Cincinnati Children's Hospital Medical Center, a retrospective cohort study was conducted in children who underwent gastrocystoplasty with inclusion criteria of more than five years of follow-up. Of 44 children identified for this study, 39 patients (89%) were continent of urine. No patient had chronic metabolic alkalosis. Two children had severe hematuria while anuric from renal failure, which was managed conservatively with bladder cycling and $H_2$ blockers. Symptoms resolved completely after renal transplantation in both cases (78,79). A significant increase in the incidence of hematuria–dysuria syndrome was reported in patients with a sensate urethra compared with those with an insensate urethra (80). Most of our patients with this syndrome have a sensate urethra as well. Therefore, our current practice is to not use gastrocystoplasty in sensate patients with an open bladder neck without performing concomitant bladder neck reconstruction. Despite negative reports concerning serious complications of gastrocystoplasty, our long-term data confirm that it remains an important option in our reconstruction armamentarium, specifically in severely compromised children such as those with chronic renal insufficiency, metabolic acidosis, or deficient bowel segments suitable for reconstruction (81).

### Autoaugmentation Combined with Demucosalized Bowel or Stomach

GI cystoplasty has potential complications and therefore a procedure that uses the advantages of autoaugmentation and GI segments was developed. Seromuscular colocystoplasty lined with urothelium involves excising the detrusor muscle from the underlying urothelium and veering it with a demucosalized segment of bowel (82). Early results demonstrated that this technique could be a reasonable alternative in a selected group of patients (83). Postoperatively, a 2.4-fold increase in bladder capacity was seen as well as a significant decrease in bladder end-filling pressures. No significant complications were reported, and 81% of the patients were continent. The use of demucosalized stomach was also studied by several groups, with less favorable outcomes (84,85). On long-term follow-up, some reports have shown continent rates of <50%, with 33% requiring an additional augmentation with an intestinal segment (86).

## Complications of Bladder Augmentation

Surgical complications of bladder augmentation might include bowel obstruction, bladder perforation, urinary leakage, and continued urinary incontinence requiring further procedures. Bowel obstruction either in the immediate postoperative period from poor technique or in the long term from adhesion carries a significant risk of up to 10% in a large series (87). Other side effects of enterocystoplasty might include stone formation, mucus production, metabolic derangements, malabsorption, and bladder tumors.

When intestinal segments are interposed into the urinary tract, metabolic and electrolyte disturbances can occur. The type and severity of abnormalities depend on the type of segment used (Table 4), the amount of surface area in contact with urine, and the renal function of the patient. The use of ileum or colon usually produces a hypokalemic, hyperchloremic metabolic acidosis (69,70). To compensate for the increased acid load, the body uses bone buffers, which can lead to bone demineralization. If a significant part of the distal ileum is used, a vitamin B12 deficiency can occur because it is absorbed into the distal ileum (88). The use of a gastric segment for urinary tract reconstruction can produce a hypokalemic, hypochloremic metabolic alkalosis. In this situation, the stomach secretes acid and potassium is lost in the gastric secretions (89,90). It must be remembered that the net acid-secreting properties of the stomach deserve special attention because they can promote resolution of metabolic acidosis in patients with endstage renal disease and may obviate the use of bicarbonate supplementation (90).

Intestinal segments continue their physiological roles when placed into the urinary tract. As a result, electrolytes are absorbed through active and passive transport mechanisms and mucus is secreted. The sigmoid produces the most mucus followed by ileum and then stomach. Patients who empty their bladder through catheterization may have difficulty in emptying their bladders. Irrigation of the bladder is recommended at least three times daily in the immediate postoperative period and once daily indefinitely. Mucus can also act as a nidus for stone formation (61).

The most severe complication that can occur following enterocystoplasty is perforation. This is a potentially life-threatening catastrophe if not diagnosed and treated promptly (91,92). One potential explanation is that chronic overdistention of the augmented bladder resulting from poor adherence to a strict catheterization schedule causes ischemia of the bowel or bladder wall and increases the risk of perforation (93,94). Other explanations suggest that detrusor hyper-reflexia can generate high intravesical pressures, leading to ischemic changes (95). Traumatic catheterization has also been a proposed mechanism. The signs and symptoms include abdominal distension, abdominal pain, fever, nausea, and emesis. Most children with myelodysplasia have impaired sensation, and therefore our index of suspicion must be high. A computed tomography cystogram is the best test to evaluate these patients for bladder perforation because a plain cystogram has an unacceptable false-negative rate (96). We conducted a retrospective review to examine the incidence of, and risk factors for, spontaneous perforation (92). One hundred and seven children (57 males and 50 females) were identified who underwent augmentation cystoplasty at our institution. The etiology for bladder dysfunction included myelomeningocele, VATER syndrome, bladder and cloacal extrophy, posterior urethral valves, and pelvic malignancy. Gastrocystoplasty was performed in 50 children (47%), ileocystoplasty in 37 (35%), colocystoplasty in 18 (17%), and gastric-ileal composite neobladder in 2 (2%). The overall incidence of bladder perforation was 5% (four patients presented with five bladder perforations), whereas a reported incidence of spontaneous bladder perforation is up to 13% (87). Although one was the direct result of blunt abdominal trauma, four spontaneous perforations occurred in three patients, for a spontaneous perforation rate of 4% in our series. All four spontaneous perforations occurred in patients with ileocystoplasty. All patients recovered uneventfully after exploratory laparotomy. We believe that the relatively low incidence of spontaneous bladder perforation encountered at our institution may be explained by the large number of patients with gastrocystoplasty, as well as our strict adherence to a postoperative incremental catheterization program (Table 5). In most of our patients, we implement this strict postoperative catheterization regiment that allows gradual distention of the augmented bladder. Only one patient in this group developed a perforation. In addition, we used a two-layer watertight anastomotic technique for bladder closure that may have helped to reduce the number of early perforations that have been reported to occur at the bladder–bowel anastomosis (94,97).

A rare yet life-threatening complication is the formation of a tumor in an augmented bladder. The majority of reported cases of postaugmentation malignancy has occurred in adults with multiple risk factors (98–106). Augmentation cystoplasty has only gained popularity in pediatric urology within the last 25 years, limiting the population being studied by statistical power and the lack of long-term follow-up regarding the incidence as well as risk factors of cancer associated with augmentation cystoplasty. Currently, the most common indication for augmentation cystoplasty in children and adolescents is neurogenic bladder. Soergel et al. (107) reported three cases of transitional cell carcinoma (TCC) of the bladder discovered 20 years after bladder augmentation without any of the routinely recognized risk factors for the development of TCC. Each of the individuals underwent enterocystoplasty for neurogenic bladder during

**Table 5** Postoperative Incremental Catheterization Regimen

| |
|---|
| A cystostomy tube and urethral or Mitrofanoff catheters are left indwelling for 4–6 wks after reconstruction |
| Endoscopic of Mitrofanoff performed to determine course of catheter passage and catheter size, and Mitrofanoff catheter removed |
| Patient admitted (23 hrs observation) for catheterization training; temporary cystostomy tube clamped to allow bladder filling |
| Patient discharged with instructions to use an every 2 hrs catheterization schedule during the day; cystostomy tube clamped during the day and connected to drainage overnight |
| Catheterization interval increased every 2–3 wk, to every 3 hrs, and then every 4 hrs; cystostomy tube disconnected when interval is every 3–4 hrs, and catheterization is continued through the night |
| Decision to discontinue overnight catheterization made on an individual patient basis |

the childhood or adolescence. The authors hypothesize that bladder augmentation appears to be an independent risk factor for TCC, with a lag time of less than 20 years. Therefore, it is strongly recommended that endoscopic surveillance of all patients with a history of bladder augmentation be performed routinely beginning 10 years after initial surgery.

Development of bladder calculi has been reported as the most common complication of enterocystoplasty (97). Stones are a difficult management problem because injury to the bowel and bladder can occur with endoscopic lithotripsy. Larger stones have generally been removed by an open operation, but more recently, a percutaneous technique has been shown to be as effective as open surgery, with the potential for outpatient management (108). The cause appears to be multifactorial, with persistent bacteriuria, mucus production, and urinary stasis playing roles. Patients with continent stomas tend to have a higher rate of stones, probably as a result of inadequate emptying with catheterization.

Chronic bacteriuria is a common finding after an intestinal augmentation. There is no statistically significant difference in the rate of UTI among the various segments used (109).

### Laminectomy and Microanastomosis of Lumbar to Sacral Ventral Root

For the first time, Xiao et al. (110) reported a surgical approach in myelodysplastic children reversing some neurological deficits. Twenty children with myelomeningocele underwent limited laminectomy and microanastomosis of a lumbar ventral root (L5) to sacral ventral root (S3). Sixteen of the 20 children gained satisfactory bladder control as well as continence within one year. In 13 of the 16 patients with areflexic bladder, average bladder capacity increased from 72 to 210 mL. Three quarters patients with hyper-reflexic bladder and DSD reverted to normal storage and synergic voiding. Average residual urine decreased from 282 to 38 mL. Four out of the 20 children showed no improvement. This surgical approach needs further collaboration with other institutions before it can be accepted a standard therapy.

## SURGICAL THERAPY FOR BLADDER OUTLET INCOMPETENCE

### Introduction

In addition to problems with bladder storage, urinary incontinence in children with myelomeningocele may occur as a result of an inadequate sphincteric mechanism. When urinary incontinence is primarily a result of low bladder outlet resistance, several procedures have been developed to manage this problem. Commonly performed procedures include the Young–Dees–Leadbetter (YDL), Kropp, Pippi–Salle, fascial urethral slings, injectable agents, and artificial urethral sphincter.

## Surgical Techniques

### Injectable Agents

Bulking agents are injected around the bladder neck and urethra to increase bladder outlet resistance in children with myelodysplasia. Different agents are used with varying results. There include Teflon, collagen, and more recently, dextranomer/hyaluronic acid polymer (111,112). Initially, Teflon® was used but recently its use was discontinued related to distal migration of particles and formation of granulomas at distant sites (113). Following its initial success in women with intrinsic sphincter deficiency, collagen use was attempted in children. Early reports were promising, with success rates of 76% (114). However, recent series have demonstrated unsatisfactory continence rates (111,112,115). Repeated injections are often required approximately every three months. Although a minimally morbid procedure, with few if any complications, endoscopic injections have a limited role in treating urinary incontinence from an incomplete bladder outlet with the exception being injection following bladder outlet reconstruction for residual incontinence.

### Artificial Urinary Sphincter

The advent of an artificial urinary sphincter by Scott et al. (116–121) in 1973 provided a reliable means of achieving continence with a single operation, with no need for self-catheterization. A device is composed of an inflatable cuff, balloon reservoir, and pump mechanism for the treatment of urinary incontinence (Fig. 5). The cuff is placed around the bladder neck in children. The pump is inserted into the scrotum in males and into the labia majora in females. This procedure is

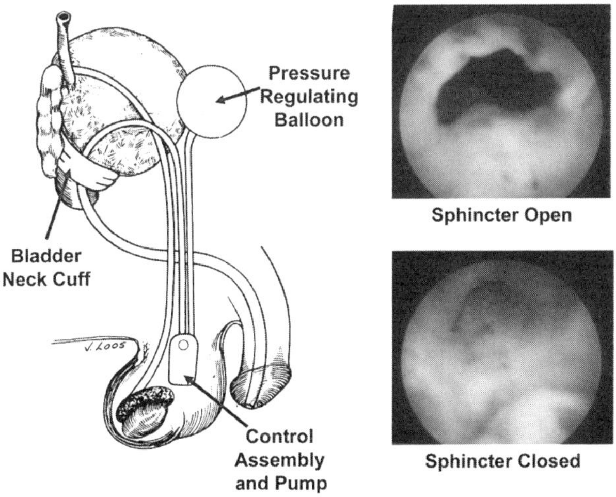


**Figure 5** An example of an artificial urinary sphincter and the endoscopic appearance after implantation.

recommended for myelodysplastic children with outlet incompetence and a large capacity, highly compliant bladder, who void spontaneously. Thus, it is best suited for those individuals with good manual dexterity who can empty their bladder just using Valsalva voiding. The sphincter has undergone several revisions since its original description in 1973, and continence rates are now reported to be 80% to 97% (122–126). This artificial urethral sphincter has been shown to be effective when used concomitantly or after an enterocystoplasty (127). Unfortunately, as a mechanical device, the artificial urinary sphincter is associated with the inherent complications of component malfunction. Erosion or infection of the device can also occur, which usually necessitates removal of the sphincter.

### Kropp Procedure

In 1986, Kropp developed a reconstructive procedure whereby an anterior bladder wall flap was tubularized and reimplanted into the posterior bladder wall (128). The Kropp procedure, while eliminating any possibility of spontaneous voiding, has demonstrated continence success rates of the reconstructive procedures, ranging from 80% to 90% in a relatively short-term follow-up (129–131). Unfortunately, the procedure has been associated with significant catheterization difficulties and virtually every patient requiring bladder augmentation (129,131).

### Pippi–Salle Procedure

In 1994, Salle et al. (132) modified the Kropp procedure in an effort to simplify the technique yet retained the flap valve mechanism of continence (132). This technique has yielded slightly lower success rates (61%–69%) than the Kropp procedure, but there are fewer reported cases of difficulty with catheterization. The most common complication of the Salle procedure has been the development of urethrovesical fistula, followed in descending order by VUR and bladder calculi (133).

### Fascial Sling

Fascial slings are an alternative method to manage urinary incontinence in children with myelomeningocele (Fig. 6). This procedure involves taking a rectangular piece of autologous rectus fascia or allograft material and suspending the bladder neck. The ends of the graft are tied together over the rectus muscle. This results in elevation and compression of the proximal urethra and bladder neck (134,135). The majority of published series demonstrate a continence rate of between 40% and 100% (136–138), and the reasonable expectation for success is approximately 50%. The urethral sling has been popular among female patients with sphincteric incompetence and has been used for neurogenic incontinence. The advantages of the sling are technical ease, preservation of bladder capacity, and reportedly good continence rates among female patients. McGuire et al. (139) reported continence rates of 100% among eight female patients with myelomeningocele, Elder (140) reported a 90% success rate in 10 female patients with myelomeningocele, and Gormley et al. (136) reported a 92% success rate among female adolescents. As seen in other bladder neck

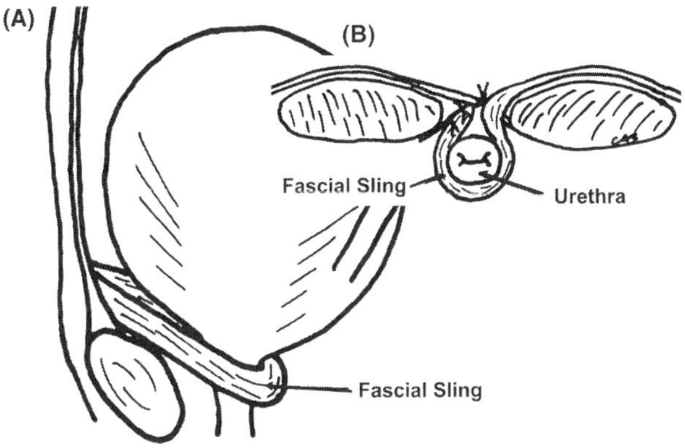


**Figure 6** The fascial sling contributes to coaptation of the urethra to increase outlet resistance.

repairs, the continence rates obtained with the urethral sling are better among patients who have undergone simultaneous bladder augmentation (141). In contrast to female patients with neuropathic bladder, male patients have had somewhat disappointing results with the sling and continence rates were reported as low as 25% (142).

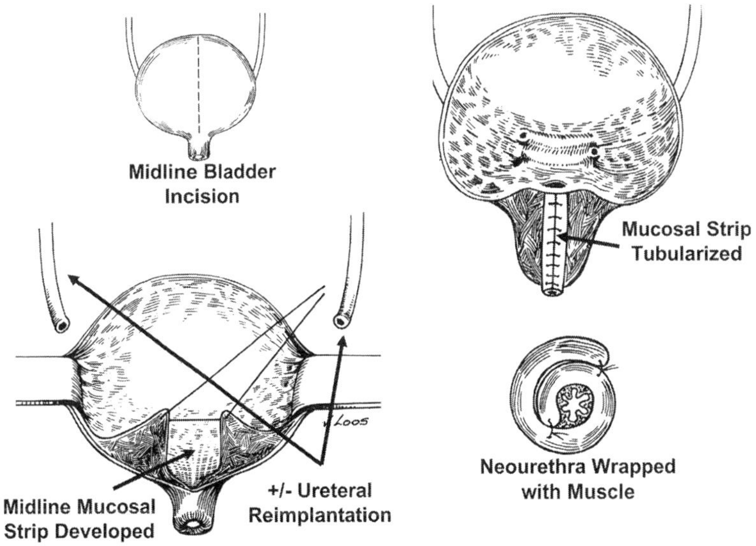


**Figure 7** An example of how the neourethra is created for increased outlet resistance for the YDL bladder neck procedure.

### Young–Dees–Leadbetter Procedure

The YDL bladder neck repair has evolved since 1922, when Young (143) first described a procedure to achieve continence in the epispadias population. Dees and Leadbetter later modified the technique, improving continence rates. The majority of experience with the YDL bladder neck repair has been in the exstrophy–epispadias population, with continence rates reported to be 70% to 86% in several large series (146–148). However, unfortunately, little information is available regarding the use of this procedure in children with neurogenic incontinence. Donnahoo et al. (149) reported reasonable continence rates using this procedure in patients with spina bifida. The majority of patients (68%) were dry after just one operation, and nearly the entire remainder of the patients (79%) was dry after one or two additional procedures. Nearly all patients required a bladder augmentation (149).

At Cincinnati Children's Hospital Medical Center, a retrospective cohort study was conducted of all children (<18 years old) with spina bifida who underwent a bladder neck procedure with inclusion criteria of at least of four years of follow-up (150). The combination of a YDL procedure and urethral sling was performed in 11 children with the mean follow-up of 5.8 years (Fig. 7). The majority of children (81%) were dry without any deterioration in the upper tracts. Therefore, it is our impression that the combination of a YDL and urethral sling procedure may be helpful in improving urinary continence in high-risk children with spina bifida.

## ALTERNATIVE CONTINENT CHANNELS

### The Mitrofanoff Principle

A wide variety of surgical options currently exist for bladder augmentation or continent urinary diversion. These reconstructions, using stomach, ileum, cecum, sigmoid colon, and/or dilated ureter, optimize urinary storage and emptying and preserve upper urinary tract integrity as previously mentioned. Catheterizable access to the reconstructed reservoir can be achieved through the native urethra or, when urethral catheterization is difficult or not feasible, through a continent cutaneous stoma.

The Mitrofanoff principle (Fig. 8), whereby the appendix or an alternative conduit is placed in the urinary reservoir in an antirefluxing manner, provides a reliable, continent, on-way access system. This technique is based on the flap valve mechanism, in which pressure from the bladder is transmitted to a conduit tube (preferable the appendix or segment of ileum) tunneled submucosally into the bladder, compressing its lumen (151). Since Mitrofanoff introduced the continent appendicovesicostomy in 1980, a variety of options have been used to achieve continent catheterizable stomas available, including the appendix, ureter, stomach, tapered ileum, and bladder flap (152–154). More recently, variations of the Mitrofanoff principle have been used to achieve fecal

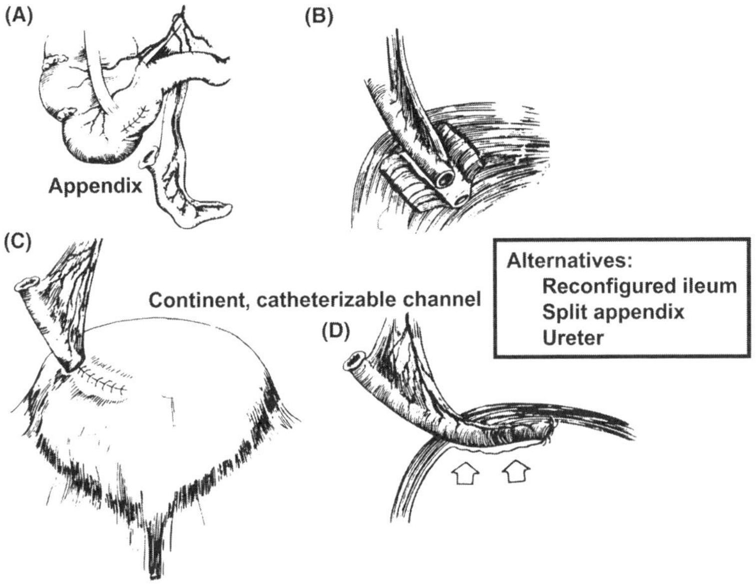


**Figure 8** (**A**) The appendix is amputated from the cecum and maintained on its blood supply. (**B–C**) A seromuscular tunnel is created for continence. (**D**) The course of the Mitrofanoff should be straight to facilitate catheterization.

continence. These tissue constructs have allowed a wide rage of patients to undergo reconstruction and maintain or assume independence and self-esteem. Umbilical or abdominal access (Fig. 9) to the urinary system provides some patients (those who are obese, have poor manual dexterity, and/or are

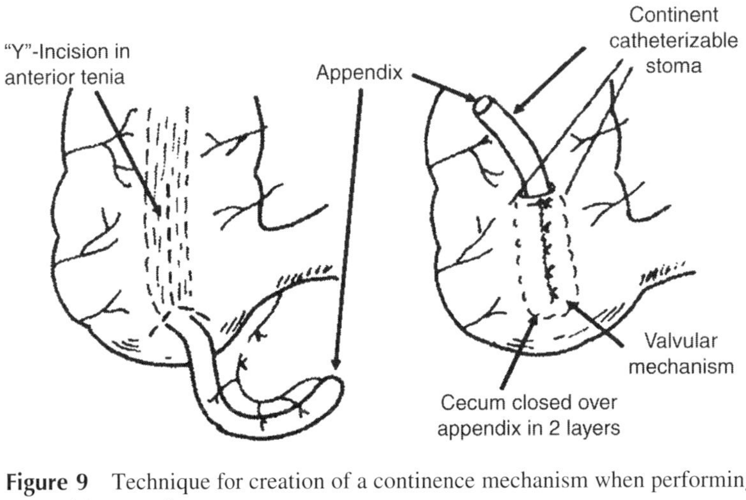


**Figure 9** Technique for creation of a continence mechanism when performing a cecostomy with appendix.

wheelchair-bound) with the means for intermittent urethral catheterization that would otherwise be tedious, difficult, or impossible through their native urethras.

The Mitrofanoff channel can serve as a safety valve when access to the urethra is difficult to potentially avoid devastating complication of bladder perforation. This is the case with the native urethra. Whenever possible, the urethra should be maintained as a second continent channel. This is particularly important in the younger population, since compliance with catheterization schedules can never be assured. Preservation of the native urethra allows some degree of safety by preserving a potential "pop-off" valve. Preservation of the native urethral also allows for bladder access when the continent stoma is inaccessible because of false passage or stomal stenosis. Thus, closure of the bladder neck is considered only in salvage situations, where multiple attempts at achieving outlet competence have failed.

## Results and Complications

The successes of the Mitrofanoff principle during creation of continent urinary reservoirs have been widely demonstrated. Published urinary continence rates associated with CIC at least every three hours ranged 83% to 100%.

In patients undergoing continent urinary diversion, complications with the catheterizable stoma tend to be most problematic in the immediate postoperative period. The most common problem is difficulty with catheterization. The incidence of stomal ischemia, stomal retraction, prolapse, and parastomal hernias can be reduced avoiding angulation of the efferent limb, fixing the reservoir to the anterior abdominal wall, and incorporating as a vascularized skin flap at the stoma (155).

The most frequent complications reported were stomal stenosis and stomal leakage (156). Van Savage et al. (157) suggested that stomal location might play a role in the development of stomal stenosis, with an incidence of 13% at the umbilicus and 4% at a lower quadrant location. Stomal stenosis usually can be corrected with a local stomal revision incorporating an inlay skin flap (155,158). Stomal incontinence typically is the result of an inadequate flap valve mechanism or inadequate reservoir capacity (or both). The former requires an open repair to lengthen the submucosal tunnel. In the latter case, bladder augmentation is indicated (159). Urodynamic evaluation of the reservoir is essential to detect the cause. Furthermore, it must be remembered that cord tethering may be etiologic.

Evidence suggests that stone formation is more common in CIC children who access a Mitrofanoff efferent limb rather than the native urethra (160). The catheterizable limb enters the bladder/reservoir in a nondependent position, and thus does not allow dependent drainage of the system. Therefore, reservoir stone formation is usually a reflection of inadequate evacuation of the reservoir with CIC. Retained mucus, coupled with bacterial colonization and nondependent drainage, most likely contributes to stone formation. At Cincinnati Children's Hospital Medical Center, augmentation cystoplasty is associated with a low rate

(11%) of bladder calculi. Our current strategies for bladder stone prevention include an early regimen of regular low-volume bladder irrigation in patients with enteric augmentation and a Mitrofanoff neourethra. In our patient population, UTI is an independent risk factor for bladder calculi (161). Patients with recurrent UTIs are placed on a sterile catheterization regimen and prescribed daily low dose antibiotic prophylaxis. If a bladder stone develops, a high-volume bladder irrigation regimen is begun after the stone is completely treated. If further stones develop despite compliance with this regimen, 20% urea solution irrigations are considered. Stones located within the conduit are easily removed endoscopically. In our hands, endoscopic management is a safe and effective treatment, and it can be facilitated by percutaneous access. Open surgical removal should be reserved for patients with a large reservoir stone burden (159).

## NEUROGENIC BOWEL

Fecal incontinence is a sequela of neurogenic bowel and affects the quality of life and social outcomes for children and adolescents with spina bifida. A variety of methods are recommended to evacuate the bowel, including voluntary bowel movement, manual evacuation, stool softeners, suppositories, or retrograde irrigation. Patients with myelomeningocele and those with spinal cord injury who lack sensation are unable to consciously initiate reflex defecation. If the lesion is above the level of the conus, the rectocolic reflex may be used to assist the patient to defecate. Digital-rectal stimulation is used to facilitate defecation by inserting a gloved finger into the rectum and applying gentle pressure in the direction of the sacrum. This relaxes the external sphincter and pelvic muscles, initiates peristaltic waves, and allows passage of stool. In patients with lesions below the level of the conus, sphincter tone is lost, eliminating reflex defecation. The bowel must be emptied by other means to prevent fecal incontinence. Digital-rectal stimulation will produce local peristalsis, but disimpaction is required to empty the bowel (162). The treatment regimen in children involves a combination of dietary manipulation, medication, behavior modification, and positive reinforcement offered in a stepwise approach. Laxatives should be avoided because although they treat constipation, symptoms of encopresis may be worsened. Stool softeners are more appropriate for the management of constipation in children with spinal cord injury or myelomeningocele. Other strategies include scheduled toileting and positive reinforcement. Toileting after breakfast uses the gastrocolic reflex and, when successful, prevents soiling throughout the day. Children should be encouraged to sit comfortably on the toilet with their feet supported on a flat surface or stool, and they should be instructed to increase the intra-abdominal pressure by bearing down. Initially children with myelomeningocele may benefit from a stimulant or glycerin suppository to promote reflex defecation. When this routine is unsuccessful in the management of constipation, more aggressive therapy with routine enemas or retrograde enemas should be implemented. If the combination of dietary manipulation, laxatives, bowel training, and retrograde enemas fails to control constipation and encopresis, a colostomy or antegrade continence enema procedure may be performed (163).

## The Malone Antegrade Continent Enema Procedure

Pediatric patients with neurogenic bowel, chronic constipation, Hirschsprung's disease, or anorectal malformations may benefit from construction of a continent stoma to manage fecal soiling. The antegrade continent enema stoma was first described by Malone et al. (164) in 1990. Another surgical option includes a button cecostomy that allows placement percutaneously but might limit future reconstructive options (165). Minor complications are reported by many patients after insertion of the button, including cellulitis, stomal stenosis, and superficial infection at the button site (166). The stoma can be created from the appendix (Fig. 10), from the small intestine, or from colonic segments but the appendix is the preferred bowel segment. After the cecum and appendix are mobilized, the tip of the appendix is brought out through a skin incision below the normal appendectomy incision (152,167) or through the umbilicus (168). The procedure is usually performed through a midline incision because of abnormal fixation of the cecum in the right upper quadrant (a common finding in children with myelodysplasia), exaggerated lordosis, and intraperitoneal adhesions from ventriculoperitoneal shunts (169,170).

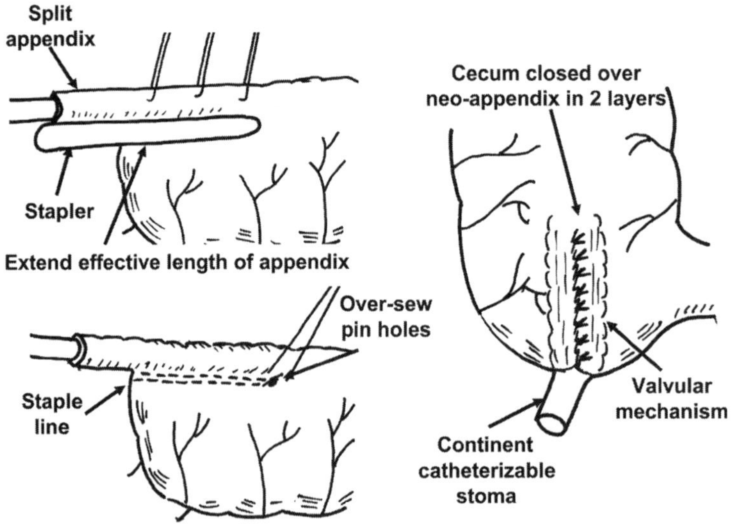


**Figure 10** The Malone antegrade continent enema procedure. (**A**) The end of the appendix is amputated so that a 12 or 14 Fr. catheter can be easily passed retrograde into the cecum. With minimal mobilization, the appendix is rotated in situ along the anterior tenia. (**B**) Using multiple interrupted permanent sutures, the serosa of the cecum is plicated over the appendix to prevent leakage.

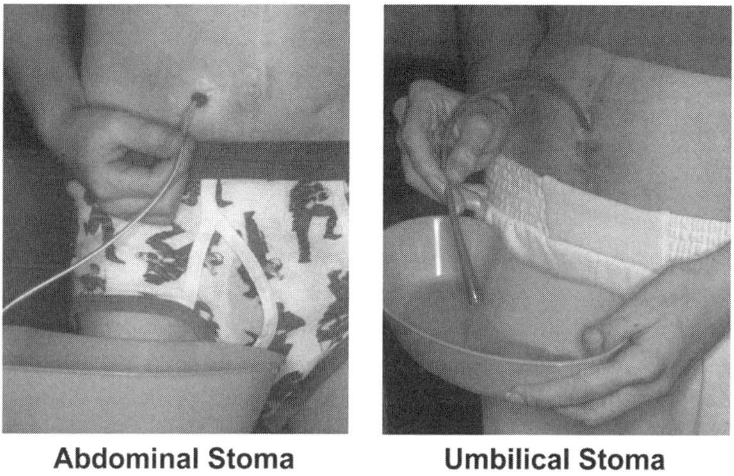


**Figure 11** Two alternatives for stoma placement.

In situations when the appendix is too short or when a concomitant appendiceal Mitrofanoff stoma is required, we now consider a stapled cecal extension technique (Fig. 11). We assessed the long-term outcome of the staple technique for constructing a Malone antegrade continent enema (MACE) conduit (153). Primary diagnosis included myelomeningocele (13), VATER (1), and spinal cord injury (1). Fecal continence was achieved in 14/15 (93%) with an acceptable low rate of minor complications (stomal stenosis in one and peristomal abscess in one).

At our institution, in selected cases, laparoscopic-guided MACE procedures have been performed in children with spina bifida (Fig. 12). Laparoscopy is mainly

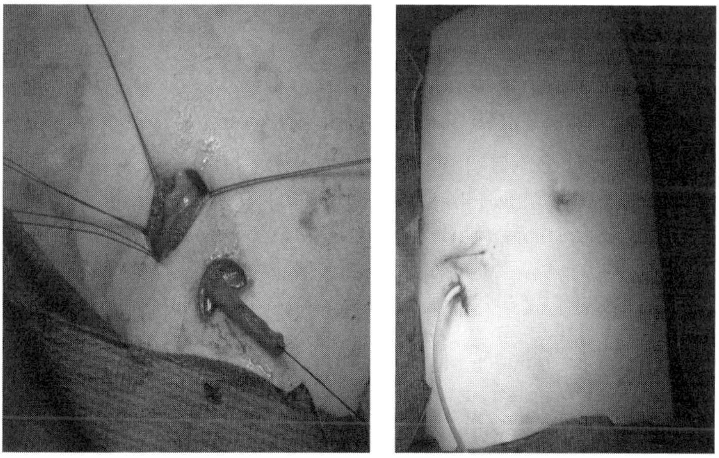

**Figure 12** Cecostomy creation using incisions based on laparoscopic findings and mobilization.

used to identify the cecum and appendix, with a single port placed at the inferior umbilical crease in order to allow correct placement of a small transverse incision overlying the cecum. The appendix and cecum are externalized to creat antireflux mechanism. Then a skin flap is fashioned in a U-configuration at a different skin incision. Our simplified laparoscopic-guided MACE procedure with extracorporeal imbrication creates a reliable and durable mechanism and an improved cosmetic appearance without a midline abdominal incision (171).

The most common complications include difficult catheterization, stomal leakage, sloughing of the conduit, and stomal stenosis. Clark et al. (172) reported that the following variables are associated with better outcomes in children with a neurogenic bowel and bladder managed with a Mitrofanoff and/or MACE procedure: compliance with clinic visits and irrigation, younger age (less than 8 years old), and smaller body habitus. The result is fewer complications and better urinary and fecal continence.

Patients are instructed to administer irrigant by means of a catheter in the stoma in the evening while sitting on the toilet. Patients are instructed to lavage at different intervals varying from 24 to 72 hours. The volume is individualized to the patient and generally ranges from 500 to 1500 mL; evacuation takes place from 15 minutes to two hours after lavage (166). Irrigant solutions vary from tap water to saline as well as laxative agents and glycerin. One of the problems encountered in some children with the MACE, particularly those with constipation, is the time it takes for the washout to work, which has let to failure and abandonment of the procedure in a number of patients (173). In an attempt to overcome this problem, some surgeons have placed a catheterizable conduit in the left colon to reduce the length of bowel that has to be washed through and thus the time taken. Preliminary result with this approach is encouraging (174,175).

In summary, patients report improved quality of life and emotional and psychosocial well-being after the procedure because of improved continence and independence (167).

## MINIMALLY INVASIVE ALTERNATIVES TO RECONSTRUCTION FOR INCONTINENCE

One of the more exciting developments in surgery for neurogenic urinary incontinence has been the application of minimally invasive techniques. The first laparoscopic bladder augmentation was a gastrocystoplasty performed in a pediatric patient with sacra agenesis (176). Since then, most of the reported laparoscopic bladder augmentations have been performed in adults (177). The current state-of-the-art for bladder reconstruction and the MACE procedure is laparoscopic-assisted reconstruction. In this technique, the umbilical stoma is prepared by creating a posterior umbilical flap and then achieving open access into the peritoneum using a radial to radial dilating laparoscopic trocar (178). Laparoscopic techniques are then used to mobilize the cecum and appendix, mobilize the sigmoid, harvest omentum, or perform nephrectomy in preparation for an ureterocystoplasty. Happily, laparoscopy appears to be safe in children and adults with ventriculoperitoneal shunts (179). The more technically demanding reconstructive procedures can then be performed through a very small lower abdominal incision, usually a Pfannenstiel. Comparison with open techniques for similar operations suggests equivalent or improved results with shorter hospital stay and time to regular diet (180).

## SEXUALITY

Now that individuals with spina bifida live well into adulthood, sexuality in this population is becoming an increasingly important issue. However, few studies are available that look critically at sexual function. It must be remembered that sexual development depends on socialization and the ability of the child to make friends and discuss shared experience and thoughts. Mental handicaps, poor manual dexterity, lack of education, and overprotective parents often prevent independent behavior and, as a result, lead to poor understanding of sexual issues (181).

It is more likely that men will have problems with erectile and ejaculatory function because the sacral spinal cord is frequently involved, whereas reproductive function in women, which is under hormonal control, is not affected. Men with neurological lesions at S1 or lower are likely to have normal or adequate reproductive sexual function, but only 50% of those with lesions above that level have adequate function (182).

Some studies revealed that 70% to 80% of myelodysplastic women were able to become pregnant and to have an uneventful pregnancy and delivery, although urinary incontinence in the latter stages of gestation was common in many, as was delivery by cesarean section (183,184). In one study, 72% of male subjects claimed that they were able to have an erection, and two-thirds of those were able to ejaculate (184). Palmer et al. (185) conducted a prospective study in order to determine the ability to treat erectile dysfunction in men with spina bifida with sildenafil citrate with a significant dose-dependent improvement (80%) of erectile function. They address that beyond just treating the physical symptoms, the improvement in sexual confidence is equally important as erectile dysfunction contributes to a lack of confidence, poor body image, and difficulty with intimate relationships, which health-care providers must also address.

The degree of sexuality is inversely proportional to the level of neurological dysfunction (181,186). Boys reach puberty at an age similar to the age for normal males, whereas breast development and menarche tend to start as much as two years earlier in myelodysplastic girls for uncertain reasons.

## SUMMARY

Urological management of the patient with neurogenic bowel and bladder is aimed at maintaining normal renal function and, when appropriate, promoting urinary and fecal continence. Lifelong follow-up is necessary for these patients, whatever their management, because of the risks of neurological deterioration, renal and bladder calculi, UTI, urinary incontinence, and renal impairment. Urological concerns were one the most common cause of death in children and adults with myelomeningocele; now these issues can be managed with the expectation of normal renal function and urinary continence in the majority of cases.

## REFERENCES

1. Patriarca P, Korniewicz DM. Latex allergy and implications for urology nursing. Urol Nurs 1999; 19:187, 91, 201.
2. Porri F, Lemiere C, Birnbaum J, et al. Prevalence of latex sensitization in subjects attending health screening: implications for a perioperative screening. Clin Exp Allergy 1997; 27:413–417.
3. Porri F, Pradal M, Lemiere C, et al. Association between latex sensitization and repeated latex exposure in children. Anesthesiology 1997; 86:599–602.
4. Cochrane DD, Finley C, Kestle J, et al. The patterns of late deterioration in patients with transitional lipomyelomeningocele. Eur J Pediatr Surg 2000; 10(suppl 1):13–17.
5. Tarcan T, Bauer S, Olmedo E, et al. Long-term followup of newborns with myelodysplasia and normal urodynamic findings: is followup necessary? J Urol 2001; 165:564–567.
6. Rai AS, Taylor TK, Smith GH, et al. Congenital abnormalities of the urogenital tract in association with congenital vertebral malformations. J Bone Joint Surg Br 2002; 84: 891–895.
7. Chan BW, Chan KS, Koide T, et al. Maternal diabetes increases the risk of caudal regression caused by retinoic acid. Diabetes 2002; 51:2811–2816.
8. Lynch SA, Wang Y, Strachan T, et al. Autosomal dominant sacral agenesis: Currarino syndrome. J Med Genet 2000; 37:561–566.
9. Muthukumar N. Surgical treatment of nonprogressive neurological deficits in children with sacral agenesis. Neurosurgery 1996; 38:1133–1137.
10. Yeung CK. The normal infant bladder. Scand J Urol Nephrol Suppl 1995; 173:19–23.
11. Yeung CK, Godley ML, Duffy PG, et al. Natural filling cystometry in infants and children. Br J Urol 1995; 75:531–537.
12. Yeung CK, Godley ML, Ho CK, et al. Some new insights into bladder function in infancy. Br J Urol 1995; 76:235–240.
13. Yeung CK, Godley ML, Dhillon HK, et al. Urodynamic patterns in infants with normal lower urinary tracts or primary vesico-ureteric reflux. Br J Urol 1998; 81:461–467.
14. Yeung CK. Continuous real-time ambulatory urodynamic monitoring in infants and young children using infrared telemetry. Br J Urol 1998; 81(Suppl 3):76–80.
15. Bachelard M, Sillen U, Hansson S, et al. Urodynamic pattern in asymptomatic infants: siblings of children with vesicoureteral reflux. J Urol 1999; 162:1733–1737.
16. Sillen U, Solsnes E, Hellstrom AL, et al. The voiding pattern of healthy preterm neonates. J Urol 2000; 163:278–281.
17. Ghoniem GM, Bloom DA, McGuire EJ, et al. Bladder compliance in meningomyelocele children. J Urol 1989; 141:1404–1406.
18. Withycombe J, Whitaker R, Hunt G. Intermittent catheterisation in the management of children with neuropathic bladder. Lancet 1978; 2:981–983.

19. Spindel MR, Bauer SB, Dyro FM, et al. The changing neurourologic lesion in myelodysplasia. JAMA 1987; 258:1630–1633.
20. Koff SA. Relationship between dysfunctional voiding and reflux. J Urol 1992; 148:1703–1705.
21. Galloway NT, Mekras JA, Helms M. et al. An objective score to predict upper tract deterioration in myelodysplasia. J Urol 1991; 145:535–537.
22. Steinhardt GF, Goodgold HM, Samuels LD. The effect of intravesical pressure on glomerular filtration rate in patients with myelomeningocele. J Urol 1988; 140:1293–1295.
23. Reiner I, Jones M, Donnell S, et al. Incidence of normal micturition in myelomeningocele patients. Arch Dis Child 1992; 67:640–641.
24. Keshtgar AS, Rickwood AM. Urological consequences of incomplete cord lesions in patients with myelomeningocele. Br J Urol 1998; 82:258–260.
25. Holzbeierlein J, Pope JI, Adams MC, et al. The urodynamic profile of myelodysplasia in childhood with spinal closure during gestation. J Urol 2000; 164:1336–1339.
26. McGuire EJ, Woodside JR, Borden TA, et al. Prognostic value of urodynamic testing in myelodysplastic patients. J Urol 1981; 126:205–209.
27. Hurley RM, Harris D, Shepherd RR. Incontinence in myelodysplasia: imipramine hydrochloride revisited. Clin Pediatr (Phila) 2000; 39:489–491.
28. Baskin LS, Kogan BA, Benard F. Treatment of infants with neurogenic bladder dysfunction using anticholinergic drugs and intermittent catheterisation. Br J Urol 1990; 66:532–534.
29. Stoneking BJ, Brock JW, Pope JC, et al. Early evolution of bladder emptying after myelomeningocele closure. Urology 2001; 58:767–771.
30. Wu HY, Baskin LS, Kogan BA. Neurogenic bladder dysfunction due to myelomeningocele: neonatal versus childhood treatment. J Urol 1997; 157:2295–2297.
31. Kaefer M, Pabby A, Kelly M, et al. Improved bladder function after prophylactic treatment of the high risk neurogenic bladder in newborns with myelomentingocele. J Urol 1999; 162:1068–1071.
32. Tanaka H, Kakizaki H, Kobayashi S, et al. The relevance of urethral resistance in children with myelodysplasia: its impact on upper urinary tract deterioration and the outcome of conservative management. J Urol 1999; 161:929–932.
33. Schlager TA. Urinary tract infections in children younger than 5 years of age: epidemiology, diagnosis, treatment, outcomes and prevention. Paediatr Drugs 2001; 3:219–227.
34. Szucs K, O'Neil KM, Faden H. Urinary findings in asymptomatic subjects with spina bifida treated with intermittent catheterization. Pediatr Infect Dis J 2001; 20:638–639.
35. Kasabian NG, Bauer SB, Dyro FM, et al. The prophylactic value of clean intermittent catheterization and anticholinergic medication in newborns and infants with myelodysplasia at risk of developing urinary tract deterioration. Am J Dis Child 1992; 146:840–843.
36. Goessl C, Knispel HH, Fiedler U, et al. Urodynamic effects of oral oxybutynin chloride in children with myelomeningocele and detrusor hyperreflexia. Urology 1998; 51:94–98.
37. Anderson RU, Mobley D, Blank B, et al. Once daily controlled versus immediate release oxybutynin chloride for urge urinary incontinence. OROS Oxybutynin Study Group. J Urol 1999; 161:1809–1812.

38. Youdim K, Kogan BA. Preliminary study of the safety and efficacy of extended-release oxybutynin in children. Urology 2002; 59:428–432.
39. Appell RA, Abrams P, Drutz HP, et al. Treatment of overactive bladder: long-term tolerability and efficacy of tolterodine. World J Urol 2001; 19:141–147.
40. Nilvebrant L, Andersson KE, Gillberg PG, et al. Tolterodine—a new bladder-selective antimuscarinic agent. Eur J Pharmacol 1997; 327:195–207.
41. Nilvebrant L, Hallen B, Larsson G. Tolterodine—a new bladder selective muscarinic receptor antagonist: preclinical pharmacological and clinical data. Life Sci 1997; 60:1129–1136.
42. Nilvebrant L, Gillberg PG, Sparf B. Antimuscarinic potency and bladder selectivity of PNU-200577, a major metabolite of tolterodine. Pharmacol Toxicol 1997; 81:169–172.
43. Goessl C, Sauter T, Michael T, et al. Efficacy and tolerability of tolterodine in children with detrusor hyperreflexia. Urology 2000; 55:414–418.
44. Hjalmas K, Hellstrom AL, Mogren K, et al. The overactive bladder in children: a potential future indication for tolterodine. BJU Int 2001; 87:569–574.
45. Kasabian NG, Vlachiotis JD, Lais A, et al. The use of intravesical oxybutynin chloride in patients with detrusor hypertonicity and detrusor hyperreflexia. J Urol 1994; 151:944–945.
46. Massad CA, Kogan BA, Trigo-Rocha FE. The pharmacokinetics of intravesical and oral oxybutynin chloride. J Urol 1992; 148:595–597.
47. Ferrara P, D'Aleo CM, Tarquini, E, et al. Side-effects of oral or intravesical oxybutynin chloride in children with spina bifida. BJU Int 2001; 87:674–678.
48. Di Stasi SM, Giannantoni A, Vespasiani G, et al. Intravesical electromotive administration of oxybutynin in patients with detrusor hyperreflexia unresponsive to standard anticholinergic regimens. J Urol 2001; 165:491–498.
49. Di Stasi SM, Giannantoni A, Navarra P, et al. Intravesical oxybutynin: mode of action assessed by passive diffusion and electromotive administration with pharmacokinetics of oxybutynin and *N*-desethyl oxybutynin. J Urol 2001; 166:2232–2236.
50. Seki N, Ikawa S, Takano N, et al. Intravesical instillation of resiniferatoxin for neurogenic bladder dysfunction in a patient with myelodysplasia. J Urol 2001; 166:2368–2369.
51. Dykstra DD, Sidi AA. Treatment of detrusor–sphincter dyssynergia with botulinum A toxin: a double-blind study. Arch Phys Med Rehabil 1990; 71:24–26.
52. Schurch B, Stohrer M, Kramer G, et al. Botulinum-A toxin for treating detrusor hyperreflexia in spinal cord injured patients: a new alternative to anticholinergic drugs? Preliminary results. J Urol 2000; 164:692–697.
53. Schurch B, Schmid DM, Stohrer M. Treatment of neurogenic incontinence with botulinum toxin A. N Engl J Med 2000; 342:665.
54. Schulte-Baukloh H, Michael T, Sturzebecher B, et al. Botulinum-a toxin detrusor injection as a novel approach in the treatment of bladder spasticity in children with neurogenic bladder. Eur Urol 2003; 44:139–143.
55. Schulte-Baukloh H, Michael T, Schobert J, et al. Efficacy of botulinum-a toxin in children with detrusor hyperreflexia due to myelomeningocele: preliminary results. Urology 2002; 59:325–327.

56. Yamanishi T, Yasuda K, Murayama N, et al. Biofeedback training for detrusor overactivity in children. J Urol 2000; 164:1686–1690.
57. Porena M, Costantini E, Rociola W, et al. Biofeedback successfully cures detrusor–sphincter dyssynergia in pediatric patients. J Urol 2000; 163:1927–1931.
58. Chin-Peuckert L, Salle JL. A modified biofeedback program for children with detrusor–sphincter dyssynergia: 5-year experience. J Urol 2001; 166:1470–1475.
59. Goldwasser B, Webster GD. Augmentation and substitution enterocystoplasty. J Urol 1986; 135:215–224.
60. Rink RC. Bladder augmentation. Options, outcomes, future. Urol Clin North Am 1999; 26:111–123.
61. Adams MC, Joseph DB. Urinary Tract Reconstruction in Children. 8th ed. Philadelphia: WB Saunders, 2002:2508–2563.
62. Hutcheson JC, Cooper CS, Canning DA, et al. The use of vesicostomy as permanent urinary diversion in the child with myelomeningocele. J Urol 2001; 166:2351.
63. Snow BW, Cartwright PC. Autoaugmentation of the bladder. Contemp Urol 1992; 4:41–51.
64. Cartwright PC, Snow BW. Bladder autoaugmentation: early clinical experience. J Urol 1989; 142:505–508.
65. Cartwright PC, Snow BW. Bladder autoaugmentation: partial detrusor excision to augment the bladder without use of bowel. J Urol 1989; 142:1050–1053.
66. Marte A, Di Meglio D, Cotrufo AM, et al. A long-term follow-up of autoaugmentation in myelodysplastic children. BJU Int 2002; 89:928–931.
67. Bellinger MF. Ureterocystoplasty: a unique method for vesical augmentation in children. J Urol 1993; 149:811–813.
68. Landau EH, Jayanthi VR, Khoury AE, et al. Bladder augmentation: ureterocystoplasty versus ileocystoplasty. J Urol 1994; 152:716–719.
69. McDougal WS. Electrolyte abnormalities as a consequence of urinary intestinal diversion. Scand J Urol Nephrol Suppl 1992; 142:30–33.
70. McDougal WS. Metabolic complications of urinary intestinal diversion. J Urol 1992; 147:1199–1208.
71. Keating MA, Ludlow JK, Rich MA. Enterocystoplasty: the star modification. J Urol 1996; 155:1723–1725.
72. Goodwin WE, Winter CC, Barker WF. "Cup-patch" technique of ileocystoplasty for bladder enlargement or partial substitution. J Urol 2002; 168:667–670.
73. Koff SA. The shape of intestinal segments used for reconstruction. J Urol (Paris) 1988; 94:201–203.
74. Cespedes R, McGuire EJ. Bladder Augmentation. Philadelphia: Lippincott-Wiliams & Wilkins, 1998:211–218.
75. DeFoor W, Minevich E, Reeves D, et al. Gastrocystoplasty: long-term followup. J Urol 2003; 170:1647–1649.
76. Adams MC, Mitchell ME, Rink RC. Gastrocystoplasty: an alternative solution to the problem of urological reconstruction in the severely compromised patient. J Urol 1988; 140:1152–1156.
77. Gosalbez R Jr, Woodard JR, Broecker BH, et al. The use of stomach in pediatric urinary reconstruction. J Urol 1993; 150:438–440.
78. Jones J, Bickeboller R, Binder J, et al. Synchronous bladder augmentation and living related kidney transplantation. Urol Int 2001; 67:84–85.

79. Sheldon CA, Gonzalez R, Burns MW, et al. Renal transplantation into the dysfunctional bladder: the role of adjunctive bladder reconstruction. J Urol 1994; 152:972–975.
80. Chadwick Plaire J, Snodgrass WT, Grady RW, et al. Long-term followup of the hematuria–dysuria syndrome. J Urol 2000; 164:921–923.
81. DeFoor W, Minevich E, McEnery P, et al. Lower urinary tract reconstruction is safe and effective in children with end stage renal disease. J Urol 2003; 170:1497–1500.
82. Buson H, Manivel JC, Dayanc M, et al. Seromuscular colocystoplasty lined with urothelium: experimental study. Urology 1994; 44:743–748.
83. Gonzalez R, Buson H, Reid C, et al. Seromuscular colocystoplasty lined with urothelium: experience with 16 patients. Urology 1995; 45:124–129.
84. Nguyen DH, Mitchell ME, Horowitz M, et al. Demucosalized augmentation gastrocystoplasty with bladder autoaugmentation in pediatric patients. J Urol 1996; 156:206–209.
85. Dewan PA, Byard RW. Autoaugmentation gastrocystoplasty in a sheep model. Br J Urol 1993; 72:56–59.
86. Carr MC, Docimo SG, Mitchell ME. Bladder augmentation with urothelial preservation. J Urol 1999; 162:1133–1136.
87. Shekarriz B, Upadhyay J, Demirbilek S, et al. Surgical complications of bladder augmentation: comparison between various enterocystoplasties in 133 patients. Urology 2000; 55:123–128.
88. Ganesan T, Khadra MH, Wallis J, et al. Vitamin B12 malabsorption following bladder reconstruction or diversion with bowel segments. ANZ J Surg 2002; 72:479–482.
89. Bogaert GA, Mevorach RA, Kim J, et al. The physiology of gastrocystoplasty: once a stomach, always a stomach. J Urol, **153:** 1977, 1980, 1995.
90. Sheldon CA, Gilbert A, Wacksman J, et al. Gastrocystoplasty: technical and metabolic characteristics of the most versatile childhood bladder augmentation modality. J Pediatr Surg 1995; 30:283–287.
91. Rushton HG, Woodard JR, Parrott TS, et al. Delayed bladder rupture after augmentation enterocystoplasty. J Urol 1988; 140:344–346.
92. DeFoor W, Tackett L, Minevich E. et al. Risk factors for spontaneous bladder perforation after augmentation cystoplasty. Urology 2003; 62:737–741.
93. Crane JM, Scherz HS, Billman GF, et al. Ischemic necrosis: a hypothesis to explain the pathogenesis of spontaneously ruptured enterocystoplasty. J Urol 1991; 146:141–144.
94. Bauer SB, Hendren WH, Kozakewich H, et al. Perforation of the augmented bladder. J Urol 1992; 148:699–703.
95. Anderson PA, Rickwood AM. Detrusor hyper-reflexia as a factor in spontaneous perforation of augmentation cystoplasty for neuropathic bladder. Br J Urol 1991; 67:210–212.
96. Close CE. Complications of Enterocystoplasty. 1st ed. London: Arnold, 2000:61–70.
97. Hendren WH, Hendren RB. Bladder augmentation: experience with 129 children and young adults. J Urol 1990; 144:445–453.
98. Ali-El-Dein B, El-Tabey N, Abdel-Latif M, et al. Late uro-ileal cancer after incorporation of ileum into the urinary tract. J Urol 2002; 167:84–88.
99. Lane T, Shah J. Carcinoma following augmentation ileocystoplasty. Urol Int 2000; 64:31–32.

100. Barrington JW, Fulford S, Griffiths D, et al. Tumors in bladder remnant after augmentation enterocystoplasty. J Urol 1997; 157:482–485.
101. Gregoire M, Kantoff P, DeWolf WC. Synchronous adenocarcinoma and transitional cell carcinoma of the bladder associated with augmentation: case report and review of the literature. J Urol 1993; 149:115–118.
102. Golomb J, Lewin KJ, deKernion JB, et al. Primary small cell carcinoma of the augmented urinary bladder. Br J Urol 1992; 70:572–573.
103. Shokeir AA, Shamaa M, el-Mekresh MM, et al. Late malignancy in bowel segments exposed to urine without fecal stream. Urology 1995; 46:657–661.
104. Nahas WC, Iizuka FH, Mazzucchi E, et al. Adenocarcinoma of an augmented bladder 25 years after ileocecocystoplasty and 6 years after renal transplantation. J Urol 1999; 162:490–491.
105. Sato M, Fukui S, Fujita I, et al. Adenocarcinoma of the ileal segment with transitional cell carcinoma of the bladder following ileocytoplasty: a case report. Hinyokika Kiyo 2000; 46:33–36.
106. Filmer RB, Spencer JR. Malignancies in bladder augmentations and intestinal conduits. J Urol 1990; 143:671–678.
107. Soergel TM, Cain MP, Misseri R, et al. Transitional cell carcinoma of the bladder following augmentation cystoplasty for the neuropathic bladder. J Urol 2004; 172:1649–1651.
108. Docimo SG, Orth CR, Schulam PG. Percutaneous cystolithotomy after augmentation cystoplasty: comparison with open procedures. Tech Urol 1998; 4:43–45.
109. Rink RC, Adams MC, Keating MA. The flip-flap technique to lengthen the urethra (Salle procedure) for treatment of neurogenic urinary incontinence. J Urol 1994; 152:799–802.
110. Xiao C-G, Du M, Li B, et al. An effective surgical treatment for neurogenic bladder in spina bifida children: results of 20 cases. J Urol 2004; 171, (suppl 4):56.
111. Lottmann HB, Margaryan M, Bernuy M, et al. The effect of endoscopic injections of dextranomer based implants on continence and bladder capacity: a prospective study of 31 patients. J Urol 2002; 168:1863–1867.
112. Caione P, Capozza N. Endoscopic treatment of urinary incontinence in pediatric patients: 2-year experience with dextranomer/hyaluronic acid copolymer. J Urol 2002; 168:1868–1871.
113. Malizia AA Jr, Reiman HM, Myers RP, et al. Migration and granulomatous reaction after periurethral injection of polytef (Teflon). JAMA 1984; 251:3277–3281.
114. Bomalaski MD, Bloom DA, McGuire EJ, et al. Glutaraldehyde cross-linked collagen in the treatment of urinary incontinence in children. J Urol 1996; 155:699–702.
115. Kassouf W, Capolicchio G, Berardinucci G, et al. Collagen injection for treatment of urinary incontinence in children. J Urol 2001; 165:1666–1668.
116. Scott FB, Bradley WE, Timm GW. Treatment of urinary incontinence by implantable prosthetic sphincter. Urology 1973; 1:252–259.
117. Barrett DM, Furlow WL. The management of severe urinary incontinence in patients with myelodysplasia by implantation of the AS 791/792 urinary sphincter device. J Urol 1982; 128:484–486.
118. Light JK, Scott FB. Use of the artificial urinary sphincter in spinal cord injury patients. J Urol 1983; 130:1127–1129.

119. Light JK, Hawila M, Scott FB. Treatment of urinary incontinence in children: the artificial sphincter versus other methods. J Urol 1983; 130:518–521.
120. Light JK, Scott FB. Complications of the artificial urinary sphincter in pediatric patients. Urol Clin North Am 1983; 10:551–555.
121. Light JK, Flores FN, Scott FB. Use of the AS792 artificial sphincter following urinary undiversion. J Urol 1983; 129:548–551.
122. Kryger JV, Spencer Barthold J, Fleming P, et al. The outcome of artificial urinary sphincter placement after a mean 15-year follow-up in a paediatric population. BJU Int 1999; 83:1026–1031.
123. Kryger JV, Gonzalez R, Barthold JS. Surgical management of urinary incontinence in children with neurogenic sphincteric incompetence. J Urol 2000; 163:256–263.
124. Castera R, Podesta ML, Ruarte A, et al. 10-year experience with artificial urinary sphincter in children and adolescents. J Urol 2001; 165:2373–2376.
125. Hafez AT, McLorie G, Bagli D, et al. A single-centre long-term outcome analysis of artificial urinary sphincter placement in children. BJU Int 2002; 89:82–85.
126. Holmes NM, Kogan BA, Baskin LS. Placement of artificial urinary sphincter in children and simultaneous gastrocystoplasty. J Urol 2001; 165:2366–2368.
127. Gonzalez R, Nguyen DH, Koleilat N, et al. Compatibility of enterocystoplasty and the artificial urinary sphincter. J Urol 1989; 142:502–504.
128. Kropp KA, Angwafo FF. Urethral lengthening and reimplantation for neurogenic incontinence in children. J Urol 1986; 135:533–536.
129. Nill TG, Peller PA, Kropp KA. Management of urinary incontinence by bladder tube urethral lengthening and submucosal reimplantation. J Urol 1990; 144:559–561.
130. Belman AB, Kaplan GW. Experience with the Kropp anti-incontinence procedure. J Urol 1989; 141:1160–1162.
131. Waters PR, Chehade NC, Kropp KA. Urethral lengthening and reimplantation: incidence and management of catheterization problems. J Urol 1997; 158:1053–1056.
132. Salle JL, de Fraga JC, Amarante A, et al. Urethral lengthening with anterior bladder wall flap for urinary incontinence: a new approach. J Urol 1994; 152:803–806.
133. Salle JL, McLorie GA, Bagli DJ, et al. Urethral lengthening with anterior bladder wall flap (Pippi–Salle procedure): modifications and extended indications of the technique. J Urol 1997; 158:585–590.
134. Woodside JR, Borden TA. Pubovaginal sling procedure for the management of urinary incontinence in a myelodysplastic girl. J Urol 1982; 127:744–746.
135. Colvert JR 3rd, Kropp BP, Cheng EY, et al. The use of small intestinal submucosa as an off-the-shelf urethral sling material for pediatric urinary incontinence. J Urol 2002; 168:1872–1875.
136. Gormley EA, Bloom DA, McGuire EJ, et al. Pubovaginal slings for the management of urinary incontinence in female adolescents. J Urol 1994; 152:822–825.
137. Kakizaki H, Shibata T, Shinno Y, et al. Fascial sling for the management of urinary incontinence due to sphincter incompetence. J Urol 1995; 153:644–647.
138. Perez LM, Smith EA, Broecker BH, et al. Outcome of sling cystourethropexy in the pediatric population: a critical review. J Urol 1996; 156:642–646.
139. McGuire EJ, Wang CC, Usitalo H, et al. Modified pubovaginal sling in girls with myelodysplasia. J Urol 1986; 135:94–96.
140. Elder JS. Periurethral and puboprostatic sling repair for incontinence in patients with myelodysplasia. J Urol 1990; 144:434–437.
141. Decter RM. Use of the fascial sling for neurogenic incontinence: lessons learned. J Urol 1993; 150:683–686.

142. Ludlow JK, Keating MA, Wahle GR, et al. Fascial slings and incontinent children—the gender gap. J Urol 1995; 153, [abstr 201].
143. Young HH. An operation for the cure of incontinence associated with epispadias. J Urol 1922; 7:1.
144. Dees JE. Congenital epispadias with incontinence. J Urol 1949; 62:513.
145. Leadbetter GWJ. Surgical correction of total urinary incontinence. J Urol 1964; 91, 261–266.
146. Lepor H, Jeffs RD. Primary bladder closure and bladder neck reconstruction in classical bladder exstrophy. J Urol 1983; 130:1142–1145.
147. Perlmutter AD, Weinstein MD, Reitelman C. Vesical neck reconstruction in patients with epispadias–exstrophy complex. J Urol 1991; 146:613–615.
148. McMahon DR, Cain MP, Husmann DA, et al. Vesical neck reconstruction in patients with the exstrophy–epispadias complex. J Urol 1996; 155:1411–1413.
149. Donnahoo KK, Rink RC, Cain MP, et al. The Young–Dees–Leadbetter bladder neck repair for neurogenic incontinence. J Urol 1999; 161:1946–1949.
150. Nishinaka K, DeFoor W, Minevich E, et al. Long term evaluation of bladder neck reconstruction in children with spina bifida. Manuscript in preparation.
151. Lowe JB, Furness PD 3rd, Barqawi AZ, et al. Surgical management of the neuropathic bladder. Semin Pediatr Surg 2002; 11:120.
152. Sheldon CA, Minevich E, Wacksman J. Modified technique of antegrade continence enema using a stapling device. J Urol 2000; 163:589.
153. Nishinaka K, DeFoor W, Minevich E, et al. Modified technique of antegrade continence enema using a staple device: our long-term outcome. Manuscript in preparation.
154. Nishinaka K, DeFoor W, Minevich E, et al. Modified technique of Monti–Mitrofanoff procedure using a Parker–Kerr stitch. Manuscript in preparation.
155. Fitzgerald J, Malone MJ, Gaertner RA, et al. Stomal construction, complications, and reconstruction. Urol Clin North Am 1997; 24:729–733.
156. De Ganck J, Everaert K, Van Laecke E, et al. A high easy-to-treat complication rate is the price for a continent stoma. BJU Int 2002; 90:240–243.
157. Van Savage JG, Khoury AE, McLorie GA, et al. Outcome analysis of Mitrofanoff principle applications using appendix and ureter to umbilical and lower quadrant stomal sites. J Urol 1996; 156:1794–1797.
158. Gerharz EW, Kohl U, Weingartner K, et al. Complications related to different continence mechanisms in ileocecal reservoirs. J Urol 1997; 158:1709–1713.
159. Kaefer M, Retik AB. The Mitrofanoff principle in continent urinary reconstruction. Urol Clin North Am 1997; 24:795–811.
160. Blyth B, Ewalt DH, Duckett JW, et al. Lithogenic properties of enterocystoplasty. J Urol 1992; 148:575.
161. DeFoor W, Minevich E, Reddy P, et al. Bladder calculi after augmentation cystoplasty: risk factors and prevention strategies. J Urol 2004; 172:1964–1966.
162. Lynch AC, Wong C, Anthony A, et al. Bowel dysfunction following spinal cord injury: a description of bowel function in a spinal cord-injured population and comparison with age and gender matched controls. Spinal Cord 2000; 38:717–723.
163. Bishop PR, Nowicki MJ. Defecation disorders in the neurologically impaired child. Pediatr Ann 1999; 28:322–329.
164. Malone PS, Ransley PG, Kiely EM. Preliminary report: the antegrade continence enema. Lancet 1990; 336:1217–1218.
165. Shandling B, Chait PG, Richards HF. Percutaneous cecostomy: a new technique in the management of fecal incontinence. J Pediatr Surg 1996; 31:534–537.

166. Duel BP, Gonzalez R. The button cecostomy for management of fecal incontinence. Pediatr Surg Int 1999; 15:559–561.
167. Aksnes G, Diseth TH, Helseth A, et al. Appendicostomy for antegrade enema: effects on somatic and psychosocial functioning in children with myelomeningocele. Pediatrics 2002; 109:484–489.
168. Glassman DT, Docimo SG. Concealed umbilical stoma: long-term evaluation of stomal stenosis. J Urol 2001; 166:1028–1030.
169. Cadeddu JA, Docimo SG. Laparoscopic-assisted continent stoma procedures: our new standard. Urology 1999; 54:909–912.
170. Hedican SP. Laparoscopy in urology. Surg Clin North Am 2000; 80:1465–1485.
171. Nishinaka K, Sheldon CA. Laparoscopic-guided Malone antegrade continence enema (MACE) technique in children with spina bifida: our long-term outcome. Manuscript in preparation.
172. Clark T, Pope JC IV, Adams C, et al. Factors that influence outcomes of the Mitrofanoff and Malone antegrade continence enema reconstructive procedures in children. J Urol 2002; 168:1537–1540.
173. Griffiths DM, Malone PS. The Malone antegrade continence enema. J Pediatr Surg 1995; 30:68–71.
174. Churchill BM, De Ugarte DA, Atkinson JB. Left-colon antegrade continence enema (LACE) procedure for fecal incontinence. J Pediatr Surg 2003; 38:1778–1780.
175. Liloku RB, Mure PY, Braga L, et al. The left Monti–Malone procedure: preliminary results in seven cases. J Pediatr Surg 2002; 37:228–231.
176. Docimo SG, Moore RG, Adams J, et al. Laparoscopic bladder augmentation using stomach. Urology 1995; 46:565–569.
177. Gill IS, Rackley RR, Meraney AM, et al. Laparoscopic enterocystoplasty. Urology 2000; 55:178–181.
178. Cuellar DC, Kavoussi PK, Baker LA, et al. Open laparoscopic access using a radially dilating trocar: experience and indications in 50 consecutive cases. J Endourol 2000; 14:755–756.
179. Jackman SV, Weingart JD, Kinsman SL, et al. Laparoscopic surgery in patients with ventriculoperitoneal shunts: safety and monitoring. J Urol 2000; 164:1352–1354.
180. Knab K, Langhans B, Behrens R, et al. The neuropathic bowel in spina bifida—a cross-sectional study in 226 patients. Eur J Pediatr Surg 2001; 11(suppl 1):S41–42.
181. Joyner BD, McLorie GA, Khoury AE. Sexuality and reproductive issues in children with myelomeningocele. Eur J Pediatr Surg 1998; 8:29–34.
182. Woodhouse CR. The sexual and reproductive consequences of congenital genitourinary anomalies. J Urol 1994; 152:645–651.
183. Bomalaski MD, Teague JL, Brooks B. The long-term impact of urological management on the quality of life of children with spina bifida. J Urol 1995; 154:778–781.
184. Decter RM, Furness PD 3rd, Nguyen TA, et al. Reproductive understanding, sexual functioning and testosterone levels in men with spina bifida. J Urol 1997; 157:1466–1468.
185. Palmer JS, Kaplan WE, Firlit CF. Erectile dysfunction in patients with spina bifida is a treatable condition. J Urol 2000; 164:958–961.
186. Palmer JS, Kaplan WE, Firlit CF. Erectile dysfunction in spina bifida is treatable. Lancet 1999; 354:125–126.

# 12

# Families that Have Children with Spina Bifida

**Marlene L. Lutkenhoff**
*Division of Developmental and Behavioral Pediatrics,*
*Cincinnati Children's Hospital Medical Center, Cincinnati, Ohio, U.S.A.*

## IMPACT ON FAMILY FUNCTION AND INDIVIDUAL DEVELOPMENTAL TASKS

All families have roles and functions that change as the structure of the family changes. Likewise, there are developmental tasks most children master as they mature. When a child has spina bifida, the structure and function of the family and the tasks of the child remain. However, successfully mastering those tasks becomes significantly more complex and challenging. Theorists such as Duvall and Erikson have classified family and individual tasks into stages that move along a continuum (1, 2). Although there are challenges in trying to fit all families or individuals into neatly defined tracts, particularly in today's culture of diverse family forms, the developmental models give professionals a benchmark for accessing family and individual functioning. The professionals' task is to support and help families and individuals achieve developmental milestones.

### Infancy

The transition of a family unit from a childless couple to one with child is significant. As well as taking on new skills and responsibilities, such as bathing, holding, feeding, and caring for a baby, the parents must learn to give up some personal freedom (3). When the infant is born with a chronic illness, parents will need tremendous encouragement and guidance as they take on the role of becoming competent parents. Most new parents have little or no knowledge of spina bifida and are faced with feelings of doubt and uncertainty. During this initial phase of adjustment, parents appreciate health-care professionals (HCPs) who will listen to their fears, answer their questions honestly, and give them hope. Connecting families to the local spina bifida support group and/or to other families in similar circumstances can help decrease their sense of isolation. Relationship building is important during this early stage (the professional–parent relationship, parent-to-parent relationship, and parent-to-newborn relationship). The parents may need help connecting and reaching out and adjusting to their new roles.

Although bonding may be delayed due to medical complications, which result in keeping the child separated initially, and due to the grieving process of the parents who will mourn the loss of the perfect child, helping the parent develop a secure relationship with their new baby is critical. Infants easily and quickly learn to trust parents who are available and consistent in their care. Forming an attachment with the new baby and giving positive stimulation is crucial to the brain development of the infant. Although brain development continues throughout life, its growth during the first three years of life is nothing short of amazing. During this time, it has more ability to rebound from negative influences, such as a traumatic birth experience (4). This is truly good news for a parent who has a child with some type of neurological impairment. Interventions that support increased stimulation by the parent and early intervention specialists should be fostered. However, in order for infants to make the most of all this wonderful stimulation, they need to be alert and feel good about their world. There is a strong relationship between emotions and learning. In fact, when the attachment between mother and baby is secure, most other areas of development will also benefit (5).

## Toddler/Preschool

Life with young children who begin to exert some of their own demands as they strive to achieve some degree of independence is exhausting. Parenting takes on new challenges as safety concerns and discipline and feeding issues emerge. In addition to these new developments, often by the time one child reaches this age, another child has been born into the family. The absorption in childcare routines can disrupt the marital relationship, making it harder and harder for the couple to find satisfying time with one another (3). Tapping into formal and informal support systems of the family in an effort to locate suitable childcare substitutes is essential for the healthy growth of the family and individual members. Providing opportunities for the young child to make choices and to engage in play dates and preschool experiences fosters the child's need for control and socialization.

Children learn through exploration and gain sensory awareness through the movement of their bodies through space. Since spina bifida affects the ability of the child to move, alternate ways for the child to experience its environment must be considered. Parents will need help accepting and finding appropriate mobility devices for their child. Physical therapy is often indicated at this time to promote the development of gross motor skills. Physically moving the child from one area to another will increase the child's awareness of its surroundings. With a little ingenuity, it is possible to provide the child with ample opportunities to see and experience the world.

## School Age

The task of the school-age child is to succeed at school and develop friendships while the role of parents is to promote optimal growth and development. Achieving success or mastery is often difficult in the academic arena due to learning issues, and in the home due to a dependence on parents for help with daily living. Establishing friendships is often difficult because of the child's learning problems, hospitalizations, medical appointments, and mobility limitations, which impact opportunities for socialization. Parents of school-aged children will need help in understanding their child's educational abilities and their rights for services within the school system. With proper support services, it is possible for children to achieve academic success. Parents may need encouragement and ideas on how to promote maximum independence in their children. They will appreciate knowing what is available in their communities in terms of recreation for their child. Seeing their child first as a child will strengthen their willingness and desire to seek out play dates, assign chores, and discipline when necessary.

In a study looking at parenting stress in families of children with spina bifida, it was found that mothers of older children had more stress (6). Parents reported receiving sufficient attention and support during the birth–preschool years, but regretted the decreased attention and loss of regular support as their children grew older (7). During the school years, the negative effects of the child's disability on the family increase (8).

## Adolescence

Parents of teenagers seek to find the delicate balance between allowing their child too much freedom and responsibility to unduly restricting them. Managing the needs of an adolescent with spina bifida, while at the same time fostering the teen's need to function independently, creates a particular challenge for parents. The medical needs of the individual with spina bifida often result in parental over-protectiveness. In a study that looked at family and peer relationships among adolescents with spina bifida and cerebral palsy, 27.5% of the respondents with spina bifida said they objected to parents' over-protectiveness evidenced by excessive assistance, reminders, and recommendations about what to do and what not to do (9). One might hypothesize that with the parents' continued close involvement in the life of the adolescent with spina bifida at a time when adolescents typically are seeking more independence, problems might ensue. However, some studies have shown that the opposite is true. The relationship between adolescents with spina bifida and their parents is characterized by one of relative harmony in contrast to the common turbulent adolescent–parent relationship often seen in families with children without disabilities (9,10). While the protection and closeness may be comforting, it may be that it delays adolescent development (9).

Since achieving an identity apart from their parents is so important for young adults, parents of teens may need help from HCPs to identify ways they can promote individuation. Developing self-skills so that the adolescents are able to assume their own care will help decrease their dependence on their parents. It is important to remember that this process of transferring responsibility from parent to child when so much is at stake is a difficult one. Ideally, it begins in childhood and responsibility gradually shifts as the child matures. Parents relate a range of parenting approaches they face when raising an adolescent with spina bifida from openly acknowledging their over-protectiveness to being able to encourage the teen's autonomy (11).

Adolescents face the task of learning acceptance and responsibility for their changing physical body. Here, too, adolescents with spina bifida face particular challenges as they come to terms with the fact that their bodies are different from that of their peers. Teens will need gentle guidance and information at this time about spina bifida and how it affects them in terms of sexual expression, fertility, and parenting. It is important to help these adolescents achieve some of the same experiences as their peers, such as driving, dating, and working. HCPs should, at this time, shift their focus from the parents to the teens, since ultimately it will be the responsibility of the young adult with spina bifida to get their own needs met.

Parents will need ongoing support, education, and understanding to foster optimal development of their child throughout all the developmental stages of childhood. The normal developmental changes of childhood are compounded by the chronic disability. Interventions that focus on anticipatory guidance and practical solutions to day-to-day problems will increase the likelihood that parents will successfully support their child's mastery of these tasks. The goal is to help parents foster as near-normal life experiences as possible for their children.

## IMPACT ON MARITAL RELATIONSHIP

The whole family will be affected by having a family member with a chronic disability. Just as a child with spina bifida has specific needs, parents and siblings of the child have needs. Promoting the needs of one member of the family over those of others will lead to imbalance in the family system (12). In a study that included a family assessment component, one-fourth of the 54 families reported difficulty with maintaining roles and boundaries within and between family members (13). Although more studies have focused on mothers than fathers, in general parents often report feeling less satisfied and competent as parents, and more isolated, with a decreased ability to adapt to change (14). A study by Heaman that looked at stresses of 70 fathers and 133 mothers of children with developmental disabilities found that the greatest stressors of both parents revolved around the child's future. Three-fourths of the mothers reported worries about money and feelings of exhaustion with all the demands on their time. Fathers stressed about the inability to go somewhere with their spouse without the child, having enough time to spend with their spouse, the child's health, and having sufficient money (15). It is unclear if having a child with spina bifida increases the chance of marital problems. It may even be that having a child with a disability strengthens a marriage. Loebig reported that of the six married mothers interviewed in her study, half reported that having a child with a disability made their relationship with their partner stronger (16). Many mothers of children with spina bifida in a study conducted by Bower and Hayes reported similar positive results (17). As with many of life's problems that married couples face, it makes sense that if the marriage was strong prior to the event—whether that event be the birth of a child with a disability or something else—it will remain strong or, perhaps, grow stronger despite external circumstances. As Duvall describes in her theory, it is the satisfying marital relationship that is critical to the functioning of the family (1).

## IMPACT ON SIBLINGS

While siblings do not have the responsibility and needs that either the child with the disability or the parents do, there is no question that there will be some impact in their lives. Since the siblings too are developing and growing, their feelings and understanding about their brother or sister will change over time. School-aged siblings may at times feel embarrassed or resentful, and older siblings may wonder about the hereditary possibilities and their future role as potential caregivers (18). A mother's mood and her perceptions about her own ability to have some control over the illness will likely have a positive effect on how well siblings are able to adjust to their brother or sister (19,20). Siblings often take their cues from their parents. If the parents are coping and doing relatively well, it is likely that the siblings will follow suit. In fact, there are reports of positive benefits—increased compassion, tolerance, and empathy—of growing up with a sibling with a chronic disability (21). The focus needs to be on fostering these positive traits versus dwelling on potential problems.

A healthy outcome for all family members faced with the day-to-day challenges of living with a chronic disability is possible. Building relationships and community supports around the family will help offset some of the difficulties that will inevitably arise. Supporting the family's need to share information and responsibility will do much to lessen any one individual member's sense of isolation and duty. Interestingly, in a study that compared mothers of children with spina bifida with mothers of children with Down syndrome and mothers of typically growing children, sibling harmony was the concern most consistently raised by all (17). Sibling harmony will help achieve a healthy family outcome as well as a satisfying marital relationship.

## CHRONIC SORROW CONCEPT

The term chronic sorrow has been used to describe the periodic episodes of sadness that many parents of a child with a disability will experience over time. While the initial feelings of sadness, anger, grief, and guilt around the time of diagnosis is expected, it is important to recognize that some of these same feelings manifest themselves later when developmental tasks are delayed or never achieved by the child, when there is an increase in symptoms, or when there is a change in the family support system (22). As parents witness the disparity between their child and others, manifestations of grief are likely (23).

HCPs will need to be especially supportive during these critical times in order to lessen the impact of these low periods on members of the family. Parents will appreciate understanding and an individualized approach. Helping the parent take a one-day-at-a-time approach instead of considering all the potential problems down the road supports a model based on strengths versus deficits. The parent has a lifetime to adjust and change. It is neither necessary, nor realistic, to expect immediate compliance to all the medical advice given, despite its wisdom.

Acknowledging the parents' right to be sad during particularly trying times as well as celebrating their success through those periods is critical to their mental well-being. Asking the parents how they are doing and then being willing to listen will provide support and verification. Chronic sorrow does not necessarily equal a diagnosis of depression, nor does it signify perpetual sadness. Parents of children with disabilities will also experience intense periods of joy and satisfaction at their children's accomplishments the same as other parents. Having a child with a disability and the feelings that accompany it is an individual experience with manifestations of a range of emotions, from despair and sorrow to optimism, hope, and joy (24). Celebrating small successes is essential to adapting to and raising a child with a disability.

## FAMILY COPING STRATEGIES

There is no question that there are stresses that exist when a family has a child with spina bifida. Some families are crushed by those stresses, whereas others successfully maneuver through them and continue to function appropriately. The concept of resiliency is that it is possible to balance out negative factors in one's life by increasing more positive ones. Numerous studies have cited some of the coping behaviors used by parents of children with disabilities. Fostering and encouraging these traits in the families served will increase the likelihood of their successful passage through the inevitable hills and valleys associated with living with a chronic illness (25).

One way in which parents cope is by stressing the normal aspects of their lives. They look on the bright side of things and use reframing as a mechanism to constantly define what is normal for them (26). Parents will often go to great lengths to help their child appear and act as normal as possible, as well as instruct others, such as extended family members and community systems, on how to interact with their child (27). Promoting and encouraging normal life experiences benefits the child due to increased social opportunities, development of self-help skills, and subsequent increase in self-esteem. The parents benefit because they are more likely to take time for themselves and engage in normal family and community activities (28).

Closely aligned with this concept of normalization is maintaining a positive outlook. Maintaining a hopeful and optimistic outlook was cited by many of the parents as a coping mechanism (29). Horton and Wallander found that mothers in a high-stress situation who report a high level of hope exhibit less distress than those with low levels. In a study that looked at coping by mothers and fathers of children with spina bifida (30), faith in God and having religious connections was mentioned frequently by both mothers and fathers (31).

Another mentioned coping behavior is assigning meaning to the illness. A parent needs information and experience to develop eventual understanding. Armed with knowledge, parents are able to build upon their confidence and believe that they are capable of managing (27).

Formal and informal social supports are powerful tools used to help parents cope (27,28,32). Social supports were also cited in the Horton and Wallander study as factors in alleviating maternal distress (30). As the number of social supports and adult companionships increase, so too does maternal satisfaction (33). HCPs can promote increased participation in social support systems by recognizing the positive value of a family's own support system and by connecting families to community support.

Positive coping styles, social support, and other resources should be promoted to offset the more negative variables of the disability. The ideal being that the more positive factors that can be utilized in a situation, the less likely that negative factors will affect the individual/family (25).

## WORKING WITH CULTURALLY DIVERSE FAMILIES

Every third United States resident represents a minority, according to the U.S. Bureau of the Census 2000. As the faces of Americans have changed over the years, so too have American values, with greater tolerance and appreciation for cultural diversity. It is imperative that the medical community also embrace this attitude of acceptance and understanding, since language barriers and culture will have an impact on health care. With so many immigrants from Mexico and Asia, and spina bifida affecting both these nationalities, it is likely that HCPs working in spina bifida clinics will interact with families of Latino and Asian descent.

Flores proposed the use of a five-component model when working with patients of various cultural groups. The HCP will need a basic understanding of normative culture values (34). For example, respect is held in high regard by Latino families. Latinos generally view providers as authority figures who should be respected; therefore, they will be respectful of their position and, in turn, will expect reciprocal respect. In practice, Latinos may nod and generally appear to agree with the provider out of respect, but not agree with what the provider is saying and thus not follow the instructions once home. Likewise, the family that feels the provider is disrespectful is more likely to be dissatisfied with the care they receive and not follow through with therapeutic regimes. HCPs will, therefore, need to identify cultural values that affect health care and adjust their practice accordingly (35).

The next issue to consider is language barriers (34). Families unable to speak or understand the language of their health-care provider will be at a significant disadvantage. Not only will the HCP have difficulty eliciting accurate medical information—which could, potentially, lead to serious medical complications later—the family will be unable to understand the medical advice given. Obviously, the use of well-trained interpreters is of paramount importance in the medical arena, where misunderstandings can be life-threatening (35).

The third consideration has to do with folk illnesses (34). Ethnic groups that adhere to folk illnesses and the prescribed treatment for those illnesses will often find themselves at odds with professionals who prescribe more traditional approaches. For example, while discussing constipation and treatment regimes, the culturally sensitive professional working with a Latino family should explore the family's beliefs around empacho. This condition is believed to be caused by something getting stuck to the walls of the intestines causing obstruction (35). The family may confuse the symptoms of constipation caused by a neurogenic bowel with empacho and may use a treatment based on that assumption that contradicts the prescribed treatments and/or is potentially harmful to the child.

The fourth issue has to do with identifying parent's beliefs and how they differ from more conventional beliefs (34). HCPs who are able to respect and listen to the families' beliefs will have a greater chance of helping the families adapt to a new practice. The family will need a thorough explanation of the cause and treatment rationale if they are to successfully change a way of thinking that is based on the wisdom of previous generations (35).

The last consideration in Flores' model is provider practices. Often individuals from different cultures receive lower quality care (34). Prejudice and subsequent substandard care is obviously a practice that needs monitoring and prompt correction. Satisfaction surveys of clients served is one method of gathering this data. The model thus described is a framework for providers to use in their desire to provide culturally competent care (34).

## CREATING PARTNERSHIPS WITH FAMILIES

Although many professionals believe in the principles of family-centered care, their ability to consistently practice that philosophy is often diminished due to constraints of time and resources. Building partnerships with families requires a considerable degree of commitment. To what degree the child's disability affects the child or the family will differ considerably from family to family, which makes working with each family, and being supportive, a unique and challenging endeavor. A study that obtained information from 124 families who had a child with a chronic illness or disability discovered that many of the unsupportive behaviors attributed to HCPs revolved around communication (36). Communication breakdown hinders both the HCP and the parent from building solid relationships. Parents have valuable information about their child to share and are frustrated when no one takes the time to listen. Appreciating their children for what they can do, maintaining hope, and respecting their opinions and decisions are critical for fostering collaboration.

Perhaps at no other time are the stress levels of parents as high as during a hospitalization of their children. Families are required to alter their routines and roles when their children are in the hospital. HCPs need to appreciate the difficulties parents face as they try to maintain their parental role within the hospital setting. Stress that is frequently cited by families with hospitalized children is difficulty in communication and coordination of care for their children (37). Families seek information about their children and the situation and may question different professionals to get the answers they seek. It is important during this stressful period to take the time to explain procedures, answer questions, and involve the parents in all-important decisions about the care of their children. Without exception, parents of children with long-term disabilities that are hospitalized emphasize the importance of clear, honest, open communication (38). With adequate information, parents will be able to learn how to modify their roles within the hospital setting. As their feelings of control increase, their stress will decrease.

Practicing family-centered care culminates in an appreciation for the medical home concept. The American Academy of Pediatrics believes that all children, adolescents, and young adults should have access to a medical home that provides comprehensive, coordinated, and family-centered health care. This philosophy includes children with special health-care needs, even though practicing this in the community may be filled with challenges. Physicians, nurses, and other HCPs need to increase their knowledge of community resources and create partnerships with these providers as well as with the parents of children they see. These partnerships will enable them to not only work more efficiently, but also to see an increase in satisfaction with the care they provide (39). The ultimate consequence is that families will have confidence that they have professionals who know them, who are knowledgeable and available, and who are willing to coordinate the services they need. This type of partnership will be a great comfort to parents and will increase their ability to cope.

## SUMMARY

With pressures and time constraints, it is tempting to deal with children and their needs only at the time of the visit to the HCP or office. However, the child with a disability will impact the family just as the family will impact the health of the child. HCPs who ignore the importance of family-focused care will deliver less-than-optimal care to their patients. Our role is to support the family in achieving family and individual developmental tasks. Our reward will be improved health of the entire family and increased family satisfaction with the delivery of health care.

Many families are able to rise to the challenge of raising a child with a disability. Researchers should closely examine the strengths and coping strategies in these families. Practitioners can then foster these positive practices in the families they work with—families that have children with a chronic illness.

## REFERENCES

1. Duvall EM. Marriage and Family Development. 5th ed. Philadelphia: Lippincott, 1977.
2. Erikson EH. Childhood and Society. New York: Norton, 1950.
3. Friedman M, Bowden V, Jones E. Family Nursing Research, Theory, and Practice. 5th ed. New Jersey: Prentice Hall, 2003.
4. Shonkoff J, Phillips D. From Neurons To Neighborhoods. Washington DC: National Academy Press, 2000.
5. Ramey C, Ramey S. Right from Birth. New York: Goddard Press, 1999.
6. Maricas M, Clifford S, Saylor C, Kreh S. Predictors of parenting stress in families of children with spina bifida. Child Health Care 2001; 30(1):57–65.
7. Havermans T, Eisnr C. Mother's perception of parenting a child with spina bifida. Child Care Health Dev 1991; 17:259–273.
8. Singh D. Families of children with spina bifida: a review. J Dev Phys Disabil 2003; 15(1):37–55.
9. Blum R, Resnick M, Nelson R, St. Germaine A. Family and peer issues among adolescents with spina bifida and cerebral palsy. Pediatrics 1991; 88(2):280–285.
10. Coakley R, Holmbeck G, Friedman D, Greenley D, Greenley R, Thill A. A longitudinal study of pubertal timing, parent-child conflict, and cohesion in families of young adolescents with spina bifida. Soc Pediatr Psychol 2002; 27(5):461–473.
11. Sawin K, Hayden M, Roux G, Buran C, Brie T, Fastenau P. The experience of parenting an adolescent with spina bifda. Rehabil Nurs 2003; 28(6):173–185.
12. Patterson J, Gerber G. Preventing mental health problems in children with chronic illness or disability. CHC 1991; 20(3):150–158.
13. Ammerman R, Kane V, Slomka G, Reigel D, Franzen M, Gadow K. Psychiatric symptomatolgy and family functioning in children and adolescents with spina bifida. J Clin Psychol Med Sett 1998; 5(4):449–465.
14. Holmbeck G, Gorey-Ferguson L, Hudson T, et al. Maternal, paternal, and marital functioning in families of preadolescents with spina bifida. J Pediatr Psychol 1997; 22(2):167–181.

15. Heaman D. Perceived stressors and coping strategies of parents who have children with developmental disabilities: a comparison of mothers and fathers. J Pediatr Nurs 1995; 10(5):311–319.
16. Loebig M. Mothers' assessment of the impact of children with spina bifida on the family. Matern Child Nurs 1990; 19(3):251–267.
17. Bower A, Hayes A. Mothering in families with and without a child with disability. Int J Disabil Dev Educ 1998; 45(3):313–322.
18. Children with disabilities: understanding sibling issues. NICHCY 1998: News Digest 11.
19. Daux Williams P, Williams A, Hanson S, et al. Maternal mood, family functioning, and perceptions of social support, self-esteem, and mood among siblings of chronically ill children. Child Health Care 1999; 28(4):297–310.
20. Gallo A, Breitmayer B, Knaft K, Zoeller L. Mothers' perceptions of sibling adjustment and family life in childhood chronic illness. J Pediatr Nurs 1993; 8(5):318–324.
21. McKeever P. Siblings of chronically ill children: a literature review with implications for research and practice. Am J Orthopsychiatric 1983; 53(2):209–217.
22. Clubb R. Chronic sorrow: adaptation patterns of parents with chronically ill children. Pediatr Nurs 1991; 17(5):461–466.
23. Teel C. Chronic sorrow: analysis of the concept. J Adv Nurs 1991; 16:1311–1319.
24. Kearney P, Griffin T. Between joy and sorrow: being a parent of a child with developmental disability. J Adv Nurs 2001; 34(5):582–592.
25. Masten A. Ordinary magic: resilience processes in development. Psyc Articles 2001; 56(3):227–288.
26. Robinson C. Managing life with a chronic condition: the story of normalization. Qual Health Res 1993; 3(1):2–28.
27. Holaday B. Challenges of rearing a chronically ill child. Nurs Clin North Am 1984; 19(2):361–368.
28. Patterson J. Family resilience to the challenge of a child's disability. Pediatr Ann 1991; 20(9):491–499.
29. Ray L, Ritchie J. Caring for chronically ill children at home: factors that influence parents' coping. J Pediatr Nurs 1993; 8(4):217–225.
30. HortonV, Wallander J. Hope and social support as resilience factors against psychological distress of mothers who care for children with chronic physical conditions. Rehabil Psychol 2001; 46(4) 382–399.
31. Samuelson J, Foltz J, Foxall M. Stress and coping in families of children with myelomeningocele. Arch Psychiatr Nurs 1992; 4(5):287–295.
32. RanTak Y, McCubbin M. Family stress, perceived social support and coping following the diagnosis of a child's congenital heart disease. J Adv Nurs 2002; 39(2):190–198.
33. Fagan J, Schor D. Mothers of children with spina bifida: factors related to maternal psychosocial functioning. J Orthopsychiatric 1993; 63(1):146–152.
34. Flores G. Culture and the patient-physicaina relationship: achieving cultural competency in health care. J Pediatrics 2000; 136(1):14–23.
35. Flores G, Abreu M, Schwartz I, Hill M. The importance of language and culture in pediatric care: case studies from the latino community. J Pediatrics 2000; 137(6):842–848.
36. Garwick A, Patterson J, Bennett F, Blum R. Parents' perceptions of helpful vs. unhelpful types of support in managing the care of adolescents with chronic conditions. ARCH Pediatr Adol Med 1998; 152:665–671.

37. Horn J, Feldman H, Ploof D. Parent and professional perceptions about stress and coping strategies during a child's lengthy hospitalization. Soc Work Pediatr 1995; 21(1):107–127.
38. Hayes V, Knox J. The experience of stress in parents of children hospitalized with long-term disabilities. J Adv Nurs 1984; 9:333–341.
39. Nickel R, Cooley C, McAllister J, Samson-Fang L. Building medical homes for children with special health care needs. Infant Young Child 2003; 16(4):331–341.

# 13

# Ethical Issues

**Linda S. Lazar**
*Division of Developmental and Behavioral Pediatrics, Cincinnati Children's Hospital Medical Center, Cincinnati, Ohio, U.S.A.*

## INTRODUCTION

The neural tube is laid down so early in fetal development that malformations, which will eventually become neural tube defects, are determined by 26 days postconception. Perhaps it is not surprising then that the issues surrounding the care and treatment of these children encompass the most fundamental of ethical dilemmas: When does life begin? When does life end? What is a life worth living? What constitutes futile therapy? Who should decide? The history of confronting these questions is replete with ethical people attempting to make ethical decisions that affect the lives of these children and their families often coming up with very different solutions. And today, within the new frontier of fetal therapeutics, these same dilemmas, and some new ones, re-emerge.

This chapter chronicles some of the abundant history of ethical issues surrounding therapeutic interventions for neural tube defects and looks at the anticipated challenges for the future. For those unfamiliar with the terminology, a basic overview of fundamental ethical principles related to decision making in health care may be helpful.

1. Respect for autonomy, from the Greek "autos" and "nomos," meaning self-rule. This is a complex concept with significance that varies among cultures, but all theories agree that it includes the ability to make voluntary, intentional action, independent of controlling

influences (1). Autonomy comes from an even more inclusive principle, that of "respect for persons," and the significance of this is relevant to pediatric ethics. Autonomy presumes competent adults, able to make decisions on their own behalf, and is the underlying principle that enables adults to make advanced directives and have informed consent. Respect for persons, however, also includes "protection of the vulnerable." This obligates those with this capacity to make decisions in the "best interest" of those without: either those who never had it, such as children, or those who lost it due to age or debility.

2. Nonmaleficence, from the Greek "Primum non nocere," meaning "first do no harm." This is often attributed to Hippocrates and is a loose interpretation of one part of the oath. This principle comes into play in issues such as killing versus letting die, withholding and withdrawing life-sustaining medical treatments, and the meaning of futility, all of which have affected decisions regarding children with neural tube defects (2).
3. Beneficence is often considered to be a more demanding ethical obligation, on the same continuum as nonmaleficence, and means the obligation to provide benefit or take steps to help others (3). It underlies many of the same circumstances as nonmaleficence and is foundational in deciding the risks and benefits of treatments and procedures.
4. The principle of justice moves into the forefront when discussing inequities in health-care access along with its rising costs. This concept is inherent in discussions about which newborns to save, how the decisions should be made, and what actions constitute the greater good to society.

This overview of ethical principles, albeit brief, should serve as a backdrop for considering historical controversies surrounding children with neural tube defects, specifically anencephaly and spina bifida, and in anticipating future dilemmas in the rapidly progressing field of fetal therapeutics.

## DEFINING LIFE AND DEATH: THE ANENCEPHALIC INFANT

### Anencephaly and Organ Donation

In the 1990s, approximately 500 children needed heart transplants, 500 needed livers, and 400 to 500 needed kidney transplants each year in the United States. Because of the shortage of organs small enough, 40% to 70% of these children died awaiting suitable organs and many more probably died before even being listed (4). This formed the setting for the controversy over using viable organs from anencephalic neonates for transplantation. This idea was not a new one; in fact, only a few days after the first adult heart transplant, a heart was transplanted from an anencephalic newborn into another infant. The recipient died within six hours (5).

Although the incidence of anencephaly is quite small, it is obviously an enormous heartache to those families affected. It was, therefore, not surprising that parents, as well as health-care professionals, viewed the possibility of these children becoming organ donors as a means to salvage some benefit from their tragedy.

To fully comprehend the dilemma presented by this situation, one must look at the legal and ethical rules surrounding organ donation and, indeed, in defining death. The ethical and legal foundation of organ donation in this country, in the 1990s and today, is the "Dead Donor Rule," which states that donors cannot be killed in order to obtain their organs; organ retrieval itself cannot cause death, even if doing so saves the lives of others (6). This rule is based on the ethical principle of respect for persons and helps to maintain the public trust in the organ donation system.

The requirement of death (cardiorespiratory or brain) prior to the harvesting of organs underlies the impasse to the use of organs from anencephalic neonates: the diagnosis of anencephaly does not in of itself equate to brain death. While these infants lack an upper brain, they do have brain stem function, and thus do not meet the ethical/legal definition of death.

As often happens with ethical dilemmas in the medical field, the controversy over anencephalic infants becoming organ donors hit the popular press and talk show circuit, arousing emotions and misunderstanding on both sides of the debate. This was the milieu when the birth of "Baby Theresa" occurred in Florida in 1992. Her parents wished to have her declared brain dead in order to donate her organs. In spite of severe anencephaly, Baby Theresa did not meet Harvard brain death criteria, and the hospital would not remove her organs under this circumstance. The parents appealed to the Florida circuit court, the District Court of Appeals, and finally the Florida Supreme Court. The infant was eventually removed from life support when her organs began to fail, though the Supreme Court eventually ruled, after her death, that "... anencephalic newborns are not considered dead for purposes of organ donation" (6).

Then in 1994, the American Medical Association (AMA) Council on Ethical and Judicial Affairs, citing the shortage of available organs for transplantation in infants and children, and the potential benefits to the parents of anencephalic infants, proposed the following guidelines:

> It is ethically permissible to consider the anencephalic neonate as a potential organ donor, although still alive under the current definition of death, only if (*i*) the diagnosis of anencephaly is certain and is confirmed by two physicians with special expertise who are not part of the organ transplant team, (*ii*) the parents of the neonate initiate any discussions about organ retrieval and indicate their desire for retrieval in writing, and (*iii*) there is compliance with the Council's Guidelines for the Transplantation of Organs (4).

The council acknowledged that transplantation could occur by first establishing brain or cardiorespiratory death, but pointed out the risk of the waiting time making the organs unusable. More notably, they advocated making organ donation from anencephalic neonates an exception to the dead donor rule, because these infants "... have never experienced, and will never experience, consciousness" (4). They recognized that current laws would need to be changed for this to occur.

This issue evoked a number of fundamental ethical problems. A key aspect of the principles of respect for persons, beneficence, and nonmaleficence is that for the incompetent patient, such as a child, medical decisions must be made in the "best interest" of that patient. Typically, it is the parent who is entrusted with making those decisions and they should do it by weighing the burdens and benefits of the treatment or procedure in question. Most agreed that anencephalics met the definition of personhood, and thus this standard could be applied. However, these affected neonates presented a unique situation. Best-interest judgments are supposed to focus on the value of a life to the individual (7), but because they have no consciousness, the value of an anencephalic's life is only a value for others (4). The AMA used this line of reasoning to validate their position of parents' rights to choose organ donation, with the assertion that this would necessitate changing definitions of personhood for this particular circumstance.

The justice principle underscored an even greater difficulty with the AMA's position statement. This argument was that the dead donor rule "... must not be applied without regard to whether its application serves its purposes" (4). In the case of the anencephalic infant, a greater good would be served for the donor's parents and for society as a whole by suspending the rule in this one circumstance. They acknowledged that the potential number of organ recipients may be small, but even 20 per year would be worth saving.

Arguments against this form of organ donation primarily related to "slippery slope" concerns. The natural history of anencephalic neonates is as described previously because most are given only comfort-oriented care. However, many could survive long enough for organ retrieval in a condition similar to persistent vegetative state, with more supportive care (8). In other words, the infants would be kept alive only for their organs. This fact concerned disability advocates and others who questioned what other groups of individuals who lack cognition may become potential organ donors; would we next consider severe microcephalics and others? Those opposing this unique form of organ donation maintained that the combination of these slippery slope matters, plus the relatively few number of potential lives saved, did not justify redefining personhood or relaxing the dead donor rule (6,9). The issue of anencephalic neonates as organ donors soon faded away from professional and lay discussions, due to these irreconcilable dilemmas and possibly also to the arrival of living donor transplantation, and improvements in surgical treatments for hypoplastic left heart syndrome.

## Anencephaly and Futility

At nearly the same time that the "Baby Theresa" case was unfolding in Florida, the "Baby K" case took the ethical center stage in Virginia. Although diagnosed with anencephaly prenatally, Baby K's mother chose not to terminate the pregnancy. She was vehemently opposed to abortion, or to any sort of withdrawal of life support, based on her religious values. Having an intact brainstem and normal organ function, the baby met the criteria for personhood in all 50 states (10), as explained in the previous discussion. Baby K presented neonatologists and ethicists with the opposite dilemma from the transplantation issue—what to do when the parents desire aggressive therapy, including feeding tube, tracheotomy, and intermittent hospitalization and mechanical ventilation in order to maintain life. This case engendered fundamental differences of opinion: the rights of parents, the role of religion and values in decision making, and the meaning of futility.

Trotter (11) referred to futility as "... a simple concept that is difficult to interpret in clinical practice." It involves a therapeutic goal, an action aimed at achieving the goal, and virtual certainty that the goal cannot be achieved by that action. Where ethicists have historically disagreed with each other, and often diverged from the legal community, is in defining what the actual goal is when deciding if some medical therapy is futile. Some have proposed a very narrow view—that a treatment is futile only if it cannot achieve purely physiologic goals, such as maintaining heart and lung function (12). Others have included quality of life determinations in assessing futility, but leave the physician to ultimately make the decisions (13). The broadest views advocate incorporating physiology, quality of life, and family values in a shared decision making between the physician and family in making futility decisions (14).

These opposing viewpoints were brought to light in the case of Baby K. During her first two months of life, each time she went into respiratory distress the mother insisted on mechanical ventilation. When she stabilized enough to be transferred to a nursing home, the mother insisted on returning her to the hospital for ventilatory support whenever the baby had breathing difficulties. The hospital went to court to prevent this aggressive treatment based on several state and federal laws, the most important being the Emergency Medical Treatment and Active Labor Act of 1986 (EMTALA), which states that physicians may withhold medical treatment that they determine to be "... medically or ethically inappropriate" (15). The case went through multiple levels of state and federal courts, and the hospital even tried to bring it before the Supreme Court, which has consistently upheld parents' rights to make decisions for their children, and to freely exercise their religious beliefs on behalf of their children, unless doing so constitutes abuse or neglect (10). The hospital's argument was that the condition being treated was anencephaly, and thus aggressive treatment was futile; the family argued that it was apnea/

bradypnea being addressed, and thus the therapy was not futile. The lower courts consistently ruled in favor of the family, citing EMTALA as well as the Rehabilitation Act and Americans with Disabilities Act (ADA) legislation that would be violated if treatment was withheld (10). It was further upheld that ventilating Baby K did not constitute abuse or neglect, and that quality of life and futility standards that are an integral part of bioethics principles do not have legal bearing in cases such as these (16).

In both the case of Baby K and the rejection of the AMA's proposal to allow anencephalic infants as organ donors, the views of medicine and bioethicists may have reflected the prevailing values in society. However, the legal system rejected creating what would essentially have been another class of individuals with diminished human rights (16).

## DEFINING QUALITY OF LIFE: THE INFANT WITH SPINA BIFIDA

### Historical Perspective

The history of treatment decisions for infants born with spina bifida can be deemed a case study in "the more things change, the more they remain the same." The questions of whether or not to treat and how aggressively to treat have vexed physicians, lawmakers, and ethicists, particularly since the 1960s. The ethical dilemmas inherent in these questions are what defines quality of life, what is a life worth living, who should decide, and how should these decisions be made? The technological advances that have steadily become more available for these children have not made the ethical questions any easier to answer.

Prior to the 1960s, it was rare to find reference to ethical dilemmas in medicine. It was the tail end of the long-standing "age of paternalism," in which physicians made most, if not all, medical decisions in the "best interest" of their patients. The technologies for pediatric anesthesia, closure of spinal lesions, and placement of shunts was absent or poor, rendering the surgical procedures as risky as no treatment at all (17). Closure was typically not attempted if children had high lesions or no lower motor function. Closures that were attempted were often unsuccessful. Only if a child survived the first year, through epithelialization of their lesion and resolution of any hydrocephalus, was restorative or preventative orthopedic and urologic treatment initiated to improve the quality of life.

The 1960s brought improvements in pediatric surgery and anesthesia and the development of the Holter valve for hydrocephalus. These changes engendered a paradigm shift in the treatment of infants born with spina bifida. All, or nearly all, were treated early with closure and shunting, and meningitis was treated aggressively with antibiotics, resulting in improvements in both quantity and quality of life (18). What did not change was the paternalism of the medical community. These treatment decisions continued to be made usually without consulting with parents, and the role of informed consent was largely perfunctory.

This "technological imperative" for treating newborns with spina bifida formed the backdrop for the groundbreaking work of Dr. John Lorber of Sheffield, England, referred to in the preface. Noting that the natural progression of the disorder meant that nearly all would be dead by the age of two and questioning the practice of aggressive and early treatment of the previous 12 years, Lorber sought to develop criteria based on probable outcomes, for deciding which newborns to treat and which to allow to die untreated (19,20). He undertook substantial retrospective reviews of 524 patients. He concluded that the current system of treating virtually all of these infants was an "untenable position" when future quality of life was considered (19). Lorber divided the children who had survived early aggressive treatment into five categories based on their degree of handicap and correlated this with the level of the initial lesion. Conditions described as incompatible with a reasonable quality of life included below average intelligence, paraplegia, urinary and fecal incontinence, and kyphosis and/or scoliosis. He considered these handicaps to be "... inconsistent with self-respect, earning capacity, happiness and even marriage," rendering only 7% of the children in his cohort having a life deemed worth living (19). He asserted that those with normal intelligence would suffer even more than others, as they would be more aware of their deficits. Believing that few would want to save children whose life would be characterized by physical deficits with multiple hospitalizations and procedures, Lorber proposed definitive criteria that could be ascertained at birth, for deciding which children to treat aggressively and which to allow to die without treatment (20). Lorber's system was put into practice in his community, and a later paper documented the outcomes for the 12 children who were treated and the 25 who were denied closure and shunt placement according to his protocol (21). All in the nontreatment cohort died within nine months, with demand feedings and comfort measures only. Of the treated group, only the one child who had initial "adverse criteria" (a high lesion) went on to have "severe handicaps" (21).

Attempts to duplicate these results in other centers, including in the United States, were unsuccessful. Untreated children did not die early; in fact, many did not die at all. It was later determined that Lorber's untreated patients were given chloral hydrate and morphine to prevent seizures and pain, resulting in oversedation and poor feeding; such drugs were not routinely used for these infants in the United States (17,22). The consequence of these later findings was that Lorber's system was effectively abandoned by the end of the decade in the United States. Pediatric facilities throughout the country formed multidisciplinary teams including neurosurgeons, urologists, and orthopedists to provide the best outcomes for children. There was one unexpected trial of "selective nontreatment" of children born with spina bifida attempted in the 1980s (23), which drew an outpouring of negative responses and was soon discontinued (17).

The 1980s ushered in a new era for medical ethics. Hospitals developed bioethics committees, the President's Commission for the Study of Ethical Problems in Medicine (24) unveiled guidelines for ethical decision making in research and clinical care, and pediatricians had a mandate to be the child's advocate (25). Paternalism was giving way to patient autonomy, and informed consent was an expectation for medical procedures. Organ transplantation, legalized abortion, and well-publicized cases about withdrawal of life support forced the public to grapple with the issues of when life begins and ends. These forces all converged upon the issue of withholding treatment of severely impaired newborns, ultimately resulting in the "Baby Doe" regulations (26).

The Baby Doe regulations, codified in 1984, essentially considered nontreatment of newborns with disabilities as child abuse, with the only exceptions being a child who is (*i*) chronically and irreversibly comatose, (*ii*) inevitably dying, or (*iii*) when treatment would be futile and inhumane. Although these regulations were the culmination of many contested cases, the nominal Baby Doe was a newborn with Down syndrome and esophageal atresia, for whom corrective surgery was withheld; the infant died of dehydration and malnutrition.

Nearly in tandem with the Baby Doe case, an infant was born in Long Island, New York, with spina bifida, microcephaly, hydrocephalus, and a damaged kidney. Dubbed "Baby Jane Doe" in the media and the courts, the infant was predicted to die quickly without surgery. The parents decided to forego shunting or closure of the lesion, opting for palliative measures only. This case went from the media (*Newsday*, October 18, 1983) to the local courts, the state appellate court, the New York Court of Appeals, the U.S. Justice Department, the federal Court of Appeals, and eventually the U.S. Supreme Court. By that point, the issue at hand had become the government's right to have access to the baby's hospital records, which the courts did not uphold. This in effect rendered the government incapable of enforcing the Baby Doe rules (27). As for Baby Jane Doe, in the midst of all the legal proceedings, the parents did treat her hydrocephalus and other conditions as they developed. At age 10, she was described as "self-aware" and able to give and receive love; at age 15, she was still living with her parents and attending a school for children with disabilities (27).

By the late 1980s, it was clear that most children born with spina bifida do not die quickly of infection or hydrocephalus, so around 95% were being treated. The model of aggressive multidisciplinary medical and psychosocial support became the accepted paradigm for producing optimal outcomes (17).

Advances in ultrasonography and alpha-fetoprotein screening followed by amniocentesis since the 1990s have meant that most fetuses with open spina bifida are discovered prenatally. It is assumed that a great many are electively terminated, but the actual number is unknown (17). In addition, folic acid fortification began in March 1996, resulting in a decline in reported spina bifida birth rates since 1997 (28). Of those carried to term, 75% can be expected to reach adulthood (29), but survival does not guarantee a life without disability. Although most attend high school or college, problems with urinary or fecal incontinence, seizures, shunt problems, kypho/scoliosis, and tethered cord not only persist, but also can worsen over time (29).

## Ethical Dilemmas Persist

Because open spina bifida is the most complex congenital disability that is compatible with long-term survival, it is not surprising that the ethical dilemmas surrounding the decisions about treating these children remain controversial. Prenatal diagnosis of spina bifida typically occurs at 18 to 20 weeks gestation and the option of abortion is offered at that time. The problem is that the child's potential and the extent of future disability is unknowable; thus, the mandates of informed consent are not met (17). Throughout the years, many have argued that if parents have the right to abort these fetuses, they should also have the right to withhold life-saving treatment once the child is born, and the extent of the defect more apparent. This position might be ethically valid if the newborn with spina bifida fell under one of the Baby Doe exceptions. Spina bifida is a nonlethal anomaly if treated at birth, and newborns with the disorder are not chronically and irreversibly comatose. But could a parent make the decision that treatment would be "virtually futile and inhumane," and thus allow the child to die following the natural course of the disorder? If not the parent, who should be empowered to make the decision that a newborn's condition is such that it would constitute a Baby Doe exception, and how would the decision be made? It is known that predictions about long-term prognosis for these children are never conclusive, especially when estimating future intelligence (27). Compounding this is the reality of parents receiving different opinions from the various professionals in the multidisciplinary health-care team, who are no doubt influenced by their own ethical framework.

If there were general agreement that these are newborns who are "inevitably dying" or for whom treatment would be "futile and inhumane," would it then be reasonable to end their lives quickly, rather than through the slow and perhaps painful death from infection or increasing hydrocephalus? In other words, is there an ethical difference between withholding treatment and euthanasia? Of course, the latter is illegal in this country, but many have maintained that it would be the more humane option for these children (27,30). Indeed Lorber's work forced us to look at that very gray area between euthanasia and palliative care.

Inherent in these dilemmas are value judgments as to the quality of life of children with spina bifida. As noted with anencephaly, best interest decisions are typically trusted to the parents and are to be made relevant to the child's quality of life, not the family's. Nonetheless, do we want a family saddled with the lifelong care of an unwanted child with complex medical needs? But imagine the slippery slope of allowing a child to die simply because their disability does not "fit into their parents' plans" (27). Parents are given substantial rights to autonomous decisions about their children, but these rights are not absolute and cannot supersede the obligations of beneficence and nonmaleficence.

Clearly, the more than 40 years of technological advances and attempts at selective nontreatment have not resolved the ethical conundrums of spina bifida. Perhaps the years have merely enabled us to understand Freeman's conclusion that "... the process for arriving at a decision is far more important than the decision arrived at" (31).

## THE ISSUE OF PERSONHOOD: FETAL SURGERY FOR SPINA BIFIDA

### The Prospects for Intrauterine Repair

In spite of the declines in spina bifida birth rates attributable to increased folic acid supplementation and elective abortions, over 1000 are born with this condition yearly in the United States today (28,32). Surviving children will require costly multidisciplinary care, often with a lifetime of surgeries and therapies. These facts provided the impetus for attempting intrauterine repair of the lesion. The rationale for this endeavor, confirmed by animal studies, is known as the "two-hit hypothesis." This theory is that the sequelae of spina bifida result not only from the initial embryologic malformation, but also secondarily from exposure of the neurological tissue to trauma and amniotic fluid, especially with advancing gestational age (32,33). The hope was that intrauterine closure of the lesion would prevent the secondary damage and lead to better neurologic and orthopedic outcomes.

Open intrauterine repairs were first performed in 1997 at Vanderbilt University Medical Center and Children's Hospital of Philadelphia, and a total of 104 of these procedures were done and analyzed (32). These surgeries produced some surprising results. Although there did not appear to be any improvements in motor or urologic function, fetal surgery produced a definite decrease in the incidence of Chiari-related hindbrain herniation and shunt-dependent hydrocephalus associated with spina bifida. The intrauterine closure seems to change the flow of cerebral spinal fluid, decreasing the Chiari and, therefore, the need for shunting; these improvements were more significant with earlier gestational ages for the surgery (33–35). These early findings led the National Institute of Child Health and Human Development (NICHD) to authorize and fund a randomized clinical trial to evaluate this surgery versus the conventional treatment (32). This trial is currently in progress.

The apparent benefits of these surgeries did not come without some major complications. Compared with controls, fetal surgery for spina bifida resulted in an increased rate of premature deliveries, in spite of the use of tocolytics. Early figures of 4% mortality and 11% morbidity rates attributed to the surgery were reported, with birth weights and prematurity complications typical for those gestational ages (32,33). Though troubled by these findings, the researchers affirmed the benefits of the procedure outweighing the risks and recommended earlier gestational ages for repair of the defect to maximize the positive effects (32,33).

While these risks to the fetuses are well documented and quantified, there is much less data about the risks to the pregnant women. Fetal surgery involves a uterine incision and prolonged tocolysis, and carries the risks of uterine rupture, small bowel obstruction, compromised future reproductive status, psychological stress, and all other risks associated with major abdominal surgery (36,37).

Inherent risks to the pregnant mother and fetus are associated with all fetal surgeries, regardless of the defect being treated. In fact, surgeries to correct congenital anomalies date back to the 1980s with attempts to correct congenital diaphragmatic hernias, in which overall mortality rates were as high as 75% (32). The difference with the current drive to correct spina bifida in utero is a crucial one. Large morbidity and mortality rates for lethal anomalies are not only expected, but are considered worth the risk when the alternative is certain death. Spina bifida, however, is a nonlethal anomaly in which the surgery is an attempt to improve quality of life through opportunities for such things as improved mobility and urinary continence. So any increase in morbidity and mortality associated with the surgery must be weighed against a highly survivable disability (36,37). In fact, a fetal surgery that ends in fetal demise essentially turns a nonlethal anomaly into a lethal one.

## The Problem of Personhood

All of the fundamental principles of bioethics enter into the controversy over fetal surgery for spina bifida, and all revolve around the issue of personhood for the fetus. To appreciate the magnitude of these differences of opinion, one need only be reminded of the ongoing debate over abortion rights in this country, as it is in essence the same debate. One side ascribes full moral status to the fetus, equal to that of the mother, whereas the other side gives the fetus no moral status and allows the pregnant female total autonomy in choosing abortion. Proponents and critics of fetal surgery run the gamut regarding this crucial issue. Some argue that moral status increases with gestational age, and the fetus attains full personhood at the age of viability. Others propose "conferred moral status" meaning that by not choosing abortion, the pregnant female is obligated to make decisions in the fetus' best interest (36). Chervenak and McCullough (38) propose that it is not necessary to define personhood, but only to define the fetus as a patient. This confers upon the fetus the rights to treatment as a condition of beneficence, even if this is in conflict with the mother's right to autonomy. Bliton (39) defines the fetus' personhood from the perspective of the pregnant mother and her partner. Noting that the expectant couple refer to the fetus as their "baby" and often give it a name and moral status, its "life" and personhood essentially begins with the fetal surgery.

What most of these professionals fail to give credence to are the woman's rights not only to autonomy, but to nonmaleficence. According to Lyerly and Mahowald (36), ". . . there is one patient: the pregnant woman." Any treatment done for or to a fetus must go through the pregnant woman, and likewise anything done for or to her affects the fetus. So, a surgery that has definite risks with unproven benefits to a fetus, and clear risks with no benefits to the pregnant woman, may not be ethically justifiable.

The authors note that there may be a psychological benefit to the woman undergoing this surgery, which could outweigh the risks, but this has not been quantified or thoroughly researched.

Another potential erosion of autonomy is in the informed consent process. It is essential that the pregnant woman and her partner be informed of all possible risks and benefits to herself and the fetus. But until the clinical trial is completed, the extent of risks is not fully known. While the protocol of participating institutions includes a two-day process of meetings with all parties, including the bioethics team, parents often come to the meetings with preconceptions. Many couples noted that the initial responses and counseling they had received from obstetricians and others were skewed toward grim accounts of life for a child with spina bifida and toward termination of the pregnancy (37). Their decision not to abort, often based on religious principles and their perceptions about the disability, can further predispose them to choosing the fetal surgery without fully considering the risks (39). Their choice of surgery could be a tacit avowal that living with a disability may be worse than death (36).

The American Academy of Pediatrics statement on fetal therapy asserts that "... a pregnant woman should be discouraged from placing herself at undue risk where the potential benefit to the fetus is remote" (40). There is some data on the benefits to the fetus in terms of shunt-related hydrocephalus and Chiari related hindbrain herniation, though the long-term benefits of these are not yet known. It is hypothesized that earlier correction of the defect could produce even greater benefits for these and other aspects of the congenital anomaly, such as urinary and motor function. But earlier surgeries run the risk of premature delivery of a previable fetus and certain fetal demise. This must all be balanced against the rights of the pregnant female to autonomy and beneficence. The NICHD-funded randomized clinical trial will hopefully iron out some of the inherent ethical dilemmas. In the meanwhile, the data that we do have in abundance is on the thousands of children with spina bifida and who have received the conventional treatment over the last 25 to 30 years. It is the feeling of professionals that these individuals are living productive and satisfying lives in spite of their disability, but this too needs further research.

## REFERENCES

1. Beauchamp TL, Childress JF. Principles of Biomedical Ethics. 4th ed. New York: Oxford University Press, 1994:120–121.
2. Beauchamp TL, Childress JF. Principles of Biomedical Ethics. 4th ed. New York: Oxford University Press, 1994:189.
3. Beauchamp TL, Childress JF. Principles of Biomedical Ethics. 4th ed. New York: Oxford University Press, 1994:190.

4. Council on Ethical and Judicial Affairs, American Medical Association. The use of anencephalic neonates as organ donors. JAMA 1995; 273(20):1614–1618.
5. Pence GE. Classic Cases in Medical Ethics. 4th ed. New York: McGraw-Hill, 2004:345–365.
6. Robertson JA. The dead donor rule. Hastings Cent Rep 1999; 29(6):6–14.
7. Beauchamp TL, Childress JF. Principles of Biomedical Ethics. 4th ed. New York: Oxford University Press, 1994:178–180.
8. Berger DH. The infant with anencephaly: moral and legal dilemmas. Issues Law Med 1989; 5(1):67–85.
9. Committee on Bioethics, American Academy of Pediatrics. Infants with anencephaly as organ sources: ethical considerations. Pediatrics 1992; 89(6):1116–1119.
10. Flannery EJ. One advocate's viewpoint: conflicts and tensions in the *Baby K* case. J Law Med Ethics 1995; 23:7–12.
11. Trotter G. Mediating disputes about medical futility. Camb Q Healthc Ethics 1999; 8:527–537.
12. The Hastings Center. Guidelines on the Termination of Life-Sustaining Treatment and the Care of the Dying. Bloomington: Indiana University Press, 1987.
13. Nelson LJ, Nelson RM. Ethics and the provision of futile, harmful, or burdensome treatment to children. Critical Care Med 1992; 20(3):427–433.
14. Lantos JD. The illusion of futility in clinical practice. Am J Med 1989; 87:81–84.
15. Capron AM. Medical futility: strike two. Hastings Cent Rep 1994; 24(5):42–44.
16. Koch T, Ridgley M. Distanced perspectives: AIDS, anencephaly, and AHP. Theor Med Bioeth 1998; 19:47–58.
17. Freeman JM. Changing ethical issues in the treatment of spina bifida: a personal odyssey. Ment Retard Dev Disabil Res Rev 1998; 4:302–307.
18. Sharrard WJW, Zachary RB, Lorber J, Bruce AM. A controlled trial of immediate and delayed closure of spina bifida cystica. Arch Dis Childhood 1963; 38:18–22.
19. Lorber J. Results of treatment of myelomeningocele. Dev Med Child Neurol 1971; 13:279–303.
20. Lorber J. Spina bifida cystica: results of treatment of 270 consecutive cases with criteria for selection for the future. Arch Dis Childhood 1972 47:854–873.
21. Lorber J. Early results of selective treatment of spina bifida cystica. British Med J 1973; 4:201–204.
22. Zachary RB. Life with spina bifida. British Med J 1977; 2:1460–1462.
23. Gross RH, Cox A, Tatyrek R, Pollay M, Barnes WA. Early management and decision making for the treatment of myelomeningocele. Peds 1983; 72:450–458.
24. President's Commission for the Study of Ethical Problems in Medicine and Biomedical and Behavioral Research. Deciding to Forego Life-Sustaining Treatment. 1983.
25. American Academy of Pediatrics, Committee on Bioethics. Treatment of critically ill newborns. Peds 1983; 72:565–566.
26. Department of Human Services. Child abuse and neglect prevention and treatment program. Fed Reg 1985; 50:148788–148901.
27. Pence GE. Classic Cases in Medical Ethics. 4th ed. New York: McGraw-Hill, 2004:216–242.
28. National Center for Health Statistics, CDC. Trends in Spina Bifida and Anencephalus in the United States, 1991–2002. [On-line] Available: http://www.cdc.gov/nchs/products/pubs/pubd/hestats/spine_anen.htm

29. Bowman RM, McLone DG, Grant JA, Tomita T, Ito JA. Spina bifida outcome: a 25-year prospective. Peds Neurosurg 2001; 34:114–120.
30. Freeman JM. Is there a right to die—Quickly? J Peds 1972; 80(5):904–905.
31. Freeman JM. On learning humility: a thirty-year journey. Hastings Cent Rep 2004; 34(3):13–16.
32. Tulipan N. Intrauterine myelomeningocele repair. Clin Perinatol 2003; 30:521–530.
33. Bruner JP, Tulipan N, Paschall RL, et al. Fetal surgery for myelomeningocele and the incidence of shunt-dependent hydrocephalus. JAMA 1999; 282(19):1819–1825.
34. Tulipan N, Hernanz-Schulman M, Lowe LH, Bruner JP. Intrauterine myelomeningocele repair reverses preexisting hindbrain herniation. Pediatr Neurosurg 1999; 31:137–142.
35. Tulipan N, Bruner JP, Hernanz-Schulman M, et al. Effect of intrauterine myelomeningocele repair on central nervous system structure and function. Pediatr Neurosurg 1999; 31:183–188.
36. Lyerly AD, Mahowald MB. Maternal-fetal surgery for treatment of myelomeningocele. Clin Perinatol 2003; 30:155–165.
37. Bliton MJ, Zaner RM. Over the cutting edge: how ethics consultation illuminates the moral complexity of open-uterine fetal repair of spina bifida and patients' decision making. J Clin Ethics 2001; 12(4):346–360.
38. Chervenak FA, McCullough LB. A comprehensive ethical framework for fetal research and its application to fetal surgery for spina bifida. Am J Obstet Gynecol 2002; 187(1):10–14.
39. Bliton MJ. Ethics: "Life before birth" and moral complexity in maternal-fetal surgery for spina bifida. Clin Perinatol 2003; 30:449–464.
40. American Academy of Pediatrics, Committee on Bioethics. Fetal therapy—ethical considerations. Pediatrics 1999; 103(5):1061 1063.

# Index